FORGED IN HARDSHIP UNLEASHING YOUR FULL POTENTIAL AS A MAN

By Jan Rudat

In this book, we embark on a journey of self-discovery and exploration of the world around us. We delve into the complexities of the human experience and examine what it means to understand and navigate ourselves and the world. Along the way, we explore the concept of manliness and male strength, and what it means to be a strong and confident man in today's society. Through a combination of introspection and observation, we aim to provide practical insights and guidance on how to live a fulfilling and meaningful life specifically as a strong & developing Man in today's world.

Additionally, we will focus on Hardships, Mental Health, Struggles, how to solve them, as well as Self-development, building discipline, solving everyday problems, acquiring Wisdom & Accepting Reality.

At the end of this book, I will also include some Extra Lessons for you.

Do you make Life, or does Life make you?

CHAPTER ONE
SEMEN RETENTION

Conquer Your Reality

This Chapter is as much about Masculinity, Philosophy, and Self-Development as its topic Semen retention.
Because this book was written, first and foremost, for Men themselves. It still is, even though its message may be rough against the nerves. I wrote it deliberately in plain, strong language as I'd say to someone, I was counseling, looking them directly in the eye.

Trust me on this. I didn't get these grey hairs for anything.

The pursuit of pleasure as a good and the avoidance of pain as an evil, constitutes as a sin. Further, anyone who fears pain will also at times be afraid of some future event in the world, and that is an immediate sin. And a man who pursues pleasure will not hold back from injustice, which is an obvious sin.

\- MARCUS AURELIUS

Greetings Gentlemen, and welcome to the very first Chapter of this fine, relatively short Book.

Today we are going to discuss the very essential and important topic of semen retention, also known by some as "nofap" in mainstream popularity these days.

In any case, in this Chapter we will discuss its importance, benefits, truths about it & also why I personally, highly preach it to every single or taken Gentleman out there to try it for themselves for a few weeks, or, preferably, a few months. It is certainly an essential first step in the right direction, becoming a better, stronger, and more appealing & attractive man, and should, under no circumstances, be skipped in any way. How long you pursue this is your own decision, and entirely depends on your very own personal progress and speed thereof.

Semen Retention is, in specifics, the practice of completely abstaining from any form whatsoever of sexual stimulation and ejaculation for a given period of time – This can be pornography, casual Sex, and ejaculation. They all fall under the said category of sexual stimulation.

Semen retention has been long discussed and implemented by every man in the world. Some found it life-changing, while others found it just a waste of time withholding your volcanic surge of not just simple, primal, and indeed natural sexual energy but also mental energy.

The main purpose of semen retention is to invert our brain's natural, primal, inclined tendencies to always pursue more and more pleasure of any kind, and in this case, it is especially for those Men who are addicted to pornography and/or excessive ejaculation to a certain degree. Of course, it is understandable that we as men have a great natural and primal tendency as well as urges to actively procreate with Women. And if those tendencies and also urges are simply totally unfulfilled, we tend to find a practical way to release those to or with some other form of activity. This can take the form of anything, even Sports or Crafts.

Unfortunately, most of us men are doing it in the wrong way - Instead of transferring that strong energy from the urges into far more meaningful we very often just end up wasting them completely to commit impulsive and mindless acts, such as watching porn and ejaculating. You do not need me to tell you that this is very, very bad and hindering any potential progress of your Life itself, and its contents - including you, your dream job, your dream woman, you name it. It is not such a seemingly steep challenge anymore once you see what it has to offer once you have conquered and mastered it to the fullest extent.

What you gentlemen have to understand is simply that your semen is, essentially, like your life force. This sounds esoteric and is rather vague, so, think of it rather like a venomous snake or a venomous spider, or a scorpion. Their enemies want to distinguish them from others of their kind, which in almost all cases, makes them more lethal, more powerful, and more dangerous. When they inject their deadly venom into their prey, they only inject a rather tiny amount of their poison that is necessary to paralyze their victims for food - Never their full dose inside their glands, which only slowly regenerates within said glands.

That is because the venom that they have is philosophically and literally their one life force which makes them more dangerous than any others of their kind. So, if they instantly empty their poison glands, it will immediately render them very weak, defenseless, and inevitably far more vulnerable to other predators. As mentioned, just like our semen, it really takes quite a long time to produce such a life force.

If you gentlemen are, however, still not yet convinced, think about this: your semen is actually powerful enough to create a new, better life. It contains so many super essential nutrients that it can actually nourish and grow another human life within a fertile woman's womb. Therefore, if you gentlemen mindlessly waste it through synthetic, digital sex, rather than real, actual, purposeful procreation, then you are basically disregarding the value so powerful which your own body produces solely for you to make that change we talk about so in-depth in this Book. That change you most likely crave so badly, that you may not even know you crave it until this Book opens your own two eyes.

Your semen, believe it or not, when not ejaculated out of your body, and actually left to mature, collect, and grow, is completely reabsorbed into your bloodstream within your body, actively nourishing it with its nutrient-dense contents, including Calcium and up to 25 Calories, giving you many strong biological benefits both short and long-term, physically & mentally. Its nutritiousness does not, however, end just there.

World-renowned and famous Dr. Reitano said in an interview for a medical research paper, that sperm contains vitamin C, B12, ascorbic acid, calcium, citric acid, fructose, lactic acid, magnesium, zinc, potassium, sodium, fat, and hundreds of different proteins.

Now, I completely understand the feeling of sexual activities, including ejaculating, gentlemen, it really does make you feel like you have conquered the world, as if you made it in the world, that you have just reached a huge, significant goal that you can now reap the rewards from, and finally relax since you have released all those urges that have been building up inside you.

However, as we know and have all experienced, this seeming sensation only lasts for a short while. Now you see what ejaculation does to you both on a physical and mental level, that it creates such a strong sense of huge accomplishment because our primal, natural instincts as men are solely and purely to procreate as much as possible to keep humanity alive.

I know this sounds deprecating, but this is what it is all about on a bigger, grander scale. And we are doing everything and anything in life to, among other things of course, achieve that very goal. We do this through many different means and things, such as our appearance and/or looks, our finances, power, and personality, just to attract women and simply procreate. In other words, to enjoy a fulfilled and fulfilling life.

In other words, what I am saying here is that, in reality, it actually takes a lot of time to build and nurture relations with a Woman and to have Sex, while Pornography and ejaculation is basically instant, with absolutely no chance of failure and no risks whatsoever involved. No matter your experience, age, appeal, looks, money, power, fame, you name it. Because after all, as I always say, good things take time.

It is only natural, therefore, that frequently ejaculating and releasing your life force cause you to be utterly depleted from its valuable nutrients that obtain if you just hold it in - both physically and mentally. Not to mention that you are also greatly energetically depleted, again, both mentally & physically. This is because your body simply lacks the Nutrients and Calories it would have if you would, again, just hold it in.

Yes, no grand, fascinating, surprise there. At least, to some.

That is also why when you excessively ejaculate you generally feel or tend to feel far less energetic for the whole day, or even fatigued and foggy in the mind, unmotivated depressed, and even more emotional than usual. Yes, we both know we all experienced this many times in the past. We just don't want to admit it to ourselves. We do not want to face ugly truths. I know it as well as you do. We have all been there and experienced it.

So that is why I want to share with you, gentlemen, information about the big benefits I personally get on a daily basis for over 3 years in an uninterrupted row from retaining my life force for a relatively long time. I hope that you gentlemen will also get inspired from this book to try this wonderful practice for yourselves for at least a few weeks, and preferably a few months before you decide whether you want to partake in it or abstain from it. It will transform your life.

However, if any of you have done this prior, you can attest that this is one-hundred-percent true.

Clarity

The first, and most noticeable benefit is definitely clarity. My mind is just clear. My train of thought was just utterly clear of all roadblocks, interferences, problems, potholes, and distractions. It is important to note, and this is just as important, that I suffer from ADD, or attention deficit disorder, as well as PTSD, or post-traumatic stress disorder, as well as quite strong tremors, all three since birth or since my childhood. This further reinforces the effectiveness of retaining your life force. Without doing this, I am simply a total trainwreck - I cannot focus, I am neurotic, my feet are restless, my hands trembling, and my mind is just foggy, taking me to all sorts of places of thought. Naturally, this makes any work requiring attention and focus utterly impossible, including writing. But it is important that I retain my life force entirely voluntarily, and that how it transformed my life has essentially made me a functional, strong, enduring, and smart young man.

So, of course, there was absolutely no brain fog. I was very adamant about what I was thinking, what I was going to do, what I was going to say, and the list goes on and on. Everything seems quite seamless, in fact, almost entirely - That is to say that things just flow smoothly, uninterrupted. You essentially just confidently know and understand what it is that you, in any instance or moment, want for yourself and others, while at the same time knowing just how to achieve that, and direct your mind nowhere else but in that direction, only.

Physical Strength

The second one is physical strength. Now, I am personally very, very much into strength training, and I am an active Powerlifter since 2020 during the well-known Lockdowns. As some of you might also know, strength training requires an active, fresh, healthy, strong, and fully aware online nervous system in order to perform at any given moment effectively and efficiently in any given field and task. Although in this case, with semen retention, my already shaken up body since childhood was just in tune with my mind, and my whole nervous system whenever I performed my daily routine, as well as exercises throughout. Every limb structure from my feet to my core or torso, to my arms, fingers, and fingertips, to my head, my individual muscle groups, just all feel solid rigid, and intertwined in action as one big unity, and most importantly, without any sense whatsoever of disconnection, lack of energy, fatigue, or weakness.

If you gentlemen are at least somewhat fond of the gym, proper sports nutrition, or hobbyist workout, you know exactly what I am talking about here. You essentially just feel like you have just never experienced this immaculate burst of physical energy in your previous fitness sessions that you would only ever see in old comic books, or in Movies with Arnold Schwarzenegger, really. It is hard to describe what an amazing feeling it is, and what a milestone it is.

Determination & Focus

Thirdly determination and focus. I would even escalate it to an unprecedented level of determination and focus, like that of the Greek God, Zeus.

Just like having a clear path of thought, my mind and body are simply completely in tune with each other at all times with what I am actively doing at any given moment. I forgot what happened 10 minutes ago, and I am surely not worried about what is going to happen in the next 10 minutes. I was simply laser-focused and locked into the dimension of my work at that moment. Whether it is working in my gardens growing food, animal husbandry looking after my chickens and goats, exercising, writing this book, being a critic, working on my car, going for a walk, or simply thinking, to the point where I just lost all sense of time, all throughout the activity until I was completely done with my work. Just like a Tiger sharply fixating its eyes on its vulnerable prey, such as a Zebra, or a smaller type of Bird, and never taking a single glance off of it until it has killed it.

Directness

The natural follow-up to having laser-guided, unbreakable focus, is, of course, the demeanor of being absolutely one hundred percent direct with everything. And when I say everything, I really do mean everything - I will not sugarcoat what I am going to say, or express. I will hesitate to do what I will do. I am not and will not waste any time trying to please anybody, even if that means slightly intimidating, or offending the person I am talking to. I am just and simply totally unbothered by how they think, feel, or what they do.

And yes, I might come across as quite rude and/or disrespectful to you gentlemen, but it is what it is. In my mind, how they think and react, is simply not my problem to solve - It is, in fact, their very own to solve for themselves.

Confidence

And finally, the fifth, and also most important benefit in addition to being a product of the accumulation of all the previous benefits is Confidence.

Now, who does not love, trust, like, and totally admire a confident man?

I personally believe that true confidence is something that you acquire over a long time through masses of success as well as failure and not just gained naturally or exuded naturally.
However, in this case, I do believe the majority of it is because of the overall shift in my mindset and transformation, in addition to my demeanor that eventually caused a huge, revolutionary evolution in my personality which gave me this confidence, and not so much the huge amounts of work, as well as time and experience that I put into myself as I was just starting out my self-development journey at the time. But, in any case, it felt utterly amazing, and it showed me that we men were naturally meant to feel in the case that pornography and ejaculation were never a thing in the first place.
At a certain point, there comes a time in similar tension when we experienced what is widely known in history as the flatline.
This is basically the one single period of time where you do not experience those seemingly magical benefits anymore. I personally found a research paper that showed the effects of testosterone when there is no ejaculation within and beyond 7 days. In essence, this research that the research paper is based on found that there is a big, dramatic increase in testosterone levels but after day 7 it simply returns back to normal levels, although at a relatively higher level than when you were constantly ejaculating.

I personally did not experience this one particular period we have just touched upon on Day 7 of my cycle. In fact, it came after around the 3-week mark for me, and I am sure that the flatline period occurs differently, and at different time spans for every respective man, but, in any case, it is completely normal to experience this and should be treated as such. Of course, after hitting this milestone, to have arrived at this flatline period, it is all the more important to not relapse. You need to retain your life force.

And now, gentlemen, we do finally arrive at the much-awaited metaphorical Elephant in the Room.
The part of semen retention that everyone in the "nofap" community is indeed most curious about – is women's attraction.
It is important to note here that I did not experience much of this, and I really could not exaggerate something in this Book that I do not experience first-hand or have extensively experienced first-hand.
I did, however, notice very strongly how the general, emotional, and personal attitude of women in my construction-related workplace changed, a relatively small amount, to be more precise. I do though think that this is far more towards my change in general and personal demeanor from being a rather quiet, introverted, and well-reserved man to a more direct, confident, social, and spontaneous man, rather than from the talked about the pheromonic effect of semen retention. Ultimately, though, it is what you choose to do with the benefits that semen attention provides to you that would eventually elevate your value as a better, stronger, more attractive, and successful man.

Semen retention is not a cure or wonder medicine - Far from it, in fact. And the benefits of it are not necessarily the definitive answer to your problems. Semen retention is merely a tool for you to take advantage of - one of many, in fact, to become a better, more successful, stronger, more attractive, and overall winning man. And in the end, you will have to act on yourself, and use the many tools this book will provide you with to become a dream man.
Use semen retention to build yourself physically, mentally, financially, socially, intellectually, personally, emotionally, spiritually, and so on, and as a long-earned byproduct, you will, eventually, receive women's attention because let us be honest,

which woman is not drawn to a good looking, confident, providing, and successful dream man?

And to help you get started, I even attached a bonus to this Chapter.

Bonus Lesson: Awareness. Become completely aware of your level of energy and how semen retention affects your behavior at all times.

Your brain tells you when it is "in the mood"; learn to monitor yourself psychologically as well. Enlist your friends if you have any. Have them tell you when you're resorting to provocative behavior patterns and ask how your energy is. Don't yell at them when they do it, either. This is a difficult discipline, especially in the face of denial and ingrained bad habits, and it may take years to get used to it.
If you do not have the discipline to not yell at valid criticism, build it up.
Still, the people around you may have a clearer view than you yourself when it comes to figuring out when you're doing it. Expect frequent Repetition to be necessary to really optimize this, Lesson.

Figuring this out is your personal, highly important responsibility.

I know very well myself that this is indeed a very difficult Lesson, and it is so easy to just brush over and past it, to forget about it and never face the Challenge it presents to you. Because it affects you personally, directly - But it is very important to your self-development to build up the Discipline if you haven't yet, to face it head-on and complete it. Trust me, you will be on your way to being a better man in no time, and it will be visibly worth it.

CHAPTER TWO
WHY EVERY MAN MUST COMMIT TO PHYSICAL TRAINING

The high strength of men knows no content with limitation.

No man has the right to be an amateur in the matter of physical training. it is a disgrace to grow old through sheer carelessness before seeing what manner of man you may become by developing your bodily strength and beauty to their highest limits.

- SOCRATES

Welcome to another chapter in this wonderful book, gentlemen. Physical training has been on the rise for the past 2 decades, and it is very encouraging to see an increase in people are taking care of their own physical well-being. However, the statistics showed differently, a combined 69% of United States citizens are either overweight and/or morbidly obese, and it is ever-increasing by the year. In this chapter, I'm preaching my case to every man in the world about why physical training is so important to one's life, and how it can translate tremendously well to other important areas of a man's life including but not limited to self-development, discipline, philosophy, successfulness, and appeal.

In this chapter, we will talk about the huge, underestimated, and underrated importance of physical to the modern man, how physical training can massively help to build mental fortitude no matter your proficiency, and why every single man simply has to actively engage in some sort of physical training in their lives in order to consistently and reliably serve their natural purpose well, in addition to their physical activity which is expected and required of them to keep their bodies as well as minds healthy and in order. This, of course, includes   you   and   me,   gentlemen.

The human body was from the day of its evolution, designed primarily for total survival, to help us survive. Whether we are or were involved in life-threatening circumstances such as starvation, robbery, a home invasion, fire, or even natural disaster, or even circumstances that are barely detrimental to our everyday life, it is in its nature to help us survive no matter what – and we cannot change a single thing about that. Unfortunately, most people still, to this very day you are reading this book, disregard their own body as some kind of disposable, cheap suit of armor or even just a host for them to exploit however they wish. They are not treating it like the magnificent gift that it truly is. Far from it, in fact. They more so discreetly and ignorantly completely destroy them over time by various means such as overworking, bad nutrition, lack of exercise or physical and mental activity, fast food, smoking, or drug use – or they simply leave them to rot, and die of old age too early, completely wasting the profound potential your body can indeed provide to you, and by extension, to others through you, especially loved ones and family. This does not limit itself to sex, of course. What you need to understand and take careful note of, gentlemen, is that your own body is the single most important, greatest, effective, strongest, and most effectively adaptive machine in this small world. Any circumstances that you throw at it every day, no matter how big or small, or how impactful they may be, your body does always, and will always have the capability to completely adapt, withstand, tolerate, and eventually overcome that. Therefore, every stimulus that your body is exposed to, will naturally help your body find feasibly possible ways to help you control them to your fullest ability.

Where you may or may not find cold weather excessively unpleasant, dreary, and a major issue to you or your health, if you simply keep exposing your body to it, your body will naturally and internally extensively reconfigure itself to one day help you be at ease   with   said   condition. This is what is so widely known as the ever-important fight-or-flight mode, present in nearly all animals, including humans. The mode where our body naturally perceives circumstances as harmful, detrimental, or even life-threatening, and will instinctually react whether to face and combat the challenge or threat or to simply flee and go into full-on survival mode tailored to the situation it actively perceives. Those of you who studied psychology or biology, or simply experienced a near-death scenario will very well have experienced this, but it may be hard for you to properly recollect that memory and analyze what precisely happened. Therefore, this chapter is just as important for you as it is for anyone else. You know what I am talking about.

But, of course, when we are talking about physical training, the situation that it itself presents by its very own nature, is completely different from being in a life-threatening situation where, for example, a gun is pointed directly at your face, as you clearly perceive this threat. However, in any case, this is the same analogy – our own body wants to help us find the best, ultimate way to survive in even the direst of circumstances and situations. Whether this is challenges at school, work, weightlifting, and training, or being in a seemingly completely hopeless street fight, this applies to all of those situations the same way.

A much simpler and also admittedly shorter example of this would be people that just cannot stand or endure spicy foods in taste and/or hotness and whose tongue would simply feel like it is covered in gasoline and set alight. Those who experienced this know exactly what I am talking about here, too. And chances are, many men experience this aversion to hot food as well, just like me. Other people can eat extremely hot chilis as a midnight snack and not break a tear or sweat. They can very well enjoy the taste and hotness of the chili they eat.

How do you think that those people have built and still build their tolerance to spicy food and even outright chilis directly? Well, they certainly did not start off just munching on those things and enjoying them first-hand. They simply gradually built up their physical tolerance by exposing themselves to this intense stimulus through their tastebuds for a very, very long time – each time gradually increasing the level of spice or hotness added to gradually improve their tolerance. It is really quite simple when you look at it like this. I know, I have tested this method myself, and have interviewed world champions in eating spicy foods. If you simply keep at it, your body will also learn to adjust your tastebuds and overcome the immense burning sensation from eating chilis.

Exactly the same principle applies equally to physical training – whether you are lifting weights, running marathons or triathlons, doing boxing, wrestling, or any form of martial arts, no matter how little, your body is slowly, but surely, making gradual adaptations to itself to suit itself around and within those situations and eventually also make you comfortable in whatever field, or practice you may be actively engaging in. Remember gentlemen, it always has the ability and capacity to do so, no matter how difficult the circumstances are in whatever you are facing. The more you gradually expose yourself to weightlifting, your muscles will get bigger, denser, stronger, and more enduring, your fast levels will drop drastically over time, and your bones will get denser and stronger to more and more help you survive, adapt to, and eventually overcome that situation so that you can move onto heavier weights and more difficult exercises in weightlifting. Many of you will inevitably see this many times a year in the Gym, or at home.

The more that you gradually expose yourself to any martial arts whatsoever, your reflexes will significantly sharpen over time, your stances will get more stabilized and pinned or glued to the ground, and your muscular density and endurance will of course also increase. Depending on how intense your martial arts training is, your bones may also benefit from it just like you would do relatively intense weightlifting. Similarly, the more you expose yourself to any other Sports of your choice, you will be able to jump stronger, farther, and higher, run faster, swim faster and hold your breath longer. Most of these benefits overlap each other within multiple respective fields. It really does not matter what kind of Sport you engage in, as long as you do it and never quit, or jump ahead of your current ability as you gradually improve. Be the slow but wise turtle, not the frantic hare. Your body is capable of absolutely amazing feats, gentlemen. And yes, some of you might just say "but some people have naturally great or god-like genetics that serve them far better than us in physical training", and I fully agree with that. However, is that not just a silly and pitiful excuse not to build your own body to its fullest potential for it to serve you so well in your life?

Gentlemen, your body wants to serve you. It wants to protect you at all times as well as at all costs, no matter how or what. And for it to do that, you must expose it gradually to situations and circumstances that allow it to grow and to properly fine-tune itself to the situations and circumstances it finds itself in, all to serve you better.

And I myself am not a genetic freak. In fact, I am far from it. I am only 173cm high with hands the size of teenagers still nonchalantly, lazily strolling along on the puberty sidewalk on the road for true and real men. And I manage to do pull-ups with 75 pounds tied to my   waist,   daily.
So listen to this very carefully, and write it down, as this is so important to note and remember.
Your body will only serve you well, if you gradually put them to a variety of increasingly difficult and detrimental tests, keep testing its current limits daily, and every day give them absolutely everything that it needs to properly achieve growth on an optimal scale. Never let it down. Speaking of giving your body what it needs – let us speak a little about the things that will inevitably gradually destroy your body, rather than allowing it to grow in any meaningful way or capacity no matter if other requirements are fulfilled and the body has everything to do so. And yes, I am indeed talking about all the things that, in this day and age, are a huge part of the widely accepted cultural norms in almost all of the world, and in most countries. You gentlemen of course know what they are or can imagine what they are. Excessive drinking, excessive smoking, drug-usage, processed and bad foods, sugar, and the one that almost everyone suffers from – the crippling lack of sleep. Now you might think "but you said that our body can adapt to almost if not really anything, so that would include drinking and smoking and that stuff". Of course, it can do that indeed. The more you drink alcohol, the more of a tolerance your body develops naturally to alcohol, and the more you smoke, the more your body develops more of a tolerance to nicotine, too. But do those activities profoundly and truly give the body what it needs to grow, which is proper, healthy nutrition, sufficient regular exercise, and sufficient & healthy sleep? No, they do not. Not to mention that drinking and smoking will someday inevitably lead to addiction because you seek your own susceptibleness of the harmful but somehow exciting contents that they provide, instead of tolerance. And naturally, the more tolerance you build, the more susceptibility you will, of course, want from them which will only lead you to consume more, and more, and more of them.
Instead, feed your body with nutrient-dense, organic, natural, and healthy foods that contain all the macro and micronutrients that are

so essential. Always keep your body hydrated and always, always allow it to recover properly and fully with a deep, good night's sleep. Especially after strenuous physical activity, such as Sports or Gardening, or simply a day's housework such as chores or repairs. I might sound like all of those pesky, fake fitness gurus that you gentlemen have heard everywhere, but that is sole because there is just no other, different, or unique way of saying it. Really, it is simply the truth about what proper nutrition entails. Your body is the engine to your dreams, your activities, your dreams, wishes, and desires, and most importantly, the key to the life that you want to lead so desperately, whether you know it or not. And the things that it requires in order to perform properly and healthily to its fullest extent,   are   its   fuel   sources.

Would you use the cheapest, worst engine oil, contaminated lubricant, dirty water, and recycled fuel for the engine of the sports car of your dreams? No, absolutely not. You would only use the best you can afford. It is the exact same as your body, with only minor differences.
Good physical training routines to make your body and you included grow to a greater potential, and good, proper, organic fuel sources for your body do not only affect you physically. It also affects you mentally, and just as much, in fact. Your mood, thoughts, demeanor, as well as energy, will tremendously influence how your own mind operates cognitively. You simply are what you do, and you are what you eat. That is why I am preaching this to you, gentlemen. I want you to succeed and be a winner, a king. The best there is and the best there can be.
A healthy body will always translate to a healthy mind unless you are suffering from a pre-existing, uncurable mental condition. But it is your task to conquer those three things.

And speaking about mentality, let us discuss how you, gentlemen, can use physical training to build a strong, dependable, and unbreakable mental fortitude. Because you see, gentlemen, the byproduct that comes from what you yourself decide to go through physically translates extremely well and precisely to what you will go through mentally. Because the narrative for facing and overcoming challenges is always, in any and every case, are always the same for everyone and for everything. Physical training is the first and simplest form of facing adversities like a ship caught in a huge storm on the seemingly endless and relenting ocean. You can almost call it as one of the main analogies to be used in facing adversities nowadays. Lifting heavy weights, for example, is in no way an easy task at all. Getting physically strong, is also, in no way, an easy task. In fact, what is it that is truly worth accomplishing and rewarding, that always comes easy? Of course, you first want to use those weights that you are lifting, and it is indeed grueling and deeply gradual to allow your body to morph into its desired state to get you comfortable with those weights. And then, when you are comfortable, you naturally progress into heavier weights as well as bigger adversities to face. A little at a time.

I'm telling you, gentlemen, it is genuinely addicting to suffer first, and then to reap the rewards after. This is self-development. It is an amazing sensation like nothing else could achieve. Physical training teaches you the genesis of discipline, consistency, commitment, persistence, and sacrifice, and the rewards that you reap off of them will lead you to trust those principles to be strongly planted or embedded within your mentality which can then be applied to other meaningful and purposeful activities and endeavors of your life, that truly matter, like building a company, a business, marriage, or writing a book and getting it published.

There is an old saying, that where the mind goes, the body follows. And that baffled me a little. I am not disagreeing with it in any way, shape, or form, but rather questioning it. Because you see, gentlemen, it is without a doubt that your mind fills in the gaps that your body feels otherwise insufficient, but what if your body is no longer sufficient – In fact, is completely and utterly ineffective in its current state? Would your mind still be able to lead your body, nonetheless?

I do not necessarily think so, myself. Therefore, I decided to properly complete the quote myself.

Where The Mind Goes, The Body Follows. How The Body Is, The Mind Accepts.

- JAN RUDAT

Now, you gentlemen can choose to disagree or agree with me on this one, but here is the thing. The state of your body is important to your state of mind as well. If your body is severely injured, no matter how much your mind wants to keep going, your body is simply physically unable to do so. The same thing goes when you are severely overweight and have very little muscle mass. No matter how much your mind wants to lift 100kg of weight off the floor, your body is physically unable to do so. It is important to also note that the word accepting does not mean conceding, gentlemen. It is just to take reality into account and realize that your body and mind are both deeply, deeply intertwined within each other and that they both serve each other in perfect harmony. One cannot be healthy, effective, or efficient if the other is not. And a great byproduct of physical training is obviously women's attraction. Of course, there is really no surprise there if you read the book so far without skipping ahead. A strong physical presence and shown capability display the competence to defend and protect, as well as good chances for a very healthy baby, in addition to the commitment to self-respect and leadership through actions and example which are some of the key qualities of a high-value man. Just imagine what you will be as the dream man, if you just complete this book in order, without skipping ahead, and with enough willpower and commitment.

And again, some of you gentlemen will probably say "well women don't care about looks at all you know". Yes, they do, gentlemen. Yes, they do.

You can always judge a book by its cover, no matter what people say, you can. And people's first impression of you is always based on the appeal of your cover. Whatever is beneath that cover, is to be discussed much later.

However, in the end, physical training should be done for your own health and well-being, you should always be your own mental point of focus in your life, and by committing yourself to do physical training, you simply showcase a great, great level of self-respect, integrity, dignity, and more, for your own character. And yes, I know some of you gentlemen still say, "oh but I don't have time to work out I have work to do and stuff".

Cut it out, gentlemen - you always have time.

It is all a matter of priorities and other priorities you currently do in life; do they deliver good, positive results in your life? Or do they just feel good, and easy, and that is why you are doing them? Scrolling down your phone and lying in bed there for hours is not an actual priority that could be called plausible, gentlemen. Hours spent on the computer on videogames pretending to be "Internal Security Department" in roleplaying is equally not, gentlemen. You all know that. Make the choice and sacrifice to improve your body that has kept you alive for so long and will continue to keep you alive for as long as possible and trust me on this, gentlemen - In the end, you will only be thanking me and yourself for making that decision. You know it is to choose between rotting away, and success.

And to get you started, I will even give you free two bonus exercises at the end of this chapter.

Bonus Exercise A: Write down all the big as well as small things you do to keep your body healthy. If you're not doing anything at all to keep your body healthy, change your habits now. You don't need to be super ripped, but the healthier your body is, the less work you'll need to keep up to standard. If you have a chronic illness, at least work on a healthier diet and as much gentle exercise as you can stand, even if only spaced in small amounts throughout the day. Take more vitamins and minerals. Adapt your routine so that when you feel tired and foggy, you replenish your body first, and wait a while. It is of vital importance to keep at it, despite eventual laziness and temporary tiredness. The first 3 months will be quite tiring for your body if it is not used to this, but after those 3 months have passed, you will noticeably grow stronger and more enduring. It is of vital importance to keep going and to keep improving your diet as well as your exercise regime. It has to be adjusted gradually, or you will most likely fail.

Bonus Exercise B: You can do this exercise anywhere where it is calm and relatively quiet. Sit quietly, become calm and collected, and let your consciousness flow through your body, area by area. Be aware of your body, and what you feel, do not force anything. Just sit and meditate, explore your mind and body in its fine, often unnoticed by most, details. Do this for at least 30 minutes in one session, and slowly work your way up. It is possible that you may not be able to do it for 30 minutes in one, single, uninterrupted session. If that is the case, simply go down to 15 minutes, or just 10, or even just 5. Whatever works for you, as long as you eventually go up to longer durations as they become feasibly possible for you.

You may also visualize your breathing like energy flowing into and out of your lungs with each breath. How the oxygen aerates your blood and body. How it helps you concentrate and maintain Meditation. This can help significantly break up and slowly reduce possible boredom that many people encounter during this exercise. It is totally normal and should be treated as such and is no reason or excuse of any kind to grow weary of the exercise.

CHAPTER THREE
WHAT TRULY MAKES A MAN

Be the man you need to be.

Men are thrifty in guarding their private property. But as soon as it comes to wasting time, they become the most extravagant with one commodity for which it is respectable to be greedy.

- SENECA

Taking action is the core of manhood maturity. Combine this with a good character and keeping one's word and any man is off with a really, really decent foundation-

- JAN RUDAT

What does it take for a man to be considered masculine? What traits must we have as men so that we ourselves can be confident enough to admit that we are masculine and high-value men? Strength?

Courage? Emotional control? Ambitions? Big, extraordinary Visions? Humility? Generosity? Great strength? They are all essential and important traits that a good man must have. But what is that "One" definitive thing that eclipses all these traits, and actually harnesses them together? This will be slightly shorter, but just as equally important chapter in this ever so important book.

Because we are going to directly talk about the very core foundations of masculinity, which, in essence, this entire book is at least partially about. It is actually by all means a very common and defining term that is used every day. But unfortunately, it has seldom been kept an eye out on in today's world and society, and, in my opinion, also massively lacked emphasizing until I wrote this book's chapter. Masculinity is an innate, natural, primal, dynamic that we as men express to the outside world in anything and everything that we show and express as men.

Although we do indeed have some feminine qualities of our own, we as men lean very strongly and heavily toward the masculine side. And this is simply the nature of our male dynamic since the human evolution of men in the historic caveman-filled stone age. Unfortunately, due to today's massively feminine-leaning social order, masculinity is currently, for some time now, at its lowest point of expression, possibly ever – causing strong imbalance and extraordinary amounts of chaos within the social and intersexual dynamics as well as a man's own identity and character, including gender identity as well as gender expression. This is by all means a very new occurrence, and, while it is not a problem, it is detrimental to the mental health of young men and women, as recent studies have shown. But these sorts of topics are for another chapter in this book.

Masculinity in and of itself is very outward-driven energy, as opposed to femininity, which is naturally inward-driven in almost all cases. Masculinity is more active than passive, more giving than receiving, more consistent rather than wavy, riskier rather than safe, more bold than shy, and more logical than emotional. It is, in essence, more objective-driven rather than subjectively driven. This is the one dynamic that we lean towards far more as men.

An example comes from the olden, long bygone days – where men were the hunters and scavengers, and women the foragers and nurturers. Men went out to seek and scavenge or harvest resources and find new land to inhabit and fight off intruders and attackers. While women took care of the children, and nurtured the community, back in the tribe, as the most important part of the community itself – the caretakers.

So then, gentlemen, what is that one, particular, definitive word that will provide the absolution of what masculinity is all about – the one word that can provide all the clarity for this outwardly driven, objectively focused, and assertively expressed, male dynamic? The one word in which we can completely be clarified as masculine men. That word is "action". Now, there is a very old saying that goes "Women talk, men do". Do not misunderstand me in any way – this is in no way to discriminate against women. It is just factual. We have more men leaders than women leaders in the history of mankind, and even still today, in companies, the military, political offices, and the list goes on. We, men, are among many other things, natural and inherent problem solvers. We thrive in challenges and challenging surroundings, rather than staying in our comfort zone. We love content rather than context. We innately love to create, develop, invent, and make things feasible, rather than wallow ourselves and others in dreams, wishes, ideas, conversations, plans, ambitions, opinions, as well as visions. It is especially important to note that this is absolutely not to say that having dreams, wishes, ideas, conversations, plans, ambitions, opinions, as well as visions is in any way, shape or form bad. Far from it, in fact. It is quite necessary, but those are the big parts of our dynamic and, whatever those dreams, wishes, ideas, conversations, plans, ambitions, opinions, as well as visions, are, we as men often get fidgety to get to work those manifests imaginations and creativity into reality. We know it.

Because, unlike women who are defined through their physical aesthetics and feminine traits, men, on the other hand, are defined in this world through work, our contributions to ourselves and the people of the world, and the legacy and value that we eventually, one day, left behind for our successors to eventually inherit and continue in our name and legacy, on and on.

When there is an idea, we want to demonstrate it. When there is a blueprint, we want to construct. When there is a plan, we want to execute it. When there is an emotion, we want to sublimate it. Whatever it is that you gentlemen have in mind is really not that important at all. What is, in fact, far more so important, is you putting those thoughts into action. Actions that do change.

Most men of today are very timid, quite fearful, and overall indecisive or unsure of their actions.

Because they are afraid of putting their identity, character, body, and soul out there, to the test, to be criticized and judged. Because they have been deeply manipulated to approach life in the completely wrong way in today's world and modern society. Men of today have been taught and convinced throughout most of their lives that the world is nice, soft, and compassionate. Wherein reality is that most of the world is very much less forgiving than it actually seems to almost every person on the planet. And men of today are having huge dilemmas of hopelessly having their own ideals crushed by reality. But again, more of that in another chapter.

Most men today would simply sit and wait endlessly for the right time to start, while letting their own ideas eat away rapidly at their own mind and overall associated mental health, unknowingly, waiting agitatedly to be executed and put into reality, to be able to be grasped and perceived in person, to reap the rewards of their success – rather than to just put them out to the test. So, try them out, and see where exactly they stand in the world, and how so. I cannot stress this enough. I have experienced this myself; I know how it feels. I have been there, too.

The more you wait, the more and more uncertain and fearful you will quickly become, gentlemen. Do not wait too long for the perfect time to act with your life – because there is no such thing as the perfect, or optimal time. If you have a vision, or a goal, or a dream, or an ambition, or a wish, or a hope, or an idea, and you have laid out a plan to reach them, why wait for the perceived, never-coming perfect time to lay them all out then and there?

Equally, if you are feeling stuck in life, no matter where you are, there will never be a magical fairy descending from the heavens that will tell you what to do and how to do it, gentlemen.

If you are feeling purposeless in life, your purpose would never just fall in front of you, or into your lap, on one lovely, sunny morning.

Never. You have to pick yourself up, think of the scenarios, lay out a plan, and execute and realize or manifest them at the end of the day. There is absolutely no use whatsoever in showering yourself in or with emotion and self-deprecating all day long. And there is most certainly absolutely no use whatsoever in you thinking of the solutions and keep on dreaming about them manifesting into your own life without you executing them, possibly ever or never, by simply acting then and there. Because, after all, actions always speak louder than words and thoughts combined, gentlemen. As cliché as it may admittedly be, it is simply the bare truth. You will not go far just thinking and explaining and contemplating about a business if you are in any way fearful to take necessary risks and actually build it, step by step, day by day. Most men fail at this. Most men also regret never even actually trying what they wanted to do throughout their entire life. With many things. In actually trying and failing in the process you will always learn something which is always going to be useful in your own future, rather than staying safe in your bedroom all day long and learning absolutely nothing along the process of staying safe in that bedroom of yours. It is a pitiful existence where you watch your body rapidly erode and rot away, affecting your mind strongly.

If you want to build a good-looking, aesthetic body, stop thinking about going to the gym – pick up your lazy ass and actually go there and work out 5 days a week, 10 hours a day. If you want to build a business, stop wallowing and dreaming and fantasizing about it and your plans – get out of the house, gather the people and the tools, and start building. If you want to write a book, like me, stop thinking about its contents and hallucinating how we can write meaningful messages – get to your desk, open up your computer, or pick up your pen, and start writing.

Whatever it is that you are fearful of, whatever questions you might have, they will all, and I mean all, be answered when you take the appropriate actions. And the beautiful thing about that is that you can learn and make adjustments along the way, however, and whenever you like, rather than wasting time never actually starting and getting your questions unanswered. So, act, gentlemen. Always keep that in mind. This book – my book, would not exist today and help you achieve great things if I kept wondering and thinking about it. That is mental self-ejaculation. In the end, we all have to get off of our ass and act. Vision without actions is merely mental self-ejaculation, and all your questions will only ever be answered if you act. It is not that you don't know what to do, gentlemen – it is that you choose not to do anything. Anything at all. Real men live through actions and examples, not just through words and thoughts. Strength, courage, and discipline are more important, essential traits of high-value men. But when there is no action, there is simply no case of proving them, and no self-improvement. People, including yourself and especially women, are far more drawn to men's manifestation of reality rather than getting lost, and enamored within one's own mind and fascination.

Bonus Exercise A: Whenever you are angry, emotional, or upset in any other way, realize it. Notice and embrace it but contain it. Be calm and let it brush and flow over you, bend, but do not break. Therefore, control your emotions and continue your way and/or activity.

Note that this exercise counts for anything and everything that makes you feel any emotion without your permission. Be a real, better man.

CHAPTER FOUR
A MAN'S TRUE REASON TO LIVE

Purpose.

Everything, a horse, a vine, is created for some duty. For what task, then, were you yourself created? A man's true delight is to do the things he was made for.

- MARCUS AURELIUS

A man's search for meaning can be the hardest task to endure and eventually accomplish. Many men of today are struggling to find that meaning, that definitive reason for a life worth living. Most men run towards pleasure and allowing the world to define who they are because they don't know who they are themselves. Materialistic possessions can offer them joy, but only temporarily, because those things are acquired out of selfish reasons, and do not properly represent a man's own greater meaning of existence. Purpose is something that you do for circumstances that are greater and more impactful than just yourself. Regardless of money, fame, or attention, you are not committing to your purpose only for the sole reason to acquire those things, you are going to do it regardless of the rewards because it represents your own integrity of your character, and the legacy that you are trying to leave behind when you eventually leave this world.

Truly a very complex term to dissect. Though, if I was to explain it in the tiniest of details it respectively has to provide, this book would be two times as large. And I will not waste your time. I will explain everything necessary here, and as such, will keep this chapter equally short but equally important as chapter two. Every man wonders, to some extent what the particular and definitive reason is, that they are on this planet. Only a very select few would, in the past, eventually understand and receive their own, respective answers. However, for most men, it is simply nothing more than a complex chasm of haze, dread, and despair where nothing seems to provide any clarity, whatsoever. Purpose, to all of us, is the reason to live, or at least, the meaning of life. What are we here for – is it just to enjoy earth's wonders? Is it only to create temporary memories until our inevitable death? Or is it solely to eventually embrace our next of kin, watch them grow, and achieve manhood like you eventually will, my dear reader? That is, of course, if you haven't yet. But that is reserved for very few people in comparison.

Well, all of those are certainly idealistic – they do not provide absolution to us at all. Many people had seen the world, experienced wonderful moments, and have many smart, talented, wonderful children – yet, after achieving all this, they still struggle to this day to be truly happy and to find fulfillment in their life. That is because they have not yet found the major thing this book offers as one of its many gifts – profound significance, in their lives. Do not get me wrong though, while traveling around the world, creating wonderful memories, and having great children are all relatively great feats to accomplish in this day and age, they do not provide the same magnitude and magnificence as the moment you realize and experience the clarification of your purpose life in life.

Human beings' natural, innate purpose is to pursue growth. And if we do not experience growth, we will eventually rot and die. That is also the reason why we get the feeling of being depressed, the feeling of our life going nowhere, being stuck and our situation being utterly helpless and pointless, as we drown in our very own dread and sorrow, emotionally. And we all crave growth and novelty in some form to relieve us from all this parasitic disease that is slowly, but surely, creeping up on us and suffocating us from the inside out. Just like an eagle, really. An eagle's purpose is to fly free and explore the continent, not being held in a cage to serve as a Zoo showpiece, being trapped for their entire life. They too, then get sick and depressed and rot and die. Growth can be in the form of many, many things such as physical strength, mental strength, skills, social ability, knowledge, experience, wisdom, intelligence, spirituality, the list goes on. But the thing is, unlike animals, growth itself is simply not enough for us. Our desires are just boundlessly greater than that of any animal on this planet. There needs to be significant growth and a feasible, applicable reason for that significant growth. Whatever form of growth you choose to be greatly significant in, be it physical, mental, wisdom, skills, or whatever, it is different from person to person. The far more important thing is why you choose to be significant in that one, particular activity or form. There must be a bigger reason, other than yourself to be profoundly significant in one of those activities or forms. Or even multiple. Now, I have probably got you gentlemen into a bit of a minefield here, but what it essentially means, is that purpose is all about the combination of doing what you love and doing what the world needs. As I have previously said in this chapter, this can be absolutely anything. And when I say anything, I mean anything. Doing what you love, will create sustainability as well as a passion for you to pursue growth unrelentingly constantly, and consistently. And doing what the world needs, will ensure that you have a greater reason or reasons other than yourself to carve your own legacy out for when you eventually leave this world, for others to uphold, remember, and continue in your name and honor, for the greater good – whatever the world needs. This will also give you and the world reasons for your own value and worthwhileness, entirely on the side, when you can be doing something entirely different altogether. That is profound significance, gentlemen. Nothing else, nothing more, nothing less than this.

Just like a king – a king pursues growth in his wealth, territory, and also influence. But does his purpose really end then and there? For a horrible king, it would. But a true, good king has a clear purpose and uses his wealth and power for greater reasons other than himself such as leading his united people to greater and greater prosperity throughout the generations by improving the general quality of life, creating new establishments within his conquered lands to create new opportunities such as overseas trading, inspiring his people with his battle-tested and battle-proven leadership character and personality and wisdom that can be continuously passed on after generation and generations and still apply and make the profound change will eventually cement his legacy as a great king for all of history, such as Richard Lionheart. That is purpose, gentlemen.

Now, I am absolutely not trying to be like other people who would just tell you to just "go for your passions man" – while you can most certainly pursue profoundly significant growth in whatever it is that you truly love doing, whether it is art, writing, business, engineering, architecture, designing, spirituality, woodworking, psychology, music, biology, physics, quantum science, virology, you name it, if there is no other reason behind it than yourself, well, you will not feel empty because you are competent, but you most certainly will feel utterly useless, which is, in fact, another form of emptiness. This is what most of those gurus very seldom tell you, gentlemen, that reason in order for you to fully realize your purpose in life.

Passion itself is not enough. Growth itself is not enough. At the end of the day, that reason will always involve other people or the world. Whether you want to help inspire, entertain, cure, fix, improve, or whatever form of positive and valuable conduct, it must involve other circumstances than yourself. I will give you gentlemen, even my own example. I love automobiles, and engineering, and I love physical fitness and improving one's own physical strength and aesthetics. But back then, the only reason I am passionate and competent in those areas, are only for my own pleasure and fascination. And that is why I always feel like things that I love and that I am also good at, are simply utterly meaningless. Because they are, after all, for selfish reasons – only for me, for no one, and nothing else, whatsoever. It was only after I got completely and brutally honest with myself for the first time in my life, and ever since then, that I can know my reason for living. What is it that gives me the greatest possible sense of fulfillment? And that reason is always and will always be, helping people become the best version of themselves that they can possibly be and ever be through the truth. Whatever your reason for living is, gentlemen, I cannot answer that. Nobody but yourself can. It is all your responsibility to know and answer. Because only you know about it, deep down within yourself.

And gentlemen, it actually takes a lot of time for you to eventually experience that clarity. Some of you gentlemen may take days, weeks, months, or even years, like me. But for some of those who might still be relatively young, it may take even a decade or two. The important thing is that, as you go through life, you have to do enough things. You have to try, fail and succeed – build up your experience level through countless encounters and activities. Build your very own character from the ground up, and maintain it for your entire life, as you adjust it finely.

CHAPTER FIVE
THE GAME OF LIFE

For all of you that are depressed and lost in life.

New beginnings are often disguised as painful endings

\- LAO TZU

Depression, confusion, perplexity, and estrangement. They are all, without a doubt the darkest experiences that every man and woman will have to face eventually, one fateful day in their lives. Because, after all, human beings are naturally emotional creatures, and it is equally natural for us to experience emotions and be overwhelmed by them – especially if we have no understanding of them, or just very little of them. This is very often found in depression and any other emotional low points in life. I completely understand that feeling – the feeling of your mind being utterly helplessly stuck, lost, manipulated, contorted, and just being completely engulfed by negative emotions and/or apparitions. Everyone has been there, gentlemen. Me included. In fact, I suffered from depression my whole life until I met my wonderful partner. They among many, many other things have given me the light, the energy, and the inspiration, that I so desperately needed and have fought for my entire life. And so, the truth about depression is that you are simply in some sort, way, shape or form, unhappy with your current situation or circumstances in your own life. You are still clinging to past actions, memories, and events that you committed, remember, or were involved in and experienced, that you have no control of, that will ultimately get you into your current, undesired, depressive circumstances in your own life. You are still wallowing in deep self-deprecation; however, it may manifest itself in your life and circumstances, or situation.

Therefore, what you gentlemen will have to understand is that for every single human being, and I really mean every single human being, life itself is an endless cycle of triumph, defeat, and rebirth – a continuous cycle of the highest of highs and the lowest of lows. Depression, or also defeat, is an inevitable sequence that life will eventually, in whatever form it may manifest itself in for you, present to you and every other human being on this planet at multiple certain points in your and their life. There are no set conditions for when this will happen, nobody knows when you or someone else will experience depression. It just happens one fateful day to someone.

The story of life itself, for every human being, is simply an endless and continuous cycle of highs and lows distributed in all important aspects of life. Career-wise, hobby-wise, relationship-wise, belief-wise, skill-wise, knowledge-wise, experience-wise, everything, gentlemen. One period in your life you could be working in your dream job, and the next morning, the company you work for goes bankrupt, leaving you jobless when you desperately need money. One period in your life you could be enjoying your days with the woman of your dreams, but the next day the relationship has to end because of different perspectives and parts. We have all been there, we know and understand what I am talking about here. My good friend Tezeracts even wrote a just wonderful and captivating essay about it.

That is why everything has a beginning and an end. Not to discourage you gentlemen, or anything, it is simply the game of life. Life is not permanent. Everything is always shifting and changing as we speak at this very moment. It is the game. And the narrative of the game is all about that cycle of highs and lows - a constant, never-ending cycle, that defines what life is all about, and will always be about. Especially when we are young, before having the chance, or option to become men, free, wild, full of energy and excitement to take on new things every day, and stupid, the gaps between the highs and lows are much, much greater than when we are olde, when we are fully grown men when we have already seen much of the world we live in, and indeed also know a lot more about ourselves and why we do what we do.

The story, or cycle, starts with enslavement, also known as subjugation. This is where the circumstances overwhelm you. It is where the challenges or the obstacles conquer you instead of you conquering and being in control of them. Breakups, unemployment, characterlessness, injury, failure, accidents, demise, and the list goes on and on. You are not ready for these situations, at all. And that is a normal life because you have not already experienced it before, you just do not know what to do - you are confused, and overcome with all kinds of emotions as well as thoughts, respectively. And that, gentlemen, is perfectly all right. There is nothing whatsoever wrong with that. Because then, you can finally start to familiarize yourself with all of these circumstances to eventually conquer and be in control of them at all times.

Then we finally move on to conceding and realization. This is where depression happens. Where the feeling of being completely, utterly lost in life, meaninglessness, helplessness, despair, dread, purposelessness, and undesirableness all kick in. This is where you, gentlemen, often wallow in defeat, failure, emotions, worry, or endlessly self-deprecate yourself by repeating all the discouraging words in your head like the usual "I am just not good enough I can't help it" or "I am a failure I cannot do this" or "she deserves better than me I am a loser" and many more. And yes, unfortunately, it takes a long time to get out of this period for some people. Then we come to reconstruction and rebirth. The transition from defeat to rebirth is probably the hardest one for all of us and it is what I will be emphasizing the most in this chapter. And I tell you, gentlemen, this is the one and only way to climb out of that pit of darkness. Anyways, here is where you finally decide to just keep going and keep pushing on in life - you have slowly unshackled yourself from the past and made the right decisions to bring yourself back to your feet, to crack on, to continue conquering life. Next up is actions and trials. And yes, I know, I have been mentioning and preaching this term for a bit already. Action is the sole term that truly defines a man's character, and it is no different here, either. The decisions you have made prior to this stage of the cycle. Well, here is where you finally put them to the test and make the necessary adjustments to face the challenges and obstacles that are ahead of you. Here is where you truly start to begin again. And finally, the cycle eventually completes with triumph and conquer. This is where you finally overcome and conquer those challenges and obstacles. Where you finally familiarized yourself with the circumstances that broke you previously, when you were once distraught by breakups, you now realize that the best thing is to move on and find a better partner if one exists. Where you were once crushed by unemployment, you not only realize that the best thing is to keep looking for another job or create a business of your own, but you actually do it. Where you were once devastated by the demise of someone that is close to you, you now realize that they are never going to come back and that the best thing you can do is to continue living your life as if nothing happened. You, of course, also now understand that the cycle doesn't only apply to major things in life, gentlemen, but also the small things, such as your minor nitpicks, or small wishes, or the challenge of lifting a heavier weight, or get a raise, or get a better living situation. You name it, it applies to it. And to realize that you have unlocked the first step towards greatness only limited by your will to achieve it is to have already completed the second step.

Realize, though, that it is far, far from over. And you have an extremely long way to go, and you are the one to make it happen. If you do not make it happen, nobody will. If you do not get off of your ass and get to work, nobody will. It is that simple, gentlemen. Decide to get out of that pit, commit more energy to your training, make plans, get out of that pit, adjust your plan, build up your willpower over your self-development journey, and slowly but gradually conquer anyone and anything that you want to conquer.

So, what is it then, the only way to get out of the pit of depression and defeat effectively, feasibly, and reliably?

You, gentlemen, have probably missed that it is simply to keep going. Keep going – that is it. In other words, it is the decision to act to just keep going in life, in whatever you do. No matter what the mainstream media says, you now know the truth. And with that, you are doing just fine, my friend. Just keep going. Trust me, it is the one and only way. You will see for yourself and thank me and yourself once you finish this book and once you have applied its teachings. Things in life will get better if you want to make life itself better, by making that decision to just keep going. The past is the past, gentlemen. It is, of course, okay to look back for some time and admire it a little bit, for what it is worth. But there is nothing you can do to change the past, ever. All you can do is keep going in life, keep on improving, to keep working on your self-development. And that is why you picked up this book and decided to read it.

CHAPTER SIX

THE BRUTAL TRUTH ABOUT LOVE LIFE

What you all must know and conceive.

The truth is not what you want it to be. It is what it is, and you must bend to its power or live a lie.

\- MIYAMOTO MUSASHI

Love is unconditional and will always prevail right? Well, think again, gentlemen. If love is unconditional or pure, there won't be breakups or heartbreaks. There won't be infidelity or cheating. The simple fact of the matter is love is built out of reasons, and underneath those reasons, they consist of values. Human beings desire and are attracted to certain values, and they can tolerate certain flaws from someone, but when those values are no longer there, or if they decline over time, or if they remain stagnant for too long, the love will inevitably disappear. Society and media have conditioned us through all the movies, stage dramas, music videos, and lyrics, that love will win no matter what, and all of us at least once were convinced that it is true, because, what works in the movies will also work in real life right? That is where our ignorance comes in, especially in today's digitalized age.

Fresh love. The oh-so-wonderful experience and delight that quite literally everyone seeks and pursues. It is truly emotionally enlightening being physically, emotionally, and mentally caressed, supported, loved, and nurtured by someone you deeply love, is it not, gentlemen? Intimacy is, after all, what everyone in this world is so enchanted by. And from the outside, what society and the media, and the wider populace portray looks really just like a magical experience that everyone is somehow fated to have all throughout their entire life once they find and attain it. However, the truth about love is not as simple as it seems. Far from it, in fact. People, generally speaking, think of love as this unconditional desire and total acceptance of another person's upsides, downsides, and flaws. That we can hold onto this person we love so deeply no matter what, and that it is in every way right to do so, without hesitation. This could not be farther from the truth. The simple, but disappointing truth about love is that it is never unconditional. It is never without reason. It is never without motive. It is never without thought.

Love is always about reasons. Just think of why you love cute little puppies or cute little kittens. Because they are cute, fluffy, and adorable. Do they not count as reasons why you love the woman of your dreams – because she is aesthetically beautiful to your liking because she is cute and adorable, emotionally pleasing, socially nurturing, supportive, caring, and feminine because she compliments your life rather than turning it completely upside down, leaving you in mess and chaos? The very same goes for the woman's point of view. She loves that man because he is masculine, assertive, dominant, and a charismatic leader. I will say it again, there is simply no such single thing as unconditional love and intersexual relationships, gentlemen.
Love is formed out of reasons and reasons are formed out of values. What other values do you have as a man, what can you bring to the table, what can you do? Physical appearance, general appeal, financial stability, wealth, power, humor, wisdom, intelligence, skills, experience, leadership value and abilities, emotional control and understanding, you name them, gentlemen.
The same thing can, of course, be said and vice versa – for women. What can that women bring to the table, to the relationship, what can she do, what does she know and is able to handle? What values does she have, does she have a nice physical appearance to please your eyes and overall body? Does she have great personality but also standards?   Again,   you   name   them,   gentlemen.

Love is not formed because of who each person is. It is fought for because of what each person is truly about. So, why do people leave their relationships and replace them with another one, which is arguably inferior to what you gave that person? The answer is simple. Because the values of the person whom they are in a relationship with, disappear or get stagnant for too long, without timely improvement. This is why I stress that you need to finish this book and take it seriously. Otherwise, you will slack off, and you will lose any partner you may get.

Think about it, gentlemen. When a woman falls in love with a man because he is strong, masculine, likable, dominant, and attractive, she would not express the same level of desire and attraction to that man if he becomes soft, feminine, weak, and submissive in the slightest. It only makes sense, gentlemen. Face it and learn from it. The same thing can, of course, be said if a woman whom you are in a relationship with, becomes confused; when she previously took care of you, her physical appearance, her submission to you, and being supportive and caring to you, now becomes lazy, ignorant of your needs and instructions to her, and stops caring for most things you both encounter on a daily basis or complains about them. Let us be brutally honest, gentlemen. Would you not fall out of love with her if she became like that? If she is not the person whom you so desire and initially truly fell in love with and became attracted to?

I completely understand that some of you gentlemen may or may not get hurt by this and are finding it very, very hard to accept at first. However, you all know, deep down, it is simply the cold, hard, manly truth. Love is simply not, and simply will never be a fantasy-based term, gentlemen. In reality, as you hopefully all remember and have realized by now, love is formed out of each person's desires, values, wishes, and tolerance for flaws. And should all those values that you are attracted to, and desire, disappear from that – Well, it will simply escalate to the worst, gentlemen. Do yourself a favor, listen to me, and trust me because I will show you the way. Now then, in summary, love is essentially made out of desire and attraction. Desire and attraction consist of core values. And to maintain attraction and desire, you have to compensate and keep adding qualities and skills to yourself. This is self-development 101 – precisely what this book is teaching you all along. This is the truth, gentlemen.

CHAPTER SEVEN
THE BRUTAL TRUTH ABOUT PEOPLE

Everyone is responsible for their own problems and challenges in life. Might have heard that somewhere, but it is rarely implemented by a lot of people. Reality is often too much for us human beings. Many wonder why when hardships struck your life, everyone around you just slowly disappears, even if you reach out for their help, most simply won't give you a time of the day. Why do people distance themselves away from you when you are struggling in life? Why do they avoid you and make themselves unavailable to you? And as much as I hate to say it, even your best friends can distance themselves from you. Humans are meant to help one another, right? So why do they leave you for dead when you need them the most?

I will tell you a little story of mine. When I was 18, a few years back, I decided not to go to college. I hated school, and I absolutely never had any intention to pursue any academic degree. You can say that I was a rebellious little bum, and I was, make no mistake. So, my dad decided to make an example out of me. He said: "Okay son if you do not want to go to college, I want you out of this house and prove to me and your mother that you can handle the real world on your own. So, get a place on your own, get a job on your own, wash your own clothes, and cook your own food. In fact, I will be generous enough to hand you these 500 bucks so that you can have a bit of a start already."
So, off I go then. To take on the real world by myself at 18 years old. All of my friends went to college, so I pretty much have no one to ask for help. I very quickly ask myself if I made the right decision, or if I should have just taken the offer of college from my dad. But I went: "Fuck it, I never half-ass things anyway, might as well go all the way and not look back ever again". I took a job as a cashier, which paid me about 10 bucks per hour. I barely had any knowledge of money, back then. And surprise, I know, by the end of the third month, I was already living on the very bare minimum of essentials

and especially money. Even when I decided to skip lunch for a day, I would not be able to properly make ends meet. I worked 9 hours a day for 5 days a week. That soon became 10 hours a day for 6 days a week in addition to making laundry, cooking, household chores, etcetera. After a few weeks, the time was just not enough for me to work 10 hours a day anymore, so I had to make a crucial sacrifice. The answer is pretty obvious, as to what I had to give up and let go. Although I loved going to the Gym, as I mostly sat at my work, I just had to give it up. The time was not there. So, I decided to restrict myself to pullups and pushups at home. And although quitting the gym saved me some much-needed money and time, it just was still not close to being enough. Especially not to save up to progress and free up time for self-development. Eventually, I had to go three days a week without lunch as well as dinner, do laundry only once every two weeks, cut down on my groceries, no entertainment, and very, very limited access to the internet. All in order to just meet my rent of 1100 bucks and save up 25 bucks a month. I know it was doomy, gloomy, grim, and bleak for me at the time, especially when I am only 18 and with absolutely zero knowledge, experience, career, and saved-up money. I had blown all my money on rent the first few months, in fact. I had to do extra shifts on the weekends to make up for my lack of cash, but it eventually took a big toll on my physical as well as mental health, and quite quickly at that. Eventually, I decided to call some of my friends who were still in college, but much better off than me - simply to ask them whether they have a place for me to stay or borrow some money, or even just some real, true moral support to get my mental energy back that my living conditions and my work completely drained me of. Well, they all pretty much turned their back on me. Some of them told me that I should have stuck with college and enjoyed my time with them, while others told me to simply leave them alone and that it is not their problem. Those were the people I genuinely thought were my friends. Friends I could rely on in most situations. So, in essence, all of them gave me a made-up and meaningless story about encouragement which I had absolutely nothing to do with purely to justify to themselves how they would abandon me and leave me to slowly starve to death. Naturally, I was completely overwhelmed with emotions at the time, but in my head, I was like: "Yeah, I have absolutely no money now, but the last thing I want is to give up". I never heard from those people I used to call my friends ever since. This is the part where I realized that when you are actually struggling, and I mean big time, really, nobody, nobody at all wants to be a part of it, even if it is your so-called friends merely to help you out even a little. Everyone, including your so-called friends, simply wants to get away from you as far as possible and stay away from you.

And in my case, most of those people whom I called my friends were well-known to me for over 5 years, having been actively hanging out with them and enjoying similar interests and hobbies with them. When you appear to look, dress, smell, and live like a bum, people would absolutely spit on you and leave you behind for dead, and literally could not care less about you. It got me so emotional and sad to realize that, And I always tried to convince myself that this just was not real, that people could not be that bad, that people like to help other people. Well, unfortunately, reality hit me extra hard back then. At first, I did not understand why, in fact, I could not even grasp the idea that people would leave a struggling person behind, even if that person is someone they know very well. I really wanted an answer to why they would do such vile things to me. A friend - someone whom they shared laughs and good times with, someone whom they shared a lot of things with, being absolutely deserted, and literally left to rot in the streets.

Then, one day, after work, my dad called me and asked how things were going with me and my job, my career. I obviously lied and said everything was going great because I did not want my ego to be crushed by his barrage of tips and help. Although, he invited me to a father-and-son football lounge on Sunday at his house, since we used to do that over the years when I was still in high school. I reluctantly accept the kind offer, but secretly, I was simply relieved to hear that my own father at least still cared about me enough to invite me to an evening Sunday lounge. So, I arrive at the house, and we start watching. Eventually, he asks me "So, my son, enjoying the independent life of a young man? You know, I never told you, but at your age, I was spending a lot of time getting drunk and getting laid. Fun times. Look, are you currently regretting that you rejected my offer of going to college?" I replied that I wasn't and that I met some cute colleagues at work. He replies that: "You asked for this life, son. I am glad you are enjoying it." I reply that I just have to develop myself and keep on going, and never stop. He just smiles at me. That is when I knew I had manifested my own key to life, and eventually saved up the money to move, and to write this book you are reading right now.

Always keep moving forwards, gentlemen. Never ever stop, or you will rust and fail rapidly.

CHAPTER EIGHT
WHY PEOPLE DON'T RESPECT AND ADMIRE YOU

Most people conceal their genuine selves in the deepest corner of their heads because the opinions and judgments of society intimidate them to a great extent, to the point where just expressing them feels utterly wrong, or even just thinking about them on their own makes them feel alienated.

- JAN RUDAT

Now, this is going to be a complete and utter shift in tonality in comparison to my previous chapters which are soft, calming, and outright boring - at least in comparison to this one. This chapter is not for the light or thin-skinned type of individual. This will probably offend you and get under your skin. If it does, you only have yourself to blame and you are not ready to move on to other chapters if you cannot apply this chapter's teachings to the fullest extent. Let us jump right into it, then.
What is the number one reason why people do not admire or respect you? The simple answer is that you are an inauthentic, pathetic, weak-willed, and weak-minded people-pleaser. People-pleasers are

those who do not have any opinions, passions, boundaries, enthusiasms, or beliefs and are just the sort of people who don't stand up for anything and just let life take them wherever it wants to take them. So now, why do people pleasers always get implied to fuck off by others? It is simply because they are annoying, pathetic leeches with little value trying to validate others and give others attention in order to fulfill a malicious agenda. Most commonly in the form of quite desperate hopes of receiving attention, validation, and acknowledgment back.

And to be honest, most people today are doing just that. They are just pathetic, blank, people-pleasers. They just follow whatever the others are doing in order to hopefully receive validation and/or attention in order to, in turn, fulfill their self-esteem, which is horribly lacking by the very nature of being a people-pleaser. Even though deep down they have their own set of opinions, beliefs, and so on, they are deathly afraid to simply express them and stand by them, to defend them, and to know what they like or do not like. All in the fear that society or other people would cast them out for being different. Disgusting, is it not?

Therefore, a man's true sense of self-worth depends upon the things that he values and defends, and truly stands by. And if you extensively, and impeccably people's opinions, validation, and acknowledgments of yourself, well, what do you really have left to value for yourself? The simple answer is plain nothing. Nothing at all. That is exactly why when those opinions of you change, you will feel completely, utterly, completely worthless as a man. People are attracted to values. I have mentioned this before but stick with me here - people-pleasers simply have no value whatsoever. And the simple reason behind this is that they give, give, and give. This is all they do. That makes sense, right?

I used to be a people pleaser myself in my youth. In fact, quite strongly. That is why I can confidently talk about this. And how I know that I am right and that you too can understand these basic principles that will decide whether you will make it or whether you will not make it. This "obviously" fictional character, Authory is one of those pathetic, worthless, leeching people pleaser that will never be anything else but that – a people pleaser.

It never ceases to amaze me: We love ourselves more than other people, but care more about their opinions than our own

- MARCUS AURELIUS

That is why you need a sense of self-gentlemen. One that is utterly and completely unbreakable. Value yourselves. Have your own opinions - stand by them and defend them. Have your own set of beliefs, dreams, wishes, everything.

CHAPTER NINE
MINDSET OF A TRUE KING

Masculinity is every man's natural proclivity. A masculine man is the king of his own life, the master of his own universe. Many are wondering what having a masculine mindset is, or how to think and behave like a masculine man. Masculinity is all about having your own set of desires, values, and goals, and then going after them on your own terms, unapologetically pursuing them regardless of what other people think. Most men of today try so hard to live other people's lives, they are lost in reality and fear that what they want in life will be rejected by people, so they simmer down their desires and just follow what other people do instead. Why? Every single one of you has the power to have your own life, create your own world, and be the king of it, why do you want to replicate someone else's life? Trying to live like how others live will most likely leave you empty because it is on their terms, not yours. Deep down, every man knows what he wants from life, THEN GO AND GET IT. MAKE IT HAPPEN. That is masculinity.

What does a true king do? He rules he conquers, he leads, he protects, and he provides. A true king is not just all about power, status, wealth, and fame - as how he is normally perceived by everyone else. He understands the rewards and consequences of power. A true king utilizes all of those things for the greater good of his kingdom The place, domain, and territory that he had built to protect and nurture because a true king is both a loyal servant and leader to his people and his kingdom. Truly, A true king's role is just not about being tyrannically abusive with the acknowledgment of his power. Because such a king will never be respected by anyone.

In fact, a true king treats his kingdom just like his very own child. He innately and carefully takes care of it at every step, just like how a skilled and experienced blacksmith carefully forges, shapes, and polishes his arsenal of deadly weaponry. Or, alternatively, precisely how an experienced master chef delicately cooks and prepares his impeccable and delicious dishes that feed both the body and the mind. You gentlemen know what I am talking about. You are more than welcome to use your own allegory in this chapter.

Therefore, a true king takes care of his kingdom wholeheartedly because it is his sole purpose. He nurtures his people and kingdom by creating a fair and stable economic system, entertainment, and all kinds of opportunities, that will all outlast him by a thousand years as his kingdom continues to prosper even long after his death. He also expands the territory of his kingdom, to explore new, promising, golden lands and create even more opportunities for his people. He protects his kingdom valiantly by creating countless impenetrable fortresses out of the strongest materials, and the ultimate strategic plan for when inevitable future attacks from opposing forces are soon imminent. He only fights when it is absolutely necessary simply because war and battle are both great inevitable courses for the destruction of his kingdom and the tragic death of his people, without any hope for recovery. And finally, a true king is always ready to wholeheartedly be willing to make great sacrifices for the greater good and future of his kingdom, so that it may prosper for a thousand years and beyond.

So, gentlemen - how can we, as the civilized, advanced, and essential men of the 21st century have a mindset like a true king to bring prosperity to our own lives, ambitions, and dreams? It is actually quite simple. It all starts with you taking the decision to take full control and responsibility and to lead your own life on your own terms. Now, indeed, this may or may not sound just so common to at least some of you, gentlemen. However, in reality in today's world, we far too much time trying to live other people's lives. A king does not imitate another king's kingdom. he simply builds his own, stone after stone. That is what all of us men should do instead - create and build our very own kingdom, once and for all. Why be in someone else's movie if we can make our own movie? Why mimic someone else kingdom when we can make our own kingdom?

Our life is our sole kingdom, gentlemen. And everything within our kingdom is part of our life. This can be a career, relationship, physical health, financial well-being, mental and/or spiritual health, really, you name it, gentlemen. Treat every aspect of your kingdom as your own little prize. Protect them, make sacrifices for them, stand by them, and make sacrifices for the greater good of your kingdom. This is how you nurture your kingdom so that it may grow to eternal prosperity in the future. So many men of today just neglect and do not take care of their kingdom. And by that, I mean that their physical health, mental health, life situation, financial well-being, beliefs, spiritual health, goals, dreams, wishes, relationships, bodily and mental hygiene, and activities are all not on point whatsoever.

How can any man be the master of his own life and the life of his female partner if he does not value his own life? How can a man conquer and control his life if he treats his life like a total and utter waste disposal site? How can a king be truly a king if he operates like that? The answer is quite simple, gentlemen. He cannot. But that is what the men of today are doing - leading their own life, their very own kingdom, into a chaotic mess that is extremely hard to get out of. As men, we are natural-born leaders. We build, we hunt, we explore, we protect our female partner, we discover, we fight, we find, and we conquer. As much as you gentlemen want to deny it, what a real man does is not different from what a king would do. With great power, comes great responsibility. Do not make these mistakes, gentlemen. Treat yourself and take control of your life and your prosperity, and be responsible for the prosperity for your own partner. Be the master of your own world and the prosperity of your family.

CHAPTER TEN
HOW TO BE COMFORTABLE ALONE

Go through it all.

Are you crushing life yet, or is life crushing you?

- JAN RUDAT

In this chapter, we will talk about loneliness. Yes, it is that annoying, silent, devious little devil that disturbs every single human being alive in this world. And, in truth, I could not agree more – human beings are, by natural evolution since the stone age, social creatures. Therefore, we, by default, require companionship, social interactions, and intimacy at certain points scattered throughout our lives, no matter the conditions. It is just a fact, gentlemen. Face it.

However, as mentioned before, the game of life is never about nonstop indulging and showering yourselves in the good times, such as the many parties, the huge amounts of great sex, the experiences, the laughter, and the excitement. The reason is quite simple. Because you will inevitably have to face the bad and very, very annoying times too - such as when you are simply financially broke, when your girlfriend leaves you a better, stronger man, and when you are severely injured, or when your friends leave you. In essence, the pain of reality. Trust me, this is just as much an integral part of life as the fun you will undoubtedly have. It is a giving and taking. And really, that is simply how life works - you cannot change that. Loneliness is just one of those shitty things in life that you will have to face eventually, and you will either succumb to it or conquer and control it. This is your only choice, gentlemen.

So, what can you utilize to mitigate and loneliness one fateful day? Now, before we start, keep in mind that this is very own personal list of methods on loneliness. And I've got to be honest - it has been very effective for me, my family, my friends, and my clients.

Now I personally experienced loneliness for most of my life by not having many friends, or ever getting close to people in my childhood to hang out with, since I was five years old. In my early teens, I was frightened to death by having countless heartbreaks, betrayals, and losing friends. And by choosing a profession that does not allow me good opportunities to actually get to know people to any meaningful degree - So, I am arguably quite experienced for the absolute majority of my life in the loneliness department, and even at the manager level, so to speak. I am not going to claim that I am the absolute, single-most-experienced expert or guru on the topic, or the wizard that will push your loneliness away from you. With that in mind, let us get straight into it. The first method is actually the simplest and really most obvious.

Work On Yourself

Really, really work on yourself. While this may or may not be a no-brainer to most of you, when you are all by yourself, you have all the time and the resources in the world at your disposal to work on yourself and to truly improve yourself - to grow as a human being, whether it is your career, your relationship, your wishes, your dreams, your goals, your knowledge, your beliefs, your wisdom, your spirituality, your looks, your appeal, your crappy appearance, you name it, gentlemen. In my opinion, this is the perfect time to make the most out of your life. Yet, almost nobody does this, and prefers to waste their time on things such as junk food, watching TV, gaming, and the list goes on. Is this still a no-brainer for you? In truth, your time is the single-most precious commodity you can ever have as a human being - it is even more important than money once it is actually spent. And the worst thing about it is that you can never get it back. No matter what you do, the time that you have spent is never going to come back whatsoever. You can always get more money, yes indeed - but you can never get any more time. So, you better make the most out of it.

Do you want life to go in your favor at all times? To be always in your control? Exercise regularly, read books every day, eat well, meditate, learn new skills, try some experimenting, invest your money well, seek spiritual guidance, explore the possibilities at your disposal, engage in new interests and newly gained hobbies, research anything you are curious about, have questions on, and/or are unsure of. These things are key to living a profound life as a modern, strong, and individualist man. Literally, everything you can imagine is in your utter, full, and unwavering control when you are alone. Especially so in today's time, where nearly everything is available online at absolutely no cost to you or anyone else. So, face this: What excuses do you have as a man? Do not be a lazy fuck with no drive, gentlemen. Just saying "hello" or "hi" in some online chat is not actual activity. It will get you literally nowhere in life - ever. And for those of you who think that I am simply mocking people who face tragedies: In 2020, I lost my one and only grandfather.
He was my life, and I had to personally while still recovering from a major heartbreak, watching my grandmother waste away and die of cancer, and facing financial difficulties. However, I never used them even once as excuses. To not carry on in life and just pathetically feel sorry for myself, complain and blame the world, others, or God for whatever happened. Instead, I use it as an opportunity to face and embrace the painful circumstances in order to eventually conquer and control those things, completely regardless of the circumstances. I use the circumstances to grow as a person, to build unbreakable mental fortitude, to build an even stronger emotional skin, and that, gentlemen, is what I always preach to every single one of you to do too.
The second method is also relatively simple.

Accommodate Yourself

I will tell you gentlemen a story. I once taught a friend in 3D-Modelling and Design. In fact, I have even gotten him a freelance work-from-home remote job in said field. For his own privacy, we will call him Authory Dushman Bullshitovich. You may also know him as Authory Dushman Kleptovich, if you are any close to him like I am.

We spent time together, had mutual interests, and even knew each other in person. I taught him for three months in 3D-Modelling and Design free of charge. At the time, I knew the hiring manager quite well and gave him a call whether he could accommodate my friend as an intern with a few months of experience, and to my surprise, he agreed on the spot. We never told my friend about our arrangements, so as to make him excited and feel good about himself that he apparently managed to get this position all on his own and did not even mention me.

After about one month of watching my friend learn the ropes in his new job, I texted him to see how he is really doing, and how he enjoys the new job that I got him. I was greeted with a warm greeting to "fuck off" and to "shut up". He had claimed that all the knowledge that I had taught him prior was his own, and that he learned it on his own – naturally, his hiring manager knew that was not true. After all, I had told him. You see, after I had gotten him this job, he got in way over himself. He thought he walked the entire road, he thought he conquered the world, he had achieved something great in life. What he did not understand is that I taught him only one step, not even the tip of the iceberg on how to be successful. How to be a good, successful, and attractive man. Now, three more months later, he is at the edge of being fired, unaware, yet still in the same delusional place in life as he was before. He is teetering at the edge of frustration, as he cannot figure out how to progress. This is because he got far, far ahead of himself, and decided to bite the hand that fed him. This is the cardinal sin you can commit when taking care of you gentlemen - do not make this mistake, ever. He will one fateful day realize that he will never become a man, that he is a worthless pile of nothingness, the kind of person that you, gentlemen will step on to take the victory. He will never achieve greatness in life, never achieve his dreams, wishes, goals, or ambitions. He will never succeed, he will never be able to build a relationship with a woman, and he will never be able to match you. If someone kidnapped, raped, and tortured him to death, nobody would bat an eye. I and you gentlemen would even celebrate that day ever so happily. Now while I educated him on his mistakes, he recently got to keep his job for another two months, but is already falling back into old ways, sure to lose his job for good. Therefore, it is truly one of the biggest mistakes you could ever make in your self-development journey. Know your limits, and slowly, gradually push and expand them. Be the wise turtle, not the anxious hare. Be the superior, modern man. Do not be Authory Dushman Bullshitovich. Respect your parents, they are the hand that feed you. Or they will abandon you, just like this.

Moving on, focus on the simple things in life for a change. Treat yourself occasionally, learn to cook for yourself and actually do it, get a new pair of shoes, buy a new and more comfortable chair for your workstation, enjoy yourself a fine vintage wine, or clean up your room and add some air freshener with fresh air, so that it is far more pleasant to lay down to rest. In essence, it is about re-engineering to mitigate the effect of the circumstance that facing at any given moment or time. This can be anything, really. But keep it simple. Now, do not get me wrong, gentlemen – it is completely different from indulging yourself in things like porn, or ejaculating. Pleasure is to sedate yourself, and to shift your mind in the totally wrong direction to escape the inevitable and ever-present harshness of reality in life. On the other hand, accommodating yourself is to simply enlighten your mind, or to make things simpler, easier, and more pleasant.

Now, in the face of the harshness of reality in life, if you gentlemen still do not get it, and still wish to non-stop escape to comfort and self-deprecate, it is, in essence, like going for a drive-by at Burger King, to get a bit of ice-cream while you are on a long, mundane, slow, and boring journey on the road. It is basically just about making all the things around you a little bit more helpful while performing your tasks or activities. It is that simple. Thirdly is the most important part.

You Are the Master of Your Own Life

Your life's biggest and most important decisions by you and you alone. You are the master of your own life. You are responsible for your own life - the career choice you made, what woman you chose as your partner, whether current or future, the money you spent, what you choose to invest in, the things you do are ultimately always your very own decisions to make, whatever anyone else may say or think or even express. You can, of course, look for some basic advice from other people, but at the end of the day, it is solely your call to make the decisions in your own life. You have to make all the calls according to your own plans, intuitions, plans, wishes, and assessments. So don't rely on other people to make decisions for you, because if you do that, you are basically disrespecting yourself in the strongest terms possible, and you are basically allowing people to control your life, your thoughts, your ambitions, your wishes, your plans, and your emotions however and whenever they may please. That would make you a people pleaser just like I explained previously in this book. If you do not remember that part, start reading the book from the start and take notes. Another thing is that people such as your friends and colleagues will inevitably exploit this weakness of yours and completely and utterly betray you when you need them the most - they will always choose their priorities over yours. That is just how it is, and it is not going to change.

Your life's biggest and most important decisions by you and you alone. You are the master of your own life. You are responsible for your own life - the career choice you made, what woman you chose as your partner, whether current or future, the money you spent, what you choose to invest in, the things you do are ultimately always your very own decisions to make, whatever anyone else may say or think or even express. You can, of course, look for some basic advice from other people, but at the end of the day, it is solely your call to make the decisions in your own life. You have to make all the calls according to your own plans, intuitions, plans, wishes, and assessments.
So don't rely on other people to make decisions for you, because if you do that, you are basically disrespecting yourself in the strongest terms possible, and you are basically allowing people to control your life, your thoughts, your ambitions, your wishes, your plans, and

your emotions however and whenever they may please. That would make you a people pleaser just like I explained previously in this book. If you do not remember that part, start reading the book from the start and take notes. Another thing is that people such as your friends and colleagues will inevitably exploit this weakness of yours and completely and utterly betray you when you need them the most - they will always choose their priorities over yours. That is just how it is, and it is not going to change.

People Come & Go

This is indeed quite a hard one for some of you, gentlemen. It is simply to embed within your mind that people come & go. Inevitably. The people who you are close with will probably not be with you in the next five to ten years, or even less. There are countless circumstances to warrant this. We simply cannot predict the future, and we need to be able to accept people leaving our lives.

Happiness and freedom begin with a clear understanding of one principle. Some things are within your control, and some things are not.

- EPICTETUS

Sit & Accept

Simply sit & accept. This is basically the one, single major reason for everyone one of you including myself back then, complaining endlessly about loneliness. It is because we simply fail to accept. Instead of accepting, we reject. This is why we fight loneliness instead of embracing it. As I said, pain is completely and utterly absolute and inevitable in life. And rejecting pain is like rejecting life itself.

This will be it for this chapter, gentlemen.

CHAPTER ELEVEN
GOING THROUGH DEPRESSION & RESENTMENT

Simply Focus

I graduated from university back in 2016. Everyone was so happy. Celebrating graduation like it is a success, or something amazing actually happened in their boring lives. College and university were merely an excuse for me to explore my youth, get drunk, and just get lost in this world without any remorse - because my parents were the ones paying the bills. Graduation was nothing to me, just a formality that screamed "Fun times over, now time to bear the burden of real life as a grown man". So, I did what everyone else did, using the stamp of my degree that I absolutely did not have any passion whatsoever in attaining, to get a mundane 9 to 5 job and be a corporate slave. Every single one of them rejected me, banks, consulting companies, online shops, and even fresh startups rejected me. And to be honest with you, gentlemen, I never quite understood the reason behind the rejections, but nevertheless, I was devastated that after three months, I was still unemployed, and that corporate people think that I just do not have it quite in me. To make matters worse, my partner decided to end the relationship because I was going nowhere in life, and they wanted someone who can get his shit together. I do not blame them, however - admittedly, my physical and mental health was already in a bad state due to my stress and anxiety, and with them leaving me, they got even worse. But I did not feel any regret, because they were already making my life a living hell, and my ideals of them being an angelic being that can comfort me, was willing to support me, and to go through whatever with me, like a true partner that is marriage material would, was nothing but an illusion. The pressure, anxiety, fear, and feeling of uselessness just kept filling my head at night, never letting me rest, dragging me down deeper into that abyss of depression. At that time, I could not sleep, knowing that everyone would laugh at me for being unemployed for this long. I isolated myself and just kept on applying for any jobs that I could see, and after another three months, no luck whatsoever - I began to lose all hope. One night, at 3AM in the morning, I decided to cook some eggs for breakfast. Then, I suddenly took a glance at the knife, which, for some reason, was not put back into the knife rack by myself. As the eggs sizzle in the pan, I glance at the knife, and just lost all sense of time and space - I imagined stabbing myself with that knife, visualizing blood coming out of my abdomen and just bleed to death to end all this suffering. I then grab the knife, and point it directly at my abdomen, slightly applying pressure. My mind and heart were racing. I then thought to myself that that this could not be the end, the end-all. I blacked out for a second, only to wake up on the floor. I caught a glimpse of myself bleeding out on the kitchen floor, I stay silent. I stare at the knife again, and put it back into the rack. I had unknowingly slightly stabbed myself in the abdomen, as I passed out and fell the floor. I inspected the wound, it was not deep, and had only pierced some fat and skin. I stuff the wound and bandage it up, eventually going back to my bedroom with my burned eggs for breakfast.

The next week eventually came by. I was driving home from a friend's dinner party. All of them had jobs apart from me, and admittedly all of them, individually, had better grades than me. I was still envious and ignorantly resent them as a result of that. As I was driving on the quiet and empty road at 1 AM in the morning again, the thought of being useless and purposeless stroke me hard as I was driving down the road. The pain was again unbearable, I was doing about 90mph, and I felt like I was going to cry, and crash the car. The pain was just too much - I was unable to bear it. So, I contemplated again to end my life. This time by purposefully and violently swerving my car into a nearby tree, hopefully piercing the fuel tank so it catches fire as a way to make sure that I died with my miserable life then and there. The tension was incredibly high, and the contemplation extremely intense, but once I again, I decided against it, this time maintaining consciousness. Then, even slower, another month went by, and I was just a walking zombie at this point, I could not cry anymore because I cried too much. My body just could not produce that many tears. I had grown emotionally numb. I was lonely, I was afraid, I was nothing but one of those many, many wandering, lost souls. But at the same time, I was also angry, and dare I say it, the last ounce of my soul was just not willing to quit just yet - even though every single other part of me was already on the ragged edge of quitting and throwing in the towel. Eventually, I came to my senses, and continue applying for jobs, which again, I had no luck on for a couple of weeks.

But then, as I was walking to my car from a job interview, I glanced at a notice board in front of a large warehouse, saying that the company running the warehouse was searching for a warehouse clerk, and fast. And me, being the angry man with nothing to lose I was, I just stepped into that building and asked for the manager, to ask for that job. Surprisingly, I was hired right away, and the other jobs I was interviewed for, as you would expect, I did not even get a call, a letter, or even a simple E-Mail back from any of them. But at that point, I did not care, because I was just tired of looking back at my failures, and so, I made the decision to keep looking forward from there on out, and capitalizing on every opportunity that is presented to me. I worked at that warehouse for 8 months before I got a proper office job as a wealth consultancy advisor, as a trustee.

Looking back, I wonder why I did not just give up after months and months of absolutely getting the door slammed into my face countless times. I guess I just hated the words "failure" and "loser" too much to carry them with me to the grave, and that I was just too attached to my failures which were all in the past already by then. I eventually just made up my mind that If I was going to die, I would not want to die lying down. If I was going to die, I would rather die of fatigue of actually making it in life, than to not even try. As poetic as it may seem, that mindset helped me overcome many, many adversities.

So stop looking back, be in the present, and never contemplate on your failures ever again, gentlemen. As painful as it is, this made me the person I am today. A better, superior, modern person. Simply focus. It will not be easy.

This is the only way, gentlemen. I have walked this path, having proven that is indeed possible. No excuses from here on out. Keep moving and never look back, ever again.

CHAPTER TWELVE
THE CONSEQUENCE OF ANGER AND HATRED

Vengeance has always been a hot topic because it is a very visceral form of conduct. Pain and suffering brought by other people onto us, we want to give them a taste of their own medicine, by committing the same act on those people who have hurt us, through hatred, resentment, and wrath. What you must understand is that the people who initially brought pain and suffering to our lives are also living with pain and sufferings themselves, it is just that they do not know what to do with it, or how to utilize those emotions in a constructive way. So they project their pain and suffering onto other people, in order for them to hopefully, feel relieved & satiated of their inferiority. And with you committing vengeance by causing the same pain to them as they've done to you, ultimately making you no different to them, you are also unable to utilize your emotions in a constructive manner.

I was a shy and quiet kid back in 11th grade, the one you usually find in the corner of the classroom - just deeply immersed in my own world, endlessly daydreaming, and more interested in his own thoughts than any lectures given by the teachers, and even conversations between fellow classmates. I never look for trouble, nor do I ever seek any confrontations. I also never display the willingness to offend anyone, nor do I even want to purposely hurt anyone in order to make myself feel good about myself. But, I also do not have any spine to rely on. And that is exactly why I became easy prey for the packs of predators who have just entered puberty and relishing the raging hormones of testosterone to their advantage.

Home & school were either boring or unwanted by them, and they needed excitement - and since there were very few entertainments other than physical exercise class, they instead found entertainment in me. Mocking my quietness, treating me like a laughing stock, making assumptions about my life, and of course, just like all bullies, took advantage of my physical weakness, and beat me up whenever they got the chance to do so. I did not fight back, because I was massively outnumbered - they were a pack of four, and I was on my own. And on top of that, they were also physically bigger, and often carrying weapons. I just had no chance. Almost every day, I went home with a new bruise, and I hate getting my parents involved because I did not trust them, as they did not have a close relationship with each other by any means. Therefore, I always made the excuse of being clumsy while playing football. I hated going to school from there on out, as I was just getting tossed around like a garbage bag for nearly the entire first semester. By the time that holiday came, I was fueled with anger, hate, and rage. But at the same time, I was also restrained by fear and lack of confidence. I simply stayed in my room for the first couple of weeks during the holiday, just succumbing to myself within my own sadness and rage, hating myself for being weak, inferior, and defenseless.

My world was just full of hatred of wanting to beat up all of those bullies who treated me like a helpless bag of dirt - I did not want to just "hurt them", I wanted to make them suffer, or better yet, their entire family, and some, I also wanted to kill. So, I wanted to know how to fight, so I signed up for an MMA class, and learned how to punch, kick, and wrestle throughout the remainder of the holiday. I was focused as absolute and utter hell in every session, the way I never did in school. I kicked every punch and kick with determination and serious intent. I was a fast learner, and always stayed late to ask my coach for extra time, and to learn new techniques even after the sessions were finished. With a week left in the 3 months of semester holiday, I already learned how to effectively ground and pound an opponent and perform a swift takedown of opponents who are much bigger than me. My confidence grew, but my hatred and rage were also amplified tenfold, with no ethics or morals to hold me back whatsoever, merely the respect for the law due to the possibility of being arrested and facing legal charges in court.

One day, after a session, my coach said to me: "You are catching up really well, but I need you to ease it off a little, all right? I know what young people can do to others when they are given the edge over others. I just want to tell you that there will be no fighting outside of the gym of any kind - because if I catch you with blood on your hands or if anyone comes to me and says that he/she saw you fighting, you are out of here for good, and for life. Remember that". I started blankly at my coach, and simply said, "Don't worry coach, I won't".
I didn't take what he said seriously, at all. That is because my focus was never being good with martial arts. I just want to have some combat abilities as military-grade Krav Maga was not available in my region. Simply to make those bullies pay for what they have done to me - if necessary, with blood or their lives. And I really, really wanted to make them pay. The real reason why I learned martial arts was never to be able to defend myself from threats, but instead, it was to cause even more pain to those who hurt me, so they would never be able to hurt me ever again and to make them an example to their families, friends, and anyone who wanted to associate with them as bullies. The first day of the second semester came, and I was determined to finish what they had started. During lunchtime I was sitting alone by the school garden, eating lunch and reading "God is dead" by Friedrich Nietzsche, when someone hit me from the back of my head, causing me to fall onto the grass.

It was them. Now my mind was blank, I did not think at all. I pulled out a knife I had packed the day before and charged at them, and within a swift second, they were all on the ground - but I was still angry, I had no control. I did not just leave them there, I kneel on top of one of them and started punching his face repeatedly until a friend of his attacked me again, which I wrestled to the ground and started stabbing, unleashing every ounce of my anger, rage, and pure hatred that I have been bottling up since the day they bullied me. As I write this, I am shaking so strongly that I can hardly write coherently - I feel like a ball of burning ice.

Blood on my fists, wrists, and lower arms, and I was breathing heavily. I still could not think straight, but when I raised my head to look around, everyone was watching me. Their faces were filled with horror and fear, no one muttered a word. I came to my senses and realized what I had done. I could not help myself and started laughing. With absolutely nothing to say and no idea what else to do, I washed the blood off my hands, wrists, and arms, packed my things, and went home. I was filled with fear of what will happen to me, how I had so many witnesses against me, and so much evidence making a self-defense claim unlikely to be believed by authorities after I had committed such a gruesome but so pleasant and exhilarating act. I could not decide whether to be scared or just smile and enjoy the breathing room that I had created by removing such human vermin from my life.

I did not know whether it was my PTSD or just pure shock, I was not sure at all. All I know is that it felt great that I was unleashing everything, and that I had done a good deed. And I regret nothing, as it made me what I am today, and brought me such a wonderful life.

Interviewer:
"So, what happened to the other kid, that you not only had beaten up badly but almost stabbed to death? He died on the way to the hospital. The other young man that you had beaten so brutally, he passed away a week later... he went into a deep coma... he got a ruptured artery and a severe brain trauma."
Myself:
"When I repeatedly hit him, I did not realize that there was a stone behind his head, so he was not just getting hurt from my punches. Therefore, I did not kill him, but he died from the stone that his head got repeatedly rammed into with my punches."
Interviewer:
"Looking back at that moment, what would you do differently? Show me on this piece of paper."
Myself:
"I just wish I had more control of my thoughts back then, even at 17 years old... I did not have any control at all."
Interviewer:

"Now... that's just stupid, tell us the truth. We are eager to listen to the real story. Your drawing or story do not make any sense."

I cannot tell you what happened after that. That is reserved for another book, far in the future.

Moral Of the Story

Vengeance is an act committed because of the lack of acknowledgment of one's own self-worth as a person. When one is hurt by another, he wants to return the favor by committing the same hurt that befell him to that person who has caused him that pain. Because he has no strong foundation of what defines him, nothing of the sort can reinforce his confidence and integrity. He was made to feel inferior, and therefore act on an impulse.

In my case, it was completely justified. I acted in the interest of the greater good, and remember this, gentlemen - anything is justified in the interest of the greater good. There is no reason to feel bad about what I did if it is for the greater good. And in my case, it was not morals, but my own self-defense and the defense of others, which is politically defined under Socialism. You can look at it like 2 worthless capitalist predators feeling lucky, and simply losing to chance. Authory, which I previously mentioned, would be one of those people that would run risk of receiving said treatment. This is because they do not apply the lessons found in this book.

CHAPTER THIRTEEN
DEVELOPING PERCEPTION AND ACCEPTANCE

In stoicism there is a famous saying that nothing is good, and nothing is bad. Although that can be very idealistic to just be very neutral about everything, we humans can never be in such robotic manner our whole lives, we are emotional creatures after all, we unconsciously will see something as either good or bad, nice or unpleasant, preferable or not preferable to a certain extent. We love the good stuff, don't we? We love feeling happy, excited, thrilled, amazed and so on, but often we don't welcome the unpleasant stuff like sadness, boredom, struggles, failures, setbacks, and unfortunate circumstances. We often don't want them to happen ever in our lives, that is why we avoid them or just completely divert our attention away from them, because our mind always want the path of least resistance. However, hardships and struggles are the essential and unavoidable parts of life, and in fact those "painful" and "unpleasant" things are the ones that will make you grow into a better human being. The only thing that is required is for people to change their point of view on simply approaching them.

Storytime, gentlemen. I once went to Ukraine as a Humanitarian Worker, after my then ex-fiancé, a wonderful Ukrainian, persuaded me not to join the International Legion for the Defense of Ukraine, as a foreign fighter. I spent 6 months in Ukraine, hopping from the cities of Lviv to Kyiv, eventually being wounded by a trip-mine left by Russian forces, watching my friend die in front of me, listening to his half-conscious moans, given an opium addiction by the army medic, just wanting to leave the country to decompress, or I would snap like a twig. I still have nightmares and increased symptoms of PTSD from that time. I shake every time I recall this, I jump to the ground anytime that I hear a sufficiently loud noise, and I developed chronic insomnia and my chronic pain only intensified and increased.

I did not surrender. I did not falter, or kill myself, or wallow in my own emotions and self-deprecate myself. I went on, I continued life, I continued working on my self-development journey. I kept walking, and never looked back since.
I made life, life did not make me.

Take another story from me.
Jan and Authory are two brothers born just two hours apart, they both have the same collection of audacious curiosities, interests &

admirations. They both love the thrill and adrenaline of competitions, and they both share the same exciting and adventurous dreams for their future lives. However, while Jan always had a profound level of wisdom and a positive outlook on his life despite all the challenges & adversities he faced. Authory, on the other hand, had always been quite pessimistic and more often than not, always rejects or runs away from adversities, and often folds emotionally in the face of unfortunate circumstances. Jan always loved challenges, even in the face of failures or setbacks, he always had a smile on his face and has always been an incredibly determined, attractive, and appealing person when it comes to overcoming his adversities. He loves breaking down the things that he did wrong, and never stops until he found an answer or a solution to his problems. And the thing that people found quite confusing, but secretly admirable about him, is that he does all of that with an extremely elevated level of enthusiasm and commitment. He once got severely injured at the gym because he bench-pressed 100 kilograms with improper form and lack of proper, gradual progression. The injury was rather dramatic and debilitating, it was a torn right rotator cuff muscle that set him back a full six months of weight lifting. Rather than wallowing in his setbacks of having to build his body from the ground up once again and throwing in the towel, he instead researched extensively about his injuries and learned from online coaches about proper form and programming his progressions properly in the gym. When it comes to Authory, though, he often got scared of challenges, almost every time he sees them as a threat that could endanger his physical or mental wellbeing. He is always anxious about the future, he fears failure and hates facing setbacks, because he thought they never made him feel any good about himself, nor do they serve any purpose other than to show that he is incompetent at the stuff that he puts his effort into. That is why when he is faced with profound challenges, or any form of downward spiral that befall him, he often avoids them or just resigns completely. When he got fired from his first job as an accountant , on which he graduated out of university with a degree of one, he took it personally and spends a significant amount of time self-deprecating himself, endlessly saying things like "I am not good enough. it is stupid to continue" and "They deserve better than me, I am just bad.", and completely abandons his accounting roots, all the while refusing to apply for jobs related to finance because he was too fearful of getting rejected again. And now he juggles between jobs of different fields without any clue of what he wanted to do, therefore feeling lost and purposeless in life, stuck, even, which only leads him into depression.

It is also a similar case for the two brothers when it comes to getting caught in the way of life's unfortunate circumstances that are simply beyond their control. When Jan was caught in a minor crash on a Saturday night, because a drunk driver rammed the rear of his car at 100mph, causing the entire trunk lid, rear bumper, and exhaust system to be replaced and eventually costing him two grand to fix them, he did not get emotional, nor did he start a fight with the drunk man who did not have the strength to even stand up. He simply said "Oh well, shit happens", and that was it for him. He then moves on with his life, never again contemplating about the accident. Authory, on the other hand, when his car accidentally ran over a huge nail and sending the front tire to go completely flat, and rendering him stuck for five hours in the middle of nowhere. While waiting for the tow truck to come over to his location, he yelled a ton of curse words and started blaming construction workers for being stupid idiots because he thinks that they purposely left some nails on the road just to flatten his and only his tires when he drove on the road. Naturally, all of that did nothing but consume his energy and pretty much made him sound like a little, pathetic, weak crybaby that nobody likes and that gets nowhere in life, ever. Eventually though, Authory realized that what he is doing is only making his life even more miserable and temporarily stopped. So, on one night at the dinner table of his brothers home, he sought advice and clarity for his own insufferable attitude from his brother.

JAN:
You should cook me dinner for once, dear brother, present it to someone whom you are going to bring home for the night. It is really not that hard and means a lot to people, even myself.

AUTHORY:
Naah... I am not a good cook by any means, I could not cook even if I wanted to. I just suck at everything. Like you, brother. Just give me

your stupid advice so I can already leave your house.

JAN:
Wait a second, why would you not even try? Embarrassment is necessary for you to take the next step in life to improve and continue your self-development journey, dear brother. No offense, of course. You know I love you no matter what, and this is just genuine help   from   me.

AUTHORY:
The reason I have come to dinner today, is to discuss exactly that. How can you be so enthusiastic about failing, about getting embarrassed? How could you still smile when everything is going south against you? When you are going through so much pain in your life? What is wrong with you? Nobody in their right mind acts like   that,   it's   impossible.

JAN:
You see, dear brother, the simple reason why I am able to push through all those adversities, and become even more enthusiastic and determined when they happened to me, is actually because my mindset and perception of them is completely different to yours. While you treat adversities and hardships like they are dead ends, and that they are things to be avoided at all costs, if I fail, get rejected, or get embarrassed for doing something, I did not close my door on them. Instead, I saw many other doors opened for me to step inside, and experience what is inside of them. As unpleasant as they may be, they are still new experiences to be relished, cherished, remembered, and worked on. Because once you have passed them, dear brother, boy oh boy how it felt utterly amazing for me, and showed me that I am far more capable than what I initially thought about myself to be. And that, dear brother, is simply how I approach hardships. Never reject adversities, always welcome them, just like peoples thoughts and opinions, unfortunate circumstances, they all will happen one way or another, whether you face them or not. And indeed, they can be a pain in the ass to endure, but, so what? Enjoy and relish the pain. Cherish it. Welcome and accept it. Do not contemplate, do not overthink, just do it. And if you want it just a

little easier, stop it with the hilariously silly insults – they only hurt yourself.

Moral Of the Story

Your perception will result in your reality. If you perceive one circumstance as bad, it will be so for you. If you perceive another as good, then it will be likewise. Perception will lead to either understanding or resentment. Understanding or resentment will lead to acceptance or rejection. Acceptance or rejection will lead to the reality that will be morphed into your perception, reality, and life. If you are distressed by anything whatsoever external, the pain is really not due to the thing itself, but actually due to your estimate of it, and this you have the power to revoke at any moment.

\- JAN RUDAT

CHAPTER FOURTEEN
CONTROLLING EMOTIONS

Being an emotional man

We've all been there, being unable to control our impulses, and in this case our burst of emotions. Things that irritate us, things that challenge us, or things that we do not expect can trigger our emotions and make us very reactive. The problem with this is that being emotional is triggered either by our negative perceptions/perspectives on circumstances, or when our egos are challenged, doubted, or proven wrong. And with the burst of emotions that come after that, it is only to negate/defend the effect or attack back the one that caused the hurt. However, being emotional can have drastic consequences, mostly unwanted ones, and give rise to problems that initially weren't meant to be created/initiated, and this can happen in any scenario. That is why learning to control them is absolutely crucial if you want your mind to remain sharp and clear in the face of pressure and provocations.

Anger is like those ruins which smash themselves on what they fall on. The mind when it has abandoned itself to anger and is unable to check itself.

- SENECA

MOM DREEMUR:
Authory, do not forget to be back by 8PM, alright? You are always so late, its dangerous outside, I worry so much about you whenever you come home so late, it is terrible, please be timely.

AUTHORY:
I know mom, could you stop telling me that all the time?!? I am no baby anymore!!

ERICK:
Hey Authory, what is up with you mate? You look like an angry baby. Did your mom tell you to stay away from the cookie jar or what? Did someone get out of bed with the wrong foot maybe?

AUTHORY:
Nothing man, I am just not in the right mood for talking right now. Can I just enjoy some time alone, my idiot clown friend who is constantly wanting to hang out with me despite my insults?

HOWELL:
Funny you say that Erick. I thought he looked like shit today, too! Where did you get that rancid hat from, authory? It looks like some cheap limited stock. Your granddad's attic from World War two?! It probably makes you so dismal all of a sudden. You dress like shit, authory.

AUTHORY:
Hey Howell, you better shut that shit up or you will land in medical because I cut your fucking tongue off and feed them to your

mothers' dogs you stupid cunt!! Fuck you bitch, get out of my sight.

ERICK:
Yo, Authory, relax man, we were just having a good old banter with you, this is why you are on the edge of being fired from your stupid remote job as a designer which does not pay real money. Oh wait, your hiring manager already found out and fired you. Well, nevermind.

AUTHORY:
I have got to go, sorry, mom calls...

MOM DREEMUR:
Oh authory, you are home early, my boy. What is the matter, dear? Is   something   wrong   perhaps?

AUTHORY:
Nothing, I am just so, so tired, mom. Can I just go to bed? I could fall   asleep   with   open   eyes.

MOM DREEMUR:
Come and sit down, I would like to have a word with you about your remote job as a 3D designer, son. It has me and your father quite concerned,   you   know?   Please   sit   down   with   me.

AUTHORY:
I am not in the mood for talking mom, you are living dangerously, mom. Just shut the fuck up and leave me alone. I have enough issues already   I   don't   need   you   nagging   on   me   now.

MOM DREEMUR:
I am just worried about you that the longer you wait to get a roper, a real job, the more they will reject you, son. You will have to get a job and one day care for me when I get old, son. You know, companies of today would like someone with genuine experience in a given field, and not some freelance remote work in 3D Modelling that some woman on the internet taught you, only for you to waste your time on this videogame website with blocks as graphic design. It does not even pay real money my dear, only this stupid virtual

currency,   something   with   "R".

AUTHORY:
Mom!! I told you not to ever tell me what to do!! This website is my real job, and I'm going to earn real money with it soon!! You can't tell me what to do!!!! Why can you not understand that I got all this experience on my own, nobody helped me, and that this 3D Modelling job is serious, and the on-site currency can eventually be exchanged at a 5:1 ratio for real money!!?! We have talked about this many times, this cannot go on with you like this, seriously! Hell!

DAD:
Authory! Did you hear all of those things that you just said?! If you do not get a real job and respect your poor mother, you are OUT of this house! Do you understand me, my son?

AUTHORY:
Ugh, whatever.

DAD:
Authory, come here and sit down, now. What were you thinking, son? Did you think getting all emotional like that would make your problems go away? This is childlike, and you are no longer a little child. You are just a toddler who got his toys taken away. Let me tell you something about an emotional man, son. It really gets you nowhere. it only embarrasses you, make yourself depressed, look immature, and be incompetent. And that is what you are, son. If you get emotional by something as miniscule as a suggestion, imagine what the cruel and unforgiving world would do to you if you had to be a man on your own - you would probably kill yourself, and none of your internet so-called bosses or friends would miss you. You cannot think straight when you are emotional. Am I understood, son?

AUTHORY:
Yes dad...

CHAPTER FIFTEEN

SOCIETY'S FALSEHOODS

The sugarcoating revealed.

My friend, the truth is always implausible, did you know that? To make the truth more plausible, it is absolutely necessary to mix a bit of falsehood with it. People have always done so.

\- FYODOR DOSTOYEVSKY

We've been told lies after lies when it comes to our real-life problems. Many social media influencers, television shows, and movies told us that we are all deserving of love and appreciation, whoever we are, what shape we are, where we come from, and what demons we are possessed by, we will all be received with open arms everywhere we go, and if we aren't, they promise that someday we will find that place regardless. Delusional, empty, ignorant, and misleading is what I would call them. The truth is, the world despises and leave people with problems, issues, miseries, and anything that doesn't please their 5 senses. If you are physically unappealing, mentally broken, financially unattractive, socially inept, and spiritually void, you will never ever be loved by others. You must be "VALUABLE" in order for you to respect and love yourself, and eventually for others to respect and love you.

Gentlemen, have you ever been told or even sold something that sounds & looks like a gleaming beacon of hope to your ears, that you cannot help but relish it all your spirit without knowing the uncomfortable and bitter truth that lies underneath the flower painted sheets? You are not alone in this. I am sure everybody has. I certainly have. You want to know what that thing is? Let me all take you back in time once again. Ten years ago, a 25-year-old me just entered the real world after quite a wild and dull ride at university. Blind, but eager to finally make something out of my life, since I was hopeful that the real world would be even more accommodating, wiser, and nicer to me, than my mostly wasted time studying for things that I am not really interested in even to this day, getting wasted, and getting walked over by almost everyone I knew. But this turns out to be the worst mindset I could ever set for myself back in the day. I was out of shape, broke, depressed, drunk, and lost with no concrete knowledge, skills, or anything to showcase to the world at the time - and I thought people in the real world would actually assist me, or love me, despite my set of deep-running miseries. But I was completely wrong. So wrong that I would eventually take the reality of it as the single, most important lesson I have ever learned the way way in my life. You see, gentlemen, the world will not come to you, tend to your wounds and problems, and save you from all of your miseries, and they will never come to save you. Everyone would run away from you and leave you for dead. My own mother always said to me every time I was slapped with that reality, "Oh son, don't you worry too much about it, everything will be fine, you are loved and you deserve to be loved, even if yo udo not love yourself. There are good people in this world that will love you for who you are, no matter the size, shape, and conditions you are in." I am sure mangy of you have heard these words shoved and rubbed onto your face countless times by those so called "influencers" on social media, or even the movies and TV shows that were released over the last decade. Those ignorant, sabotaging, manipulating, delusional, and empty set of words that was sold to us countless times - and we would ignorantly buy into them because they offer us an easy chance to feel alive again someday in the future, catering to our needs, and making us feel at ease and hopeful that there is a place in the world that can actually love us.

Those sugar-coated lies absolutely don't relate to anything that you or me are experiencing in the real world and the harsh reality that it brings - but we buy into them because we are having trouble accepting and dealing with the wolf in the sheep's clothing, and hearing those words is like giving us slabs of meat to temporarily keep the wolf at bay, until they eventually ran out and the wolf starts to think of eating us for supper again. Those words never provide any logical and rational solutions to the problems we had dealing with ourselves and the real world that ignores them. Those words are just false hopes and temporary lies that soothe our brows and serve us tea for a while, but never cure our pain permanently, and we ended up bathing ourselves in them even more, because we are trying to hide ourselves from the pain that we want to, and must solve. We were promised, promises that never came, and they leave us alone with our shattered remains. The bitter truth is this: the world will not reward or give love and appreciation to anyone who does not have any values to bring into it. You will never be loved and appreciated, unless you bring something of value to the table - whether it is physically, mentally, financially, intellectually, and/or socially. Both love and appreciation do not exist without respect, and respect does exist without values. As much as you want to deny it, the world will judge you on everything, and I always thought the meaning of "Loving yourself" was to constantly tell yourself that you deserve to be loved, and giving yourself a million pats on the back every time you got bruised by a sniff of reality.

But we all know that those things are just empty promises deep down and eventually, reality will catch up to us and give us a huge slap of awakening. For those who are still defending that idea of you deserving to be loved and appreciated unconditionally, here is another dose of reality. The mainstream quote of "If you don't love me at my worst, you don't deserve me at my best." is basically a definitive confirmation and admission to yourselves that no one has ever loved you at your worst. Because you have experienced those circumstances before in your life, and now you are just lying to yourselves by sugarcoating that reality, with your delusional hopes and ideals to save your own broken heart, ego, and self-esteem instead of accepting it. If unconditional love and appreciation truly exist, those empty quotes won't ever exist in the first place.

In order to truly love ourselves, we must respect ourselves and in order to respect ourselves, we must add value to ourselves, and the only way to add value to ourselves is by embodying and showcasing competence in all important areas of our lives, that we all value to a high extent. And through the process, we wash away the worst version of ourselves. That is the only way we truly develop self-worth and self-actualization. It is to develop values for ourselves, independent of everything else that exist outside of that. Nowadays, we relish ourselves too much in the empirical truth rather than the objective truth. We start to believe things that we want to hear, rather than the things that we need to hear. We put a blindfold on the things we see that don't cater to our emotions and put a magnifying glass on the things that fulfill our ideals & fantasies, rather than the things that disrupts our illogical and delusional cognitive dissonance.

Never assume that love and appreciation is freely given - a healthy form of love and appreciation is always deservingly earned. Unconditional love is both a myth and an illusion, and it will always be that way. To earn respect and love from others, you must first earn respect and love from yourselves. There is absolutely no use in self-deprecating yourselves in between the cracks of your own broken heart, because you are unable to face the consequences of believing false promises that has been conditioned into your lives for years. Weakness does not thrive, and will not thrive, in a power evolving universe, gentlemen. You have to patch yourselves up, see the world as it is, and bend to the truth that it brings, so that you can take advantage of it.

CHAPTER SIXTEEN
PURSUING YOUR DREAMS

What will you be willing to give up to achieve your goals and dreams? A very Cliché question, but it is definitely true. Every man in the right mind has his own set of goals and ambitions he wants to achieve in life, and those achievements require years of blood, sweat, and tears to accomplish, and certainly will take out the most important and precious commodity of the human life, which is "Time". We all are born with a limited amount of time on this planet, what we choose to utilize that time for, is what we will eventually become. And if you want to achieve your goals and dreams, you must make sacrifices allocating the time that you spent on things that will drag you away from your goals to the things that will help you achieve your goals.

With pursuing your goals and dreams, comes challenges you've never come across before, but that you must face and overcome in order to eventually achieve those goals and dreams. And it is normal to be anxious and fearful, because only then can a man be brave and displays his courage to come out of hiding (his comfort zone) and take the risks necessary for him to move forward toward the life he wanted to live and the man he wanted to be. Failure, setbacks, anxiety, injuries, wasted money, embarrassment, and rejections will come your way, and it is up to you whether you want to keep going or if are you going to quit and go back to the life that you were promising yourself to get away from.

When I was a little boy, I was always in love with clothes, and still am to this day. I would always ask my parents to buy me clothes worn by superheroes like Spiderman and Superman. I would wear them all day long and pretend that I was Spiderman or Superman themselves. Fast forward to when I was a young adult, and that feeling never changed for me. Wearing the right clothes on the right occasions just makes you feel confident and unique to your own personality and style. I just feel like one with the clothes that I am wearing, almost like I am wearing a personalized piece of armor for me to take on the world. Whenever I had free time after work, I would always spend the rest of the day sketching and designing clothes, experimenting, and just getting lost in my own imagination and pouring out whatever ideas my brain had forged - even the crazy and unrealistic ones. I also never hesitated to manifest them into a design. I was obsessed and enthusiastic beyond measure, but I was still lacking the discipline the dedication required for me to manifest my dream into reality. I was still easily distracted and was afraid to reject people's situations. Such as whenever my friends asked me to go to the cinema together after work, or the bar. I never rejected their offer even once and was always eager to come with them, even if I had made a promise to myself early on that I was going to work on my dream for that particular day. The same thing happened on the weekends, where I would have all the time and effort in the world to commit to my dream - but instead, I found myself drinking beer at the bar in the afternoon with my friends, when I could have just said "no" and use the much-needed time to put in extra hours to my own project. And then, in the evening, I would find myself getting absolutely wasted at the nightclub, busting my ears, and getting my clothes all wet, wasting a bunch of money, and wasting my time and health. Naturally, I woke up the next day feeling like shit and having absolutely no energy to do anything else for the entire day but to let my precious liver recover and get the much-needed extra hours of sleep. I was basically slowing myself down on purpose and letting my dreams slip away from me bit by bit. And the worst part is, it was my own decision - I could have just refused my friend's offer to hang out, but I was too afraid that they might hate me for it, or they may kick me out of the group or ban me from the clubs we went to at the end of senior year.

But I had enough of it, I have different priorities now, I am done wasting so much time, energy, and money on stuff that does not get me anywhere near to who and where I want to be in life. I finally mustered up the courage to say "No" to my friends whenever they invited me out to have fun. I also gave up on my videogaming habits which also robbed some much-needed time to work on my dream. I realized that I had to make necessary sacrifices in order for me to get anywhere close to where I wanted to be, after all, I only have one brain, two arms, and two legs. So, I cannot be everywhere all at once. I have to make crucial decisions in life because every choice you make has both rewards & consequences. If I went out to bars, get wasted in nightclubs, and play videogames, I will get the reward of having fun and enjoying life, but getting the consequence of rapidly rotting away bodily and mentally, while getting nowhere in life and letting my dreams, ambitions, and wishes slip away.

You lack the courage to be consumed in flames and to become ashes: So you will never become new, and never young again! The courage of all one really knows comes but late in life.

- FRIEDRICH NIETZSCHE

So off I go then, onwards to my journey of climbing the ladder towards the mark that I set out for myself to reach. Now, do I have any idea of what I am going to come across on my journey? Some idea, yeah, but most of the time it was just the indomitable will to go through. I actually have no idea how those challenges will present themselves to me, how I will react to them initially, or what it will take. I was afraid, very afraid internally, to be honest. Because, while I might have some idea of what to anticipate along my journey, I absolutely have no clarity of how everything will turn out. Will I fail? Will I succeed? Will I create dreams that are appealing and competitive? I have no idea. The anxiety was killing me at the time, and the thoughts of quitting and thinking that everything was a bad idea always haunts me to the forefront of my head every single moment. Just the jarring scenario of me being a laughingstock and a disgraceful failure to my people, my friends, and my family never cease to bother me. But thankfully, my definitive decision to not go back to the life that I once lived, of going out to bars, getting drunk in nightclubs, playing videogames, and such, always kept me levelheaded throughout the journey. Because I realized that with all the fear and anxiety of the mountain of challenges ahead of me, I simply have to press on, never look back, and overcome the challenges to eventually conquer and control them. You just need to act and just go for it, no matter what happens. Take risks, learn from people thinking they are smart by telling on you, let them think they are in right, while you conquer them and use them for your success.

CHAPTER SEVENTEEN
BUILDING UNBREAKABLE WILL

The ultimate measure of a man is not where he stands in moments of comfort and convenience, but where he stands at times of challenge and controversy.

- MARTIN LUTHER KING JR.

Having a strong mental fortitude is probably the wish of every man of today. Being able to handle confidently & comfortably painful, arduous, irritating, and even dangerous circumstances is personally extremely appealing and inspiring. However, humans are emotional creatures by default and love the path of least resistance, and should circumstances don't cater to our emotions, we flip out and try to mitigate the negative effects by expressing their opposites. But through expressing those emotions, we release ourselves from control and let those circumstances control us instead of the opposite. We become emotionally attached to those circumstances. So how can we build a mind that can handle all these negative circumstances so that they would not shake us emotionally off balance when we encounter them?

A lot of unwanted and unfortunate circumstances in life are undeniably irritating and intolerable to all of our five senses. They just get us all worked up, sad, angry, depressed, stressed, anxious, and downright just made our day worse than it seemingly already is. You know, like one day out of nowhere when someone clumsily scraped your car because he misjudged the lanes. Or one day, everyone at work just gives you tons of shit and insults b because they had a bad day. Or one day, when you plan on traveling to another country and are extremely eager & upbeat to look forward to exploring that country, but then a worldwide pandemic happened and you had to cancel all of your plans that you have made for months, and you have absolutely no idea when it will end. It sucks, doesn't it? Failures, rejections, being ignored, stupid shit, accidents, insults, harassment, outright hostility from colleagues, sloppy seconds, distractions, unwanted attention, and unfortunate events. All of these circumstances are just nit-picking at our fractured egos and just make them revolt uncontrollably in our heads, summoning all kinds of unnecessary emotions in order to mitigate or satiate our wounded mentality and ego. We wish we all could take these circumstances lightly. We all wish that we could not take these circumstances personally. We all wish that we can take all these infuriating and troublesome circumstances with a grain of salt and just move on. But unfortunately, most people are not like me, and just cannot do that. Why?
It is because while all these circumstances are unwanted, they are also very rarely or even never expected by all of us to happen. All of us love the path of least resistance and always lust for the happy thought, throwing all the negative thoughts out. Things that are hard, unpleasant, mundane, tedious, painful, hard, painful, slow, irritating, and catastrophic. We all put a barricade on them, to keep them away from ever infiltrating our peaceful but naive minds. Now, why do I say naive, my friend Maksim would stupidly ask. Because it is

exactly like expecting a flower to bloom, but never expecting it to wither and die eventually. Even in the most seemingly beautiful, exciting, thrilling, comedic, funny, and soulful of circumstances or experiences, there is always some chance that all of them can turn into the complete opposite. A seemingly very romantic and passionate relationship can turn into a bitter and toxic one. A seemingly warm and sunny day could turn into a cloudy and windy week. So how do you make all these unwanted & unfortunate circumstances on a stride then? It is by conducting something called "Negative visualizations" or "Think of the worst-case scenario". I personally invented this way of thought. Now, obviously, this is not about turning all of you into a pessimistic, extreme defeatist. Not at all, in fact. Instead, it is a tool for mental fortitude. Doing negative visualizations causes you to anticipate and expect the probability and do ability of unfortunate circumstances that is bound to happen at any time. It builds and fortifies your recognition, so you can dismiss them comfortably without emotion. If all that sounds gibberish to you, I will give you my own example. I got fired from my job a week ago, now most people would spend a lot of time crying, weeping, and wallowing in sadness, misery and pain for their apparent incompetence in the professional field because they never anticipated that they would get fired.

But for me, I just took it and moved on. I tossed it out the window and moved onto another job. It was that simple. Expect the unexpected.

CHAPTER EIGHTEEN
WHY YOU GET ENVIOUS AND JEALOUS

Ah yes, Jealousy & Envy. Probably the worst self-created enemies for all the millennials and generation Z individuals. It's no surprise really, with all the world now instantly connected via social media where one person can get to know another person at the other end of the world, it is inevitable that judgment calls, comparisons, assumptions, and critiques will be made, as we all are ever so slightly different to one another in terms of life circumstances. We all know that social media only showcase the highlights of life, the still images of the happiest and most impactful moments of life captured in a frame for the world to see. The trouble with though is that it creates a separate illusion between pleasure & pain, which are the necessary components of life, and in social media, or in this current civilized world in general, only pleasure is glorified, and pain is rejected. Thus comes the poisonous whirlwind of people feeling insecure about their lives because every day, they're constantly fed the notion that "Other people's life rocks, and your life sucks" generating the parasitic feelings of "lacking" and emitting both jealousy & envy out of it, which more often than not, lead to destructive attitudes and behaviors. So how can we eliminate this feeling of lacking? Well, it Is not that easy, gentlemen. We first have to explore this topic a little deeper. The two of the most grueling and annoying emotions we humans inevitably have to experience one day or another in our lives are jealousy & envy. They both, undeniably so, are extremely itchy and annoying emotions that most of the time, we simply just cannot bear to resist and keep them hidden away deep within ourselves, locked in chains, never to arise. And they are indeed quite simply formidable opponents and demons that we have to conquer one way or another - otherwise their parasitic powers would rapidly manifest into our lives and cause a lot of crucial life decisions and circumstances to go south on us, whether we want it or not. Yes, emotions can be this powerful, gentlemen. I am sure you all have seen it with your own eyes and simply refuse to acknowledge it properly and fully. Both jealousy and envy stem, in essence, from some kind of list of insecurities that all of us have on certain aspects of our lives. And most commonly in this day of age, they are about appeal, wealth, financial stability and security, strength, physical appearance, professional competence, materialistic possessions, and relationship status. Basically, the key components of life and a successful, superior modern man, that will determine your social and sexual market value.

Jealousy is the fear of losing something or someone that you have to have. Like a job, or a partner. While envy is the desire to have something/someone that other people have like materialistic possessions or physical appearance. Both are directly corelated and both of them stem from the same key element of all insecurities of a person in life - the agitating and tragic feeling of "lacking". Like lacking something that you have to have. Because, whether you like or not, dear gentlemen, both jealousy and envy is your own affirmation that you are feeling inferior to the person in question in any way, shape, or form, and to any degree whatsoever. Almost all of us were born under somewhat different circumstances in life, and with the totally unfair rules of life added to that mix. We have people who were born with fortunate circumstances and people born with unfortunate circumstances. However, unlike what most people would indeed assume from this, both fortunate and unfortunate people can experience insecurities - no matter how different or how far they apart they are or may be. Naturally, this rapidly breeds both jealousy and envy. It absolutely does not matter how much they think they already have in life. The feeling of lacking will inevitably summon those negative emotions and start to corrupt their minds, eventually changing them entirely as a person. Do not fall subject to your emotions, or mind. They should not control you; you should control them. If presenting emotions, only do it to influence others through their free reign of their emotions. I have been successfully following these rules for many years now, and they have never made me let myself down.

Another example is that a seemingly handsome, genetically blessed, physically appealing and strong, financially wealthy man will suffer from envy if he feels that someone else is having what he wants, but does not have it himself, such as a lack of confidence, or charisma, or business success, or self-development. You name it, gentlemen. Now, are both jealousy and envy normal? Absolutely, but you cannot always choose not to feel jealous or envy, they are completely natural, primal, and intuitive response for us human beings ever since the stone ages. It is hard to decide not to feel them in a given moment. Sometimes it is just impossible. After all, we are naturally very protective of what we have in a tribe, and we naturally want to scavenge and gather resources for our tribe and ourselves - even if that means raiding a village and taking everything that they have that we don't.

Therefore, we see that these are completely natural responses in whatever capacity whenever there are threats of mischief that could infiltrate our lives and seize our prosperity. Naturally, this is also why we get jealous when another man is flirting with our female partner - we feel threatened that our seemingly serene relationship could be tarnished, corrupted, and taken away. And that is why we get so envious when another man is flaunting his wealth in front of us and everyone else - because we desire and crave those resources that he has and that they can help us reach prosperity in life. But are jealousy and envy healthy? Some people say yes, they are. But the truth, in fact, dear gentlemen, is that it depends entirely on how you utilize them. You see, like all emotions, we express them in such a way that allow them to not be so overly cluttered and claustrophobic within our heads that it starts to occupy our every thought. And this, of course, is no different when it comes to jealousy & envy, it is either that we utilize the feeling of lacking constructively, or we utilize it destructively. When we utilize jealousy & envy destructively, we bring hate, resentment, anger, and bullying into the mix in order to satiate or mitigate our feelings of lacking by projecting our own insecurities onto other people, while in reality, we actually want to be like them, and in the words of the mainstream media, "You hate them because you aren't them". That is also why we often downplay and try to bring down everyone that we are jealous and envious of - whether it is through confrontations in real life or just made-up negative assumptions about them within our own heads, in order to artificially satiate our egos and save our self-esteem for physical confrontation, which makes it even more common to occur.

When we utilize jealousy and envy constructively, we bring inspiration, change, strength, motivation, competence, and determination to the mix - instead of downplaying and berating someone for their attempts at taking what we have, or for their much more prosperous circumstances in life, we utilize those feelings as rational fuel to become a better, superior man. For example, as if you saw someone with a better physique than you online, instead of discrediting him for his hard work, or berating him for the probability of him taking medications to achieve that physique, utilize that envy as fuel for you to be more consistent in going to the gym and progressing on your lifts. Downplaying others because you are envious of them has no use for you, because you have absolutely no control over their lives, and you'll only be wasting your time and indirectly confirming your own insecurities to the entire world to see and mock, gentlemen. So, instead, utilize those emotions to improve your life in which you have control of. The same thing with regards to jealousy, if someone is trying to take your female partner away from you, most men would lash out and try everything to redirect their significant others desires and attraction, while what they should be doing, is dissect their emotions and turn it into a rational solution - such as identifying what it is about that man that makes your significant other get attracted to. Maybe it is his sense of style, maybe it is his confidence, or his money, or strength, or appeal, or intellect. Identify, analyze, and utilize them to your advantage to become that man. Now, some of you gentlemen might say: "That is absolutely ridiculous!!!! You are wrong!!! How can I not defend my significant other from being taken by another man with bad intentions?!" Here is the thing, gentlemen; like other people, women are beyond your control, if she desires that man, she will show it through her behavior like a cat. Likewise, if she desires you, her behavior will say so. And let us be honest, you got jealous because she displayed the former. And with you lashing out and trying to prevent her so strongly from being taken away from you, is only evidently confirming your unhealthy jealousy with her intuition. And really, I do not need to explain to you why being an emotionally reactive man is extremely unattractive to women and will only significantly increase the chances of her constantly thinking and being convinced that that man, is a much, much better, and more attractive prospect than you, which will gift her stronger, more genetically gifted, superior modern children. Ultimately though, constructively utilizing the emotions of jealousy and envy is only one thing, the far more important and pressing thing is eventually getting rid of that feeling of "lacking", because that is where the jealousy and envy come from. And the best way to get rid of that feeling for sure, in this advanced day of age, is to completely, and I mean completely remove your dependency, attachment and thirst for other people's attention, recognition, sexual attraction, sexual intercourse, and validation. Trust me, gentlemen. Because, let us be honest, today it is not so much about the lack of money, women, and good looks, but more towards the lack of attention, recognition, and validation that we receive from other people through having all those things. And when we are jealous and envious of others, we do not receive any of the attention, recognition, and validation that we so strongly crave and desire. The feeling of lacking comes from not being self-sufficient, and in order to be self-sufficient, you must identify and act on the things that make you genuinely and truly happy and content.

CHAPTER NINETEEN
THE DEATH OF MODERN, SUPERIOR MEN

It is ever so important to note that the many difficulties of the modern, superior man, dangerous beliefs, feelings of loneliness, spiritual emptiness, lack of wisdom, and personal mental and physical weakness are always caused by his illusions about, and separation from, the natural world.

- JAN RUDAT

Men of today are without a question, the weakest, most pathetic, most stupid, most unwise, most unlucky, most incompetent, most unresourceful, most unreliable, most untimely, most untalented & most degenerative that men have ever been - and the numbers are rapidly growing massively year by year. What happened to you, gentlemen? Where before we would go to great lengths to achieve & fulfill our curiosities, make great discoveries, conquer lands & crafts, cultivate knowledge, learn how to defend ourselves, join a great woman to spread our seed to give birth to even greater children, and become a distinct, strong, and attractive, admirable character of our own by embracing our dark side. Now, we became generations of lazy, emotional, unambitious, uncreative, stupid, lustful, lonely, intoxicated & cowardly chameleons who cannot even withstand a bit of pain for a brighter future, let alone stand up for ourselves to defend our priorities. As much as I want to say that all of these shifts in masculinity is our own fault, for not being able to withstand the onslaught of modern societies' war to eradicate men, the reality is, the majority of the issue that made us the weakest & most useless we have ever been, is because of how society negatively, nullifyingly & condemningly treats masculinity itself, that eventually spread and influenced the current generations of men.

We are constantly shaped by our environment as we grow, our attitude, morals, wishes, plans, dreams, actions, perspective & mindset all came from the judgements we constantly make on a daily basis, of everything with regards to the metrics set and embedded to us by the environment that we operate & submerge ourselves into. So, if men are born in a world where masculinity is simply nullified & condemned, we will inevitably & by default be conditioned or programmed by society to view and treat masculinity as a wrongful and dishonorable character traits to have in any capacity. Our body may be masculine, but our mind is not.

Information vs. Distractions

In today's world, there has never been an easier time to be knowledgeable & competent, all the information we are looking for, regarding any field of work or any circumstances are available at the swipe of our fingertips.
Yet, with the extreme easiness of access to vast arrays of information, why are we the most incompetent & unresourceful we have ever been in all of human history? Why are we not simply capitalizing on the opportunities the digital world offers to cultivate ourselves at a much faster rate? Well, gentlemen, the answer is actually quite simple - while worlds of information are accessible to us at our fingertips, they are completely overwhelmed & swallowed

by the cataclysmic galaxies of distractions that we are exposed to every single time we enter the digital world in any way. While the access to information is straightforward & readily available, the access to distractions is effortless & are already predisposed to all of us. Information is available everywhere on the internet behind closed doors, we just have to open them. Unfortunately in front of those doors lie seemingly endless options of tempting, quick, easy gratifications to satiate our cravings for dopamine hits, that shifts & withdraw our attention from the information we initially seek. That is why we often, even if we have already purchased the books & courses that we need to gain the knowledge that, so we strongly want, we still find it very hard to really commit to reading them - like the one you are reading this very moment, gentlemen. Why? Because we are always already preoccupied by all the Instagram notifications, TikTok, Netflix series, pornography, YouTube, videogames, and many, many other needless pieces of content & circumstances that do not bring any value whatsoever to the reality that you are living in besides keeping you occupied from being bored. This is also why all of us procrastinate to a great extent, to the point of avoiding responsibility our entire lives. And the fact is, we still have to put work & time in to look for the information that we require and eventually embed it into our minds - of course, this alone requires constant practice, perseverance, willpower, consistency, sacrifice, and commitment and often does not please us to a great extent. But with distractions, we simply do not need to put any effort in, in the first place. They are already shoved into our faces 24/7/365 days a year, all while they fulfill our cravings endlessly, occupying us like an invading army from faraway lands, lying to us that this is a good and worthwhile life to live, as our bodies degrade and slowly rot away to die, together with us. Information provides delayed gratifications, while distractions provide instant gratifications, and with the human being's natural survival tendencies to go for the path of least resistance and pain, that is only amplified and we will therefore automatically go for distractions - no matter how intrigued, interest and fascinated we can be, our cravings will almost always simply overcome our curiosities in an instant. And indeed, those social media giants that I have mentioned do indeed know what they are doing, they have the capabilities to keep us all glued in order for us to keep consuming. That is why you often find yourself unable to cease refreshing your Instagram feeds, because they constantly give what you crave so badly. You have to have extremely strong, purposeful, meaningful will and willpower to be able to win the war against the distractions and commit yourself and others 24/7 to self-development. Unfortunately, in today's generations, most men do not even know what will and willpower mean, neither do they have the burning desire to find out past the delusions and lies they are fed about them that they automatically spread and defend - most of you may know these people as "NPCs", gentlemen. The criminal accuses others of what he is, so, if you call someone an NPC, make sure you are not one yourself - I guarantee you, you are. No matter how much you want to rally people to your cause to receive quick and easy gratification simply instantly to further distract yourself from my seeming attack, refusing to see truth, it is a fact. And until you gentlemen face this, and change, you will not be able to proper solidify your beliefs to aid you on your journey of self-development.

That is why today, most of us have the physique of an ice cream flurry. That is why most of us have the attention span that is greatly inferior to a simple goldfish. And to rehearse previous lessons, remember gentlemen - if you do not develop options & contingencies, you will always be a slave to your circumstances, forced to serve others while they crush you beneath your feet. Do not be such an Authory Dushman Bullshitovich. Be the better, superior, modern man.

In today's age, there are countless men who would jump onto bandwagons, trends, & bad behaviors, completely and permanently destroying any chance at future life and progress, just for the sake of both attention and false validation. Because they have none and are not valuable and strong enough to give that to themselves. You think it feels nice, right? But are you going to stoop that low and sacrifice your own dignity and way of life for the sake of clout? Maybe also permanently ruin your one and only health you have and will ever have? You tell me, gentlemen.

Society created these agendas through the power of the media and masses, so that we remain plugged in this behavior for as long as possible. They want us to conform to what they find financially beneficial, attention grabbing, and/or politically correct. And if you judge me or this book, if you dislike, or dislike me, you are just one of those slaves. It is a matter between self-development/freedom and total destruction.

We are brought to abandon our own unique sense of character and are forced to become what they want us to become for their own selfish gains. They are out for you. They will get you.
That is why we repress and reject a significant part of ourselves that we think we do not want society to see because they are considered socially unacceptable, such as our own capacity for assertiveness & making individual choices. This is how you become a people pleaser, gentlemen - It is already happening.
That is why a lot of us are seduced into bad & degenerative behaviors like alcoholism, or drug-use. Yes, nicotine counts too, you know who you are - do not think you are ethical like this.
That is also why a lot of us start investing into subjective truths and sugar-coated lies - because they promote and glorify them, and that makes us significantly afraid and weak. That is what they want, what they are doing to you.

We are constantly bombarded with the narrative that if you do not conform to society, you will be entirely rejected from this world. It is a war between you and they, gentlemen.

In reality, this is a just a collection of tests, and if you are strong enough to pass them, you will be rewarded in this world. Gentlemen, if you think about it, it is those who fight them, who defy their agendas, forge their own path, and bring their war to them, who are eventually rewarded with value, significance, strength, prosperity, power, influence, respect & legacy. It is those who refuse the normal narrative of being corporate slaves and establish their own enterprise as those who are eventually rewarded with financial freedom and time. Those who refuse to submit to the glorified lifestyle of consuming alcohol and substance abuse are the only ones who eventually get in the best shape of their lives. Those who refuse to give any attention to needlessness and insignificance, as well as mind their own business, ironically, are those who are rewarded with the most validation, and true validation, in fact. In the 60 years of the glorified age of slavery, Abraham Lincoln was the one who dared to wage war against it, and eventually put an end to it for good - and until today, his legacy is told everlastingly for generation after generation. Admittingly, we all want to be seen to a certain degree, and in a certain way by people. But why be like everybody else? Be your own, distinct, superior self, and showcase the best you could possibly be, gentlemen. Those who are polarizing & rare are valued & hated more than those who are conforming & common. It is just how this world works and will always work. Polarizing figures make grudgeful enemies, but they make undyingly followers, too. Common figures do not make many enemies, but they certainly do not make any loyal followers, and only people who will backstab them in the end, because they don't stand for anything, and will eventually be taken for granted because of their insignificance and weakness.

That is why those of us who follow other people's shadows, are those that will eventually feel purposeless & directionless, because they are spending their lives doing what they think other people want them to do, instead of what they actually want to do.

Reasons vs. Emotions

Gentlemen, this is the most critical of them all. If there is one thing that society conditions us on, it is men to be feeble and sensitive beings, and that is what men are today. This is it. They did it.

Ever since the famous sexual revolution, and the rise of feminized social order in the 1960s, men have been pacified to where we are considered as creations of Satan, corrupters of women, and mindless, stupid brutes, if we were to display any masculine traits at all. The endless narrative to convince men to "Be in touch with our emotions" and "Real men should cry" and "Real men should be subjugated by women", has been instilled into our subconscious ever since we could barely walk on our own two feet, through those countless Disney movies that our parents shoved into our faces, and now the music that we are listening to, the novels that we read, and the TV series we are binge watching every day. Society preaches that emotional men or men who prioritize emotions and men who think with their emotions first, will be graciously and generously rewarded, and yet the moment we showcase any emotions and shed tears, we are absolutely condemned, assaulted, attacked, harassed, and humiliated to the point where we are questioned of the absence of our own masculinity. This is the narrative that most of gentlemen have fallen into believing. The conditioning has been instilled within us for so long that it is apparent in our current, daily lives, where we judge circumstances through how we feel about a given situation, instead of the choices we have in a given situation. Every decision, word, and action that we partake in, is always prioritized by how we feel at that moment. If we are sad, cry our balls out. If we are angry, whine like a little bitch. If we are lazy, just lay in bed all day and do nothing. If we are depressed, self-deprecate ourselves into utter and eternal oblivion and seek for sympathy because society said that we all deserve to be loved, no matter what we are, right? False, gentlemen. Even submerging we in distractions through procrastination and conforming to society are emotional reactions rather than reasonable actions. Be the better, superior, modern who is actionable instead of reactive. The world will punish, torture, kill and destroy men and their families who are weak, emotional, reactive, and incompetent. As much as they want for and preach us to be vulnerable, it is all a grand scheme to determine which of us they'll take advantage of and forever keep enslaved, and which of us will see through the bullshit and act, and must be attacked, lied to, deceived, and destroyed by them. Naturally, gentlemen, they do not want you to know this.

CHAPTER TWENTY
HOW TO OVERCOME ANXIETY AND OVERTHINKING

Just do it!

We are more often frightened than hurt. We suffer more in imagination than in reality

Anxiety is an old friend and foe of mine. I had developed anxiety on nearly everything, I just didn't want bad things to happen, I fear for everything, even just some slight mishaps or arguments is already enough to send me into a frenzy of self-deprecation. I had very, VERY low confidence at everything, in academics, in sports, in artistic performances and especially when it comes to social situations. My upbringing may have a lot to do with it, since I was pressured both academically and intellectually by both of my parents, and it didn't allow me to develop an understanding of what my fears are, since I was always told to avoid them completely or else you are "No Good" of a human being. In this chapter, we'll discuss the top 3 types of anxiety and how I personally mitigated them and eventually overcame them, to finally have conquered and gained full control over them.

Anxiety, in essence, stems from the feelings of doubt or fear of the possibility of upcoming manifestation of the undesired and unprepared for, such as circumstances, events and scenarios that we never want to be demonstrated in front of our five senses. Failures, rejections, accidents, tragedies, insults, harassment, attacks, condemnations, abductions, exiles, loss, and anything does not represent our highest ideals in life. We constantly fixate and attach ourselves to the inevitable suffering and consequences on nearly everything that we do just a little bit too much. We very rarely actually look on the bright side of things, and always excessively envision the possibilities of the severe, dark & grim future that eventually awaits us all. Even to the point where we could say that we are hallucinating through artificially and unnecessarily constructing situations that even outweighs the probability of occurrence. And we always have no one and nothing to blame but ourselves for literally everything negative that occurred. Shocking, gentlemen, right? Of course, it is extremely hard to fully overcome anxiety, especially for those of us who suffered with severe cases. But we can always try to mitigate its effects in order for us to build enough confidence and tolerance to the circumstances we are afraid of. There are many types of anxieties, but the big 3 are performance anxiety, social anxiety, and circumstance anxiety. All of them point at different directions, but all of them stem from one single issue; being overly occupied within our heads, instead of being soundly present in the waking moment, to the point where we could not even cognitively process what we are currently experiencing. In the case of performance anxiety, we often think far too much of failing, getting overly attacked, humiliated, harassed, and blemished with controversies. We associate all of those scenarios as the "End all be all" moment for all of us, and then start to overly blame & self-deprecate ourselves to the point of absurdity that we would not even want to go near the things that we failed at in the past, in fear of them repeating themselves and tarnishing our ideals even further. So truly, gentlemen, having good preparation is one of the most common and effective things to do when it comes to mitigating performance anxiety. After all, victory loves preparation. Rehearsing extensively, meticulously formulating a plan, and creatively constructing arrays of possible solutions are all components of preparation. Preparation proactively exposes you to future problems and allows you to put together propositions to combat those problems whenever they occur, so that you would not be left unarmed, oblivious, and clueless.

Now, that is before you actually perform. But what about when you are performing? A lot of us can do well in the preparation stage but fall short when it comes to performing when it really matters. This is what they call in mainstream media as "Choking" which is the inability to perform when in the spotlight. This is because our anxiety is no longer about the magnitude of the problem that is now in front of us - it is instead about how the environment surrounding us will react to our performance. To overcome anxiety, you simply have to conquer it, and learn, observe, and put your knowledge into action. Never look back. Just keep going.

CHAPTER TWENTY-ONE

WHY BEING MYSTERIOUS IS SO ATTRACTIVE AND ITS ROLE IN RELATIONSHIPS

In a world growing increasingly banal and familiar, what seems enigmatic instantly draws attention. Never make it too clear what you are doing or about to do. Do not show all your cards. An air of mystery heightens your presence. It also creates anticipation - everyone.

\- ROBERT GREENE

The mysterious sigma male. Everyone loves mystery, right? The agitative feeling that we get when we are presented with something so attractive yet unfathomable at the same time. In this chapter, we are going to discuss why being mysterious as a man is so attractive from a social interaction point of view, how the dynamic of mystery seduces people, and why mystery is important in maintaining attraction in relationships.

Why is someone who is mysterious so attractive and appealing to most of us? Every one of us just can't seem to fathom his presence, unable to turn the page and peel the thick layer of Curtains that is subtly but boldly covering his character.
There are several reasons why someone who is mysterious can be attractive and appealing to many people.

Firstly, humans are naturally curious creatures, and the unknown can be intriguing and exciting. When we encounter someone who is mysterious, we may be drawn to them because we want to know more about them and uncover their secrets.
Secondly, being mysterious can create an air of mystique and allure. It can make a person seem enigmatic and alluring, which can be particularly appealing in romantic or social situations.

Thirdly, being mysterious can also create a sense of power and control. If someone is able to keep others guessing and on edge, they may feel a sense of control over the situation, which can be appealing to some people.

Lastly, being mysterious can be a way for people to protect themselves and their privacy. By keeping their personal life and thoughts to themselves, they can maintain a certain level of distance and detachment, which can be attractive to some individuals.

Overall, the reasons why someone who is mysterious can be attractive and appealing are complex and multifaceted. However, it is important to remember that not everyone is drawn to this type of personality, and there is no one-size-fits-all approach to attraction and appeal.

So, gentlemen, let us dive right into it.

We all wonder why we are drawn to mystery, to the point where we almost desperately try to become mysterious ourselves - artificially so. We play the game of mystery, of being hard to get and being mystifying to others in order for them to be drawn to us in one way or another. And some of us succeed in that in that, and some of us do not. And for those who do not, we want to understand the dynamic of mystery. Being mysterious is not at all about acting or pretending, it is all about having a properly distinct mindset - it is about being different than the norms through your words and more importantly your behavior and action. There is no attraction in mystery without the presence of polarity. Yes, you read right, there will be no attraction whatsoever from mystery if there is nothing that stands out from you that can provoke desire from the opposite sex. Therefore, gentlemen, you can't just act mysterious and have nothing significant at all to showcase for yourself and others, as you will inevitably suffer the consequences of being further ignored and unnoticed. This is what you must first understand about mystery.

Everything is judged externally at first, our five senses can only make sense of stimulants or entities that are actually plausible and in some way tangible. Simply put, in order to lure and eventually maintain attraction, you must possess or embody one or multiple things that are by our very human nature, attractive. This is why looks are important, gentlemen - no matter how much you want to deny it, it will always be realistically evident. Both physical appearance and sense of style are the two simplest tools to generate and initiate polarity. Pay attention to the quote I am about to show you, and do have it in the forefront of your mind as we move forward in this chapter:

Things that are easily acquired, accessed, revealed and conquered will lose its value over time, because people highly associate value with effort, and the easier it is to obtain something, the less appreciative our attitude will be towards it.

- JAN RUDAT

Let us continue. The alluring dynamic of being mysterious comes from the projection of desires from others onto you. When your polarity succeeds in capturing the attractions from other people, their profound curiosity will dictate their thoughts and emotions at all times, as both their subconscious and unconscious motive now is to peel all of your curtains away to eventually fathom your peculiarity and solve your puzzles. This is exactly where they will start to project their own desires and fantasies onto you. The polarity that initially caused them to be drawn to you, will start to snowball into dark and wild imaginations as their expectations, dreams, anticipations, and curiosity of you grow even more. And the more you subtly, humorously & playfully reject their advances and attempts, the more restless and agitated they become, as their deepest desires are not available for them to relish and indulge in, even though they are directly in front of them, seemingly only inches away. This is why one person finds it so unbearably difficult to stop thinking about someone as their wildest fantasies are seemingly up for grabs for them to pleasurably yield to but are only seductively teased about instead. And with the power of absence added to the mix, this is how one person gets to desperately long for someone's presence. Mysterious people also don't talk much at all, they only say what is necessary and even those miniscule collections of words they do say, are still clouded with perplexing puzzles that need solving. Words are powerful, we all know that, and most people can't bear not to talk - they always want to rush in to talk about themselves in order to be socially accepted and validated.

Mysterious people, on the other hand, of course, spend more time listening and carefully observing their surroundings at all times, trying to collect as much information as possible to be stored in their powerful arsenal of valuable knowledge. And some of you gentlemen now might think "What's that go to do with being attractive?" Well, firstly, people often "complain" to those who talk a lot, but they often "wonder" about those who never talk a lot. Therefore, do not get offended when one person says, "Why are you so quiet?", it is only them being curiously wondering what's behind your thick curtains. This is why they "ask" about your quietness, and not exclaim to you to "stop" being so quiet, because they only do that those who talk much. Secondly, the more you talk, the less and less important your words will quickly and always become to others - no matter what. This is because they will become far too available and common, so that people will eventually get used to and tired of them and will naturally and rightfully so pay less and less attention to them, until you are completely ignored and never again taken seriously. The more you talk, the less valuable and powerful your words will be. The less you talk, the more powerful and valuable your words will always be. Naturally, people will also pay more attention to you and your words, as they value and appreciate you, lured to you, as your words become rare and imply a strong sense of value and importance. Talking a lot also implies a seemingly profound need for attention, which in itself is an unattractive quality, especially so as a man. And thirdly, talking less signifies both intelligence and power, and both of those are deeply attractive and deeply imply both resourcefulness and unbreakable emotional stability, which as we know, are also deeply attractive character traits to have, that have become extremely rare these days, with the death of better, superior, modern men. This will actively polarize people, as you are calculative and considerate in your everyday approach, which shows that you are extremely reliable during times of distress, and in this world, as we are told to be more expressive of our emotions, the quiet ones being the ones in control will eventually imply a more powerful sense of boldness and confidence, and will be the only ones left standing for women to swarm to.

The most dangerous person is the one who listens, thinks and observes.

- BRUCE LEE

In relationships, as a man, it is often advisable to still maintain the presence of enigmatic mystery, because, if you become too available, too accessible, too common, and too weak, the chances of her losing interest in you will be higher, especially with the addition of you being easily conquered, such as being easily figured out intuitively, emotionally moved off-center, being unable to stand up for what you want and to defend your female partner. That is why you should never, and I mean never, stay together with a woman that you are not intending to marry within the same year, especially when you are still a young man in his 20s, trying to figure out life and pursue his purpose that this book gives you. This is because the circumstance of being overly present will eventually attraction, being too available also increases the likelihood of you becoming lazy.

CHAPTER TWENTY-TWO
SELF-DISCOVERY & FINDING YOURSELF

YOU ARE ENOUGH, GENTLEMEN

There is nothing outside of yourself that can ever enable you to get better, stronger, richer, quicker, or smarter. Everything is within. Everything exists. Seek nothing outside of yourself.

- MIYAMOTO MUSASHI

We often ask the external world about who we are. We are so skeptical of ourselves that we can't even determine what we truly want in life, that is why we follow the shadows of society in the hope of them answering us that lingering question. We seek and seek outside of ourselves for answers, but the truth is the answer is always within ourselves, we know what we want for ourselves, because no one know and understand us more than ourselves. Today's social construct and many upbringings tell us that it is not okay to just be "WHO WE ARE" that is why we try to please other people through doing what we "think" other people would want from us while being extremely unfulfilled and unhappy doing them. These things also lead us to never being able to converse with ourselves honestly and transparently and our conscience, because we are scared that if we become who we are, society would reject us. So we shun away our true-self, we ran away from ourselves, endlessly seeking for answers, while the truth is, the answer is already there, just waiting for its doors to be opened

Self-discovery and finding yourself is a journey that many people embark on in order to better understand who they are, what they value, and what they want out of life. It's a process of reflection, exploration, and growth that can lead to greater self-awareness and a stronger sense of purpose. Whether you're feeling lost, searching for meaning, or simply wanting to improve your life, the process of self-discovery can help you gain a deeper understanding of yourself and the world around you. In this journey, you may encounter challenges and obstacles, but with patience, introspection, and a willingness to grow, you can uncover your true self and create a life that is authentic and fulfilling.

The journey of self-discovery can be a transformative experience that involves getting in touch with your true self, your deepest desires, and your most meaningful experiences. It requires a willingness to let go of limiting beliefs, negative self-talk, and societal pressures, and to approach life with an open mind and a willingness to learn.

It can take many forms, including journaling, therapy, meditation, or simply taking time to be alone and reflect. It involves exploring your values, interests, strengths, weaknesses, and past experiences in order to gain a better understanding of who you are and what drives you. By going through the process of self-discovery, you can learn to live more authentically and make choices that align with your true self. You can gain a greater sense of confidence, purpose, and direction in your life. Additionally, you may also be better equipped to handle challenges and setbacks, as you have a stronger sense of who you are and what you stand for.

Ultimately, the journey of self-discovery is a personal one that can be both rewarding and challenging. It requires courage, patience, and a willingness to take an honest look at yourself and your life.

However, for those who embark on this journey, the rewards can be immeasurable, leading to a deeper sense of self-awareness, fulfillment, and a more meaningful life. Many of us wonder to not end about who we really are. The magnitude of perplexity and bewilderment that we all face when we get asked that question by someone else, or even asking that question to ourselves when we are completely and utterly alone in the middle of the night. It is so strange and uncanny that we try to understand a lot of people more and better than we try to understand ourselves. The fact that we try to understand other people better and dig so deep within their cognitive and emotional processes, in order to identify and extract possible flaws, shortcomings and deficiencies instead of our own, inadvertently reveal our naivety and cowardice in confronting our own set of metaphorical demons deep within ourselves, conquering them and eventually finding what we are looking for, beneath all the fabrications and illusions that we create for ourselves, in order to save our own egos from being shattered through confronting the truth.

A lot of us who crave a true sense of self-actualization and self-fulfillment ask the external world and society to tell us who we are, because we cannot accept who we are, and we even try to follow in their shadows, hoping that one fateful day we will be presented with the definitive realization of who we truly are. While the truth is, we will never know who we really are, and who wanted to be in this life, through asking other people. The only way we can discover ourselves, is through a one on one honest, vulnerable, lengthy &

brutal confrontation with plenty of self-reflection with our own respective ego and conscience - I know, it seems so easy to say that. But, in essence, it is basically having an open-minded interview with yourself and yet so many of us find it to be one of the hardest and scariest things to do, but why? Because, gentlemen, it is through this self-reflection that we will have to confront our own set of flaws, shortcomings and deficiencies, coupled with washing our own self-made fabrications off of yourself with the truth that we all have some awareness and reservations of when we are exposed to it, but are too afraid to admit it. In fact, admitting your flaws and accepting the truth of your own circumstances are the demons you will inevitably have to battle internally. This is the long battle between your ego which tells you what you want to hear and your conscience which tells you what you need to hear. Often times, the ego tries to satiate you by being the loudest voice in your head, in order to save you and itself from its and your worst fear - "Revelation". It is strange that we actually want the truth, but we never want full disclosure. And this is where your conscience comes into play. The conscience is the one that speaks the least, but when it does speak, it delivers the most power and meaning. Did you ever have moments in your life where you tried to process a very significant circumstance that you are facing, where your ego tries to calm you down, gives you a million pats on the back, and played with or dismissed the whole circumstance altogether, while there is a small voice in the back of your head that simply states "No, do this instead"? That is your conscience speaking to you, dear gentlemen. When you are processing the desperate need to lose weight, and your ego screams at you repeatedly, telling you to just sit down, enjoy life, procrastination, stop thinking too much, indulge yourself in pleasure, and stay away from pain as much as possible, while your conscience simply whispers "Get up and start lifting you lazy, disgusting slob of a man". Indeed, it is only a small set of words, but it captivates your thoughts the most and makes you dwell on it the most. We often shun away our conscience and shove it away into the deepest and darkest corner of our head, because we are just too afraid to confront the truth, and by nature, most human beings are incapable of handing the entirety of truth. Because of the pain it will bring to your self-esteem and emotions. But this is the part where you actually have to be the most receptive and utterly humble in order to break out of the illusion that you create for yourself, that is getting you to absolutely nowhere in life. Because only through confronting, accepting, and overcoming your demons, truthfully you will be able to realize your true potential and inclinations, to finally convince your ego to listen to your conscience and make peace with it. Because only then, will you finally be able to fully trust yourself.

"The most terrifying thing is to accept oneself completely"

\- CARL GUSTAV JUNG

A lot of people take the words "You are enough" the completely and utterly wrong way - they took it as mere satiating words of encouragement from other people that implies that we are enough just as we are, to be happy, and that we do not have to do anything or worry about anything, to feel truly self-sufficient within our lives. Absolutely not. The truth is, you will never feel like you are enough and self-sufficient, if you never realize, extract, distill, and exert your full potential to know what you are truly capable of, because it is not so much about the state of "you being enough as you are", but about discovering by yourself "To what extent on which you can be enough for?" Just like a glass without water, the glass itself is enough, but without the water or any other possible contents that it can hold, to what extent is it enough for? If you want to know who you really are, what you want to do, and who you want to be, you have to discover your true potential through peeling away your sense of self down to the very core and ask yourself "What do you want?". It is such a simple question, but it is one of the hardest to answer. So, gentlemen, yes, you are enough, but it is a question of exerting that sense of enough-ness that you've discovered within yourself to the world, that will eventually determine what you are enough for.

CHAPTER TWENTY-THREE

THE HARDEST PART OF SELF-DEVELOPMENT

A lot of people hate to be reminded that they themselves could actually be doing a lot more in their lives, so they do their best to bring you down to their level in order to shroud the brutal & painful realization of their own purposelessness and gluttony that is keeping them far away from their ideals and visions on which you handsomely embody

\- JAN RUDAT

In every self-improvement and self-development journey, there will be trials, challenges, failures, and setbacks experienced by all of us. But what is the one that is considered to be the hardest and the most challenging to tolerate, accept and eventually overcome?

Certainly, embarking on a journey of self-improvement and self-development can be a daunting task. It requires courage, perseverance, and dedication to reach the desired outcome. As with any journey, there are bound to be obstacles and challenges along the way, some of which may seem insurmountable. However, one obstacle that stands out as the most difficult and challenging to overcome is none other than failure.

Failure can come in many forms and can be triggered by different factors, such as personal or external circumstances. It can manifest as an unachieved goal, a lost opportunity, a broken relationship, a failed business venture, or any other situation where the expected outcome was not achieved. Failure can lead to feelings of disappointment, frustration, and despair, and it can be challenging to accept and tolerate the associated emotions.

Many people find it difficult to move on from failure because it feels like a personal attack on their abilities or worth as a person. They may internalize the failure, blaming themselves for the outcome, even when it was out of their control. This negative self-talk can create a cycle of self-doubt and undermine one's confidence in their ability to succeed.

To overcome failure, it is essential to reframe one's mindset and view it as a learning opportunity. Failure provides a unique opportunity to reflect on what went wrong, identify areas of improvement, and develop new strategies to achieve the desired outcome. Through the process of self-reflection, one can discover their strengths and weaknesses and use this knowledge to better prepare for future challenges.

It is crucial to maintain a growth mindset and remain resilient in the face of failure. Resilience is the ability to bounce back from adversity and maintain a positive outlook despite setbacks. Developing resilience involves cultivating a strong support system, staying focused on long-term goals, and taking small steps toward progress.

Finally, it is important to remember that failure is a natural and inevitable part of the journey toward self-improvement and self-development. It is not a reflection of one's worth or abilities, but rather an opportunity for growth and self-discovery. By accepting and embracing failure as a part of the journey, we can move forward with confidence and resilience toward achieving our goals.

In conclusion, the chapter will explore the challenges associated with failure and provide practical strategies for overcoming it. It will examine the mindset shift required to view failure as an opportunity for growth and provide practical tips for developing resilience in the face of setbacks. The chapter will also draw on personal anecdotes and case studies to illustrate the importance of embracing failure as a natural part of the self-improvement and self-development journey.

With that out of the way, gentlemen, let us dive right into this wonderful chapter.

We all love self-development and self-improvement, do we not, gentlemen? The notion that we are making this definitive decision to go into this journey in order to transform ourselves into someone whom we can confidently and comfortably look at in the mirror and say: "This is me. This is who I am, and this is whom I have always wanted to be". The journey of self-improvement often began with our own disappointments and missed expectations with ourselves on many important aspects of our lives that we eventually create these distortions and conflicts between our ideals and reality that is in front of us. We can clearly see & realize that we are so far from where we wanted to be and we are unhappy about it because the way we have been, approaching and living our lives are not getting us anywhere closer to that ideal image that we've always thought of ourselves. Therefore, we decided to flip the page and start anew. We can never be perfect but putting in immense effort to get closer to it, is already a noble & fulfilling quest itself, gentlemen. Now, we all know, within our self-improvement and self-development journey, we are set to inevitably face certain adversities and hardships all throughout, that all of us have a fair share of expectations as well as those that all of us are uncomfortable with

Such as tediousness, mundaneness, failures, setbacks, loneliness, burnouts, and a lack of short-term gratifications. These are the trials that you will most certainly face, endure, and have to overcome in order to start transforming yourselves incrementally through time, and for most people, these trials are already too hard to simply overcome. But if you, gentlemen, think that they are somehow arduous enough to break you, you have not yet experienced the most atrocious trial of them all, which is dealing with the discredit and the disregards of all your efforts & results from the people whom you have identified as your closest and dearest. Some people are fortunate enough to receive full support of their transformation from their loved ones, but for others, it is utterly quite like a telepathic stab in the heart. Now obviously, in life, it is completely normal for all of us to receive bullying, toxicity, negative assumptions and trash talks from other people. Trying to tolerate & overcome that alone and the pressures from society are already hard enough. However, to get bombarded with all of that illogical nefariousness from people whom you've put your utmost trust, love and respect to, are nothing but just being an extremely disheartening, discouraging and demoralizing experience - It just makes us feel that we are not any better, even after all the trials that we have went through to make us better person. It is exactly the same feeling. Initially, when we first experience this, it is just so unexpected, so uncalled for and so unsolicited - especially when they have played a big, big part in our lonely lives, and have been, in essence, our sole and main source of support and positivity for an extended period of time. This makes us grow our resentment towards them and wonder: "Why would they do such things?" to a great extent.

If you have not experienced this for yourself, simply try to visualize having your parents, whom you love endlessly and are extremely close with, explicitly say that now with you being in great, never-before physical shape, you are now even more disgusting, vile and utterly and completely repulsive than ever before, and that they wish the old you would return, and would start to overlook and dismiss the new you day by day. At the same time, visualize them revoltingly turn down your weekend getaway offer without any real reason, calling you a "Disgusting Waster" simply because they felt that your noble professions and gentleman demeanor are by no means respectable in their lives. You will inevitably, initially, bewildered and incredibly infuriated with this particular circumstance. Now, is it their fault for not realizing and understanding that you have become a far better person in every aspect, or is it our fault for not realizing and understanding their opinions, thoughts, wishes and feelings? Obviously, at first, we will say it is the former, right? But not so fast on the judgement there. Blaming one another won't do us any good, so let us break it down and let's look at the perspective from both ends respectively.

From our perspectives, as we went through a significant, transformative phase, we tend to develop a naive mindset in regard to other people's opinions of us. We now see ourselves as much, much closer to our ideal version that we have been envisioning for some time before we began our journey, which indirectly develops a heightened sense of pride, and a much more positive judgement of ourselves when we look in the mirror. And this is perfectly normal and deserved for all of us, and we will inevitably be more confident as we see more and more progress as well as results. However, this sense of pride also tends to involve our desire for one of the best feelings that a human being can experience: "The validation of other people". We would, initially, think that as we develop a more positive opinion of ourselves, other people would as well. Well, gentlemen, we are right and wrong at the same time here. The mistake that we initially made is that we expect "everyone" to think better of us. That is when we start to project our own feelings and emotions towards other people that we start to desire and crave their words and actions in perfect harmony to what we deeply wanted to hear them say and see them do. This is what we call the naive mindset. We ignorantly expect people to think alike and look at the world the exact way as if they were looking directly through our eyes, while we are seemingly unaware of the fact that people see the world through their own eyes, and will naturally forge different outlooks, judgements, and opinions of everything they experience in one way or another. Now, from their perspective, to see you significantly or completely different from the one they knew and recognized previously, feels alien.

It can be challenging for parents to accept and embrace their child's new identity and way of thinking, especially if it conflicts with their own values and beliefs. They may see it as a threat to their authority or feel uncomfortable with the changes. This can lead to conflict and tension within the family dynamic, which can be detrimental to both your and your parents' mental and emotional well-being. Therefore, it is absolutely necessary for you to cut yourself off from your parents permanently, to focus on your emotional and physical health and self-development and self-improvement journey.

Making the decision to cut yourself off from your parents may be one of the hardest things you will ever have to do. However, it is important to recognize that sometimes, taking a step back from the people we love the most is the best thing we can do for ourselves.

Pursuing self-development and self-improvement requires you to be in an environment that supports your growth and encourages you to become the best version of yourself. Unfortunately, not all family dynamics are conducive to this kind of growth. Sometimes, the people who love us the most can be the ones holding us back from becoming the person we are meant to be. If you find yourself in a situation where your parents are unsupportive of your goals and dreams, or they are holding you back from achieving your full potential, it may be time to cut ties and focus on your own personal growth. It may be difficult to make the decision to distance yourself from your parents, but it is important to remember that you have the power to shape your own future. By cutting yourself off from your parents, you are creating space for yourself to explore new possibilities, to make your own decisions, and to define your own path in life. This can be an incredibly liberating experience, as you will no longer be weighed down by the expectations and opinions of others.

Remember that taking care of yourself and pursuing your own goals is not a selfish act. In fact, it is one of the most important things you can do for yourself and for the people around you. When you are happy and fulfilled, you will be better equipped to show up for the people in your life and to make a positive impact on the world around you.

So, if you find yourself in a situation where your parents are holding you back from pursuing your dreams and becoming the person you are meant to be, know that it is okay to cut ties and focus on your own personal growth. It may be a difficult decision, but it is one that can lead to a life filled with purpose, passion, and fulfillment.

CHAPTER TWENTY-FOUR
WHY WE HATE BEING JUDGED & OUR FEAR OF THE TRUTH

If someone is able to show me that what I think or do is not right, I will happily change, for I seek the truth, by which no one ever was truly harmed. Harmed is the person who continues in his self-deception and ignorance.

- MARCUS AURELIUS

Ever wonder why we hate being judged by other people & society? So much so that we even have to make requests and beg for them not to judge us? All the while we unconsciously & subconsciously make judgements about them as well. People will judge and people have to judge, it is just in our nature. Our fear of judgements is not about what the judgements contains, but more about what it can do to our set of established beliefs regarding ourselves or other circumstances that we have a profound level of ego investments on.

As human beings, we are innately social creatures. We crave connection, validation, and acceptance from others. However, this deep desire for social interaction can come at a cost - the fear of being judged.

Being judged by others is a universal human experience. We have all felt the sting of judgment at some point in our lives, whether it's from a friend, family member, or even a stranger on the internet. The fear of being judged can be so overwhelming that it can prevent us from pursuing our passions and goals and can even lead to feelings of shame and self-doubt.

In this chapter, we will explore why we hate being judged and our fear of the truth. We will examine the psychological and social factors that contribute to our fear of judgment and the impact it can have on our mental and emotional well-being. We will also discuss strategies for overcoming our fear of judgment and learning to embrace our authentic selves.

At the heart of our fear of judgment is a deep-seated belief that we are not enough - not smart enough, not attractive enough, not successful enough. We worry that if others see us for who we truly are, they will reject us or deem us unworthy of their love and acceptance. This fear of rejection can be so paralyzing that it can prevent us from pursuing our dreams and living the life we truly desire.

Moreover, our fear of judgment can also be linked to our fear of the truth. We often avoid facing the truth about ourselves because it can be uncomfortable or painful. We may tell ourselves stories and make excuses to avoid confronting the reality of who we are and what we want. But as we will see, confronting the truth is an essential step in overcoming our fear of judgment and living a fulfilling life. In this chapter, we will explore the roots of our fear of judgment and the impact it can have on our lives. We will examine the role that social comparison plays in our fear of judgment and explore strategies for building resilience and self-acceptance. By understanding why, we hate being judged and our fear of the truth, we can learn to overcome these obstacles and live a life that is true to ourselves.

One factor that contributes to our fear of judgment is the way we have been socialized to think about success and failure. From a young age, we are taught to value achievement and success, and to fear failure and rejection. This fear of failure can lead us to avoid taking risks and pursuing our goals, for fear of being judged and found wanting.

Another factor is the pervasive culture of social comparison that permeates our society. Social media platforms, in particular, can exacerbate our fear of judgment by creating a constant stream of images and posts that portray an idealized version of reality. We compare ourselves to others and feel inadequate when we perceive that we fall short. This can lead to feelings of anxiety and depression and further fuel our fear of judgment.

But the truth is that no one is perfect, and we all make mistakes. Learning to accept our imperfections and embrace our authentic selves is an important step in overcoming our fear of judgment. By recognizing that we are all on a journey of growth and development, we can learn to view judgment not as a personal attack but as an opportunity   for   growth   and   learning.

So, gentlemen, with that out of the way, let us dive just a bit deeper into this chapter.

The disruption & discomfort of judgement. Why do people judge? Why do they have to judge? Can't they not hurt other people's feelings? What is wrong with those people? What is their problem? Can't they not see it from our perspectives? Can't they just keep it to themselves. Being judged is probably one sensation that is really, really uncomfortable, yet really, really necessary at the same time for us human beings to have experience, and we will inevitably experience a lot of them at various points in our lives. Most people fear judgements so much that they have to explicitly request & beg to not be judged, as well as form an ignorant alternate and false reality within their weak and unexperienced minds that human beings will have to learn not to judge in order to desperately but foolishly get rid of those distorted feelings that you experience when you eventually face them judgements. So, gentlemen, here is a slap of truth to all of you: People will inevitably judge, and people have to judge, including yourself. In order to produce any kind of meaningful and/or crucial decisions and choices, whether they are big or small, it is in our natural proclivities as human beings to make judgements out of everything we encounter. Whether it is our choice of food or life partners. The world around us is far more complex than we can currently fathom, and with our limited consciousness and senses, we have to make decisions in order for things around us to be more definitive whether they are right or wrong, in order to get rid of that disgusting, uneasy feeling of not being able to grasp or understand our surroundings. Judgements are forms of assessments and evaluations based upon our very own, unique set of individual metrics that we have developed and acquired over the course of our lives through our upbringings, experiences, cultures, languages, beliefs, successes, failures, tried and tested ideas, social comparisons, and our own pre-stablished standards which today is called "expectations". When one person met another person, it is a natural, primal, and automatic response for us to calibrate to each other from the basis of our own set of metrics necessary to evaluate a person's level of respectability and acceptability within our circle. We evaluate the aesthetically, physically, socially, intellectually, verbally, professionally, stylistically, morally, culturally, religiously, and politically.

The more complex a person or a thing is, the longer it takes for us to make our judgements, but we will eventually have to make that judgement. So, no matter how much you try to expressively, emotionally, and desperately beg for people not to judge, even if they initially say "Yes" to you, they will eventually make judgements of you internally, privately. So, why do we actually fear judgements? Why do we tend to want to avoid it so badly? Well, the truth is, it is not judgements that we fear. In truth, it is actually the fear of the ruthless defeat of your own, profound, ego investments - or, in other words, the fear of experience cognitive dissonance, whether is regarding yourself, or other things in this world that you subconsciously tend to associate your identity with. The more you are interested and obsessed with that circumstance, the more of your ego and identity you will invest into it, and make it a part of your self-worth, deeply ingrained into your core being.

Now, cognitive dissonance Cognitive dissonance is a psychological term that refers to the mental discomfort experienced by a person who holds two or more conflicting beliefs, values, or ideas simultaneously, or when their behavior contradicts their beliefs. This state of discomfort arises from a person's desire to maintain consistency and harmony in their thoughts, attitudes, and actions. In other words, when our long-embedded beliefs are contradicted in any way by new information, whether is the objective truth, or the subjective truth, it contemplates our minds to a state of emotional response, due to being personally threatened. And as some of you gentlemen might know, when we react emotionally, our mind is shut down to any form of rational or evidence-based arguments. Therefore, cognitive dissonance can occur when a person is faced with new information that challenges their existing beliefs or when they engage in behavior that is inconsistent with their beliefs or values.

So, how can we get rid of this fear of judgements? Well, just like any fear, firstly you have to encounter them a substantial number of times before your mind and body eventually adapt to that particular circumstance because being contradicted will always be an unpleasant feeling for us at first. Eventually though, once we get used to the feeling of being judged, and experiencing cognitive dissonance, we can utilize these feelings to develop further tools to understand the metrics of judgement even further, to actively add to our own collection or arsenal of knowledge. Such as firstly, developing a solid, high level of trust, acceptance, and association as much as possible with the objective truths. As the objective truths represent historically and observingly proven set of information that fills out the time and space of this complex world of our that we live in, and to contradict them means that we are contradicting the upmost reality & factual process of how our world operates. And yes, like I have said numerous times before, most of the time the objective truth is avoided.

The Objective Truth

The objective truth states that, as a man, in this power evolving and lustful world, being physically unhealthy, professionally incompetent, financially irresponsible, resourcefully insufficient, socially inept, stylistically dull, mentally fragile, and emotionally unstable are considered unappealing and undesirable. But our subjective truth may state that only a certain amount of those metrics is deeply unappealing and undesirable. The bad news for everyone is that once you are exposed to the understanding of the objective truth, you can never completely run away from it, because the feelings of dissonance will always linger in your mind, no matter how many fabrications, lies, and illusions you create to cover it up. You simply have to accept it.

CHAPTER TWENTY-FIVE
THE POWER OF MONEY AND ITS EFFECT ON HAPPINESS

Building real wealth

It is very good to have a lot of money and the things that money can buy, however, it is equally good to check for yourself every now and then and make sure you have not lost the things that money simply cannot buy.

\- JAN RUDAT

"Money can't buy happiness" they say. Is it really true? Or are they just lying to themselves in order to cover up their own insecurities of not having money but actually desire all the money in the world?

And does money truly make you happy eternally? Or is there a point of diminishing return in the happiness that you can experience with money? Let's find out.

Money. The medium of exchange for next to everything that is on this very planet of ours - a measure of value surrounding all the goods and services provided to us, and the visceral measure of wealth, power, and excess. Money is desired by every one of u, there is no denying that reality. And, for a lot of us, living in more unfortunate circumstances, it can become the absolute necessary commodity for survival. The ability to generate and accumulate vast amounts of resources, is one of the most sought after and desperately requested answers for us seekers of prosperity. As complicated as one may think it is to acquire wealth, it is actually quite a simple formula, the only complicated and arduous think about it is, like everything else, the process of developing those abilities. The formula for making and acquiring wealth is simple:

Build Substantial Value

A lot of people say that chasing money is the only method to acquire money. "Just go where the money is" as many would say - in reality, it is more of an "opportunity" to make money, and not an "ability" to make money. And we all know opportunities do not last forever, no matter what. And yes, you could argue that there is always an opportunity to make money, and to an extent I agree, but the issue that comes after that is whether those opportunities are feasible for all of us, or whether we have the desire to monitor or keep up with the trends and capitalize on those opportunities. Developing and mastering ability, or even several, to make money based on our own potential inclinations is a far more effective and efficient way of acquiring wealth, as we will always have them at our disposal, and won't need to rely too much on external factors that are out of our control. This is also the point where need to stop chasing money and start chasing value instead.

What Is Value?

Now in business, what is value? Value is the measure of benefits within a trade. Where do those benefits come from? They come from the long-acquired and fine-tuned set of skills, knowledge, experiences, craftsmanship, creativities, and connections that are collectively integrated and implemented. When we chase money or focus our attention only on the financial gains of every transaction, we inadvertently stopped caring or paying careful attention on the actual value of what we are selling. Naturally, this is where major errors are made and crucial trusts are broken between us and the buyers, eventually leading to a corrupt, inconsistent, meritless, and inevitably dissolving system of exchange. But when we chase value, we instead direct our focus on the core essence of what we are offering, providing, and embedding quality to their intricate details, and not allowing any form of compromise in order to fulfil cheap agendas. This way people will notice the profound set of benefits they will be receiving and will be more than willing to part ways with their money. For example, will you be willing to part ways with more money in a restaurant that serves their food with a sloppy presentation, poor service, uneven cooking, mediocre taste, unaccommodating atmosphere, and bad reputation? Or a restaurant that serves their food with delicate touches, proficient cooking, lovely mannered waiters and waitresses, beautifully fitting decorations, and an excellent social proof? Therefore, money is, without a doubt, very, very important in life. Anyone who explicitly said that "money is not important at all" are those people who are afraid of money, do not have any ability to make money, and do not have enough money to get out of the circumstance that they are in. And they are just saying that in order to shroud their own insecurities, incompetence, and lack of grit. Money is important because of its ability to solve a lot of our problems. However, it is important to recognize that money is not everything. It should not be the sole focus and purpose of our lives. We should strive to find a balance between our financial pursuits and our personal goals, relationships, and well-being. Money should serve as a means to an end, not the end itself. It should be used to provide us with opportunities and resources to achieve our dreams and live a fulfilling life.

In conclusion, the formula for acquiring wealth is to build substantial value. To do so, we must focus on developing and mastering our abilities to create and provide value to others. By prioritizing value over money, we can build a sustainable and trustworthy system of exchange that benefits everyone involved. While money is important in our lives, it should not be our sole focus or measure of success. Ultimately, our success should be determined by our ability to create value, make a positive impact, and live a meaningful life.

CHAPTER TWENTY-SIX
THE REASON FOR A FRIEND BACKSTABBING YOU

Be wary of friends. They will betray you more quickly, for they are easily aroused to envy. They also become spoiled and tyrannical. In fact, you have more to fear from friends than from enemies. Believe me, gentlemen.

\- JAN RUDAT

Wonder why your best friend betrayed you? Why they disappeared all of a sudden without saying a word? Why they talk bad about you behind your back? Why they decide to humiliate you in front of your other friends? And I'm sure you also want to know how you can spot the cues leading to that betrayal so that you can avoid it. And also, how you can betray someone yourself without even noticing that you have betrayed them.

Betrayal from a friend is one of the most painful experiences that one can go through. It can leave you feeling hurt, confused, and even angry. However, before you jump to conclusions, it is important to understand why a friend may have betrayed you in the first place.

One reason for a friend to betray you is envy. Envy is an intense feeling of wanting something that someone else has. Your friend may have felt envious of your success, your popularity, or your achievements. This envy can then turn into resentment, and eventually lead to them betraying you.

Another reason for a friend to betray you is a change in their personality. Sometimes, people change and become different from who they once were. Your friend may have become spoiled, entitled, or tyrannical, which can lead them to behave in ways that are hurtful and harmful to you. Furthermore, it is important to recognize that friendships, like all relationships, can be complex and fragile. There may have been underlying issues or misunderstandings between you and your friend that led to the betrayal. Communication breakdown, unmet expectations, and unresolved conflicts can all contribute to a friend betraying you. However, it is also important to note that sometimes people betray others without even realizing it. Your friend may have made a decision that hurt you, without considering the impact it would have on your friendship. In such cases, it is crucial to have an open and honest conversation with them, in which you express how their actions have affected you and try to work through the issue together. Betrayal from a friend is a painful experience, but it is important to understand that there are often underlying reasons behind their actions. By recognizing these reasons and having open communication, it may be possible to salvage the friendship or move on from it in a healthy way. And as for betraying someone without noticing it, it is important to always be mindful of our actions and their potential consequences on others.

To spot the cues leading to a friend's betrayal, it is important to pay attention to their behavior and any changes in it. If your friend starts to become distant or avoid spending time with you, it could be a sign that something is wrong. They may also start to talk badly about you behind your back or criticize you in front of others. If you notice any of these behaviors, it is important to address them with your friend in a non-confrontational way.

It is also important to trust your instincts. If something doesn't feel right about your friend's behavior, it is okay to ask them about it. And if you feel like you can't trust them anymore, it may be time to reconsider the friendship.

Finally, it is important to recognize that friendships can come to an end, and that is okay. Not all friendships are meant to last forever, and sometimes it is healthier to let go of a toxic or unhealthy relationship. With story time over, let us dive a bit more into detail of this chapter.

It hurts, does it not? To be double crossed, deceived, and made into a foolish realization by someone whom we have and gave our utmost respect, energy, time and love to, at all times of the day. A huge rush of extremely negative and detrimental emotions simply encapsulates our minds - the feelings of disappointment, disgust, regret, despisal and disbelief dominates every part of our senses as we stood there, frozen in despair. Out of all the cluster and whirlwind of words that we want to say, we could only mutter one single world: "Why?" as we become too disoriented and bewildered by all the unanswered questions that simply ever increasingly flood our heads and minds of what that specific person just dared to do to us. Since the dawn of time, betrayal, deception, and treachery are all too common in this world.

It is really nothing new, and as common as a sack of apples falling over. It is just that, as humans, we all tend to be naive to some degree, whether we want to be or not. It is not our choice, gentlemen. Why? Because as I have said, we naturally love the path of least resistance that is presented to us. Just picture your girlfriend as she broke up with you, author in my case, or the fateful assassination of the famous Julius Caesar, to name a few of the countless examples I can give here. So, we almost always rapidly generalize everything in our minds, and put far, far too much trust into, and emphasis on what is happening, rather than what could happen. This is especially the case in friendship - one of the many positive sensations we can experience, one that lightens our emotions and makes us feel at home, in good company, and generally relaxes us. And we all know that emotions are the most powerful force in a human being, going as far as often blinding us, and we will become disillusioned by how we perceive everything in our physical surroundings. After all, I have taught you so myself in this book, and as you know, this book is your only way to become a better, superior, modern man and to conquer and rule this world like a king. Therefore, remember this carefully, gentlemen: The state of our emotions will always, no matter what we do or in what kind of circumstance we find ourselves in, inevitably determine our way of perception. The more negative we feel, the more we tend to dwell in sorrow and self-deprecation, eventually leading us into deep depression. Likewise, the more positive we feel, the more we will ignore negativity, dangers, and risks. Too much reliance and/or dependency on one side of the scale will inevitably blind you of what lies on the other side of the scale. So, with regards to friendship and good company, too much indulgence in positive experiences and fun will inevitably blind you entirely of the possibility of envy, treachery, deception, and betrayal that can occur within friendship. This is specifically why when it happened, you are completely and emotionally and mentally unprepared for it, having been taken by utter and complete surprise, gentlemen.

Betrayal can be both non-personal and personal at the same time. A non-personal betrayal occurs because of only one reason: "An offer of opportunity for better life circumstances" - it is hard for anyone to initially accept this, so you are not alone in this, but, instinctually and naturally, we human beings are only as loyal as our opportunities. If one opportunity does not serve us to the full extent, or we find an even slightly better, more loyal one, we will naturally and instinctually replace that old opportunity with the new one. Uncoincidentally then, this applies to everything in our world, even relationships. Now, we will discuss relationships in a later chapter. For now, here is another example: When the food we eat does not satiate us, we move on and look for a more satiating option. When the clothes we wear do not fit us properly, we throw them away and find other clothes that fit us better. The same principle applies to social bonding, including friendships - if one person does not serve us anymore, we slowly grow apart and throw them into the trash where they belong, and look for someone else. After all, the more we invest into someone, the harder it is to move on from them, but our priorities will naturally overpower our empathy which makes us weak. It only makes sense this way, now that you look at it from the true angle, from a higher point of view, does it not, gentlemen? You would be ignorant to deny yourself this teaching, so write it down. To deny my teachings is to deny yourself your future and your potential power that you need every single day.

This is why some of the friends you have made gradually over many years, will slowly move away from you, and daily contacts as you all grow older will slowly dry up entirely. They reject my teachings. They want you weak, they want to use you. Many, many people, unaware of this phenomenon, find it very hard to accept it at first, and I was, truthfully, one of them. I was finding out that a long-time friend had suddenly stopped regularly contacting me, and that he found a new circle of friends, baffled me at first. Of course, it did also hurt my feelings because of the amount of time we have spent together over many years, due to his lack of upfront communication, and due to my lack of strength and understanding of this event. But, as time passed, I began to understand that that betrayal was non-personal, and more so circumstantial, and he did not say a thing upfront because he was afraid that I would find out and expose him. People change, and so do their priorities and intents, and it makes logical sense that he slowly shifted from noble aims towards self-destructive and negative aims. These are your "friends", as you used to call them. You are now in a better state of mental awareness, thanks to my works in this book. It is important for us to understand this, and to not take this natural phenomenon of betrayal too personally, and simply stuff such people in the trash and move on from them.

Betrayal

Betrayal is the one personal thing that will indeed cut a deep and gashing wound into us. It will hurt, and it will hurt a lot. It will also most certainly cause us to be far more careful in social situations and/or circumstances. Personal betrayal is caused by two reasons, the first is "Hatred caused by envy", the second being "Vengeance caused by to prior non-personal betrayal" taken personally. Dangerously envious and vengeful people naturally have a very low sense of self-worth. Envy is without a doubt a parasite that can turn into an uncontrollable monster, should you let it consume you or your partner. When a person close to you envies you profoundly, they will try their best with all their might to please you, whenever you are physically with them. However, they will continuously plan your downfall whenever they are alone or within the presence of other people you know, by spreading false information about you, generating black PR, speaking ill about yourself, discrediting your achievements and works, and doing their best to convince everyone that they are the only one telling the truth about you and what is associated with you. The best thing you can do to avoid personal betrayal, is to identify and test the level of inferiority of anyone you know. The more inferior a person feels about oneself, the more one will take everything personally and emotionally. This is because the weaker their pride and/or self-worth are, the more sensitive they will be to insults and provocations. So, if anyone you know easily gets emotional over a small insult, or even natural provocations involving yourself, such as your looks, achievements, and your being, just be aware that they are envious of you and are already actively planning their betrayal of you, behind your back. Vengeance due to non-personal-betrayal is what I was talking about before, people who do not have a clear understanding of non-personal-betrayal or other types of betrayal, and people with very low sense of self-worth will tend to hold grudges for long periods time on those who choose their life priorities over empathy relating to their social bonds. And if you have betrayed someone before in the past, do not ever feel sorry for them. Forget about them. Do not take it too personal. Do not reconcile with a broken past, because the past itself cannot be fixed, no matter what you do, gentlemen.

CHAPTER TWENTY-SEVEN
WHY WE COMPARE OURSELVES TO OTHERS

Can we stop it?

For it is a matter of daily observation that people take the greatest pleasure in that which satisfies their vanity; and vanity cannot be satisfied without comparison with others.

"Stop comparing yourself to others" as they say it, and when I say "They" I mean everyone who is trying so desperately hard to be a positive figure online and have absolutely no clue why we even compare ourselves to other people in the first place. Well, the answer is because it is an inevitable, innate and instinctual response for us human beings to compare. But comparing ourselves to others is very unhealthy right? How can we stop it from impacting our mental health?

All of us absolutely hate it when our comparison with other people backfires, making us feel inferior, and putting us in the awkward spot of really being on the receiving end of our very own reality check. It causes us to be hateful, vengeful, and lackluster. But on the other hand, all of us celebrate and enjoy and even cherish it when the wind is blowing in the direction of our opponent in whatever it is we are doing to make a case for the ever so delighting feeling of superiority of ourselves, especially in comparison with other people. In other words, we hate comparing ourselves to others when we are on the losing side, but we absolutely love it when we are on the winning side. The ironic thing is, we almost never realize this phenomenon occurring. We only notice and complain about how bad it is to compare ourselves to other people when we are losing. But when we are winning, we throw all the morals and ethics out of the window and start to celebrate our sense of superiority. This is because the sensation of defeat will always raise questions and debates to be answered and make sense of for the defeated. So, we then come to the naive mainstream conclusion that comparing ourselves to other people is not healthy at all, and that it makes us feel dangerously envious and start to to compromise our own mental and physical health. That it is an abomination of a behavior to be included in our day to day lives, and that it must be removed completely and replaced with something "Healthier". But the brutal truth is, you cannot and will never be able to stop comparing yourself to others - it is an inevitable occurrence for all of us human beings. it is one of the basic, primal methods of us trying to make trying to make sense of the circumstances we find ourselves in. We have to make assessments and judgements out of everything we encounter, and those assessments and judgements are made from our own set of personal metrics. And our own set of personal metrics come from our own embedded perception of ourselves and our environments.

So, if we cannot completely avoid socially comparing ourselves, how can we easily and quickly utilize comparisons to our own advantage, or remove the negative mental health impact of comparisons?

Easy, gentlemen. Here is how:

Focus on self-improvement: Instead of comparing ourselves to others, we can focus on our own progress and growth. We can set goals for ourselves and work towards achieving them, without worrying about how others are doing. This way, we can use comparisons as a motivator to become a better version of ourselves.

Practice gratitude: Comparing we to others can lead to feelings of envy and dissatisfaction. Practicing gratitude can help shift our focus from what we lack to what we have. We can appreciate our own strengths and achievements and be grateful for the opportunities and resources we have.

Recognize our own unique qualities: We all have our own strengths and weaknesses, and comparing ourselves to others can make us overlook our own unique qualities. Instead of trying to fit into someone else's mold, we can embrace our individuality and celebrate our own strengths and talents.

Limit social media use: Social media can be a breeding ground for comparison, as we often see curated versions of other people's lives. It is important to remember that social media is not a reflection of real life, and to limit our use if it starts to negatively affect our mental health.

Surround ourselves with positive influences: We are often influenced by the people around us, so it is important to surround ourselves with positive influences who encourage and support us. We can also seek out role models who inspire us, and use their success as motivation to achieve our own goals.

Understand the limitations of comparisons: Comparing ourselves to others can be helpful in certain situations, such as when we are setting goals or seeking inspiration. However, it is important to recognize the limitations of comparisons, such as the fact that everyone's circumstances are unique and that we often only see the surface-level of other people's lives.

Practice self-compassion: Comparing ourselves to others can lead to feelings of shame and self-criticism. Practicing self-compassion can help us be kinder and more understanding towards ourselves, especially when we fall deeply short of our own expectations.

Reframe comparisons in a positive way: Instead of viewing comparisons as a negative behavior, we can reframe them in a positive way by seeing them as a way to learn and grow. For example, we can use comparisons to identify areas where we can improve, and use this information to create a plan of action.

Be aware of the impact of comparisons on others: Just as comparisons can affect our own mental health, they can also impact the well-being of others. It is important to be mindful of how our actions and words might affect others, and to avoid making comparisons that are hurtful or unhelpful.

Seek support when needed: If comparisons are impacting our mental health and well-being in a significant way, it can be helpful to seek support from a mental health professional or trusted friend or family member. They can provide us with guidance and support as we work towards finding a healthier way to navigate comparisons.

Use workouts as a form of self-improvement:

Working out or exercising regularly can have a significant positive impact on our physical and mental health. Instead of comparing ourselves to others, we can focus on our own progress and celebrate small improvements. Here are some ways to incorporate workouts into our daily routine and use them as a form of self-improvement:

1.   Set achievable goals: Instead of comparing ourselves to others, we can set achievable goals for ourselves. For example, we can aim to run a certain distance, do a certain number of push-ups or lift a certain amount of weight. Setting realistic goals can help us stay motivated and feel a sense of accomplishment as we make progress towards our goals.

2.   Track our progress: Keeping track of our progress can help us see how far we've come and motivate us to keep going. We can use a workout app or a fitness tracker to track our progress and set new goals.

3.   Focus on the process, not the outcome: Instead of comparing ourselves to others or focusing on the end result, we can focus on the process of working out. We can pay attention to our form, our breathing and how our body feels during the workout. This can help us stay present in the moment and enjoy the process of working out.

4.   Find a workout buddy: Working out with a friend or partner can be a great way to stay motivated and accountable. We can encourage each other and celebrate each other's progress, instead of comparing ourselves to each other.

Incorporate meditation into our daily routine:

Meditation is a practice that can help us develop greater awareness and clarity of thought, and can have a positive impact on our mental health and well-being. By incorporating regular meditation into our daily routine, we can reduce stress and anxiety, and learn to approach comparisons in a more mindful and balanced way. Here are some tips for incorporating meditation into our daily routine:

1.   Start small: We don't need to meditate for long periods of time to reap the benefits. Starting with just a few minutes a day can be a great way to build a meditation practice.

2.   Find a quiet, comfortable space: Find a quiet, comfortable space where we can sit or lie down without being disturbed. We can use a meditation cushion or chair if it helps us sit more comfortably.

3.   Focus on our breath: Focusing on our breath is a simple yet powerful way to meditate. We can pay attention to the sensation of our breath as it enters and leaves our body, and bring our attention back to our breath whenever our mind starts to wander.

4.   Use a guided meditation app: There are many guided meditation apps available that can help us get started with meditation. These apps provide step-by-step guidance and can be a great way to learn different meditation techniques. Use them, gentlemen. They do help.

5.   Be patient and non-judgmental: Meditation is a practice that takes time and patience. It's important to approach meditation with a non-judgmental attitude and not get discouraged if our mind wanders or we find it difficult to focus. With regular practice, we can develop greater mindfulness and awareness, and learn to approach comparisons in a more balanced and healthy way.

Read to broaden our horizons:

Reading is a great way to learn about different perspectives and experiences and can help us broaden our horizons. Instead of comparing ourselves to others, we can focus on learning and growing through reading. Here are some ways to incorporate reading into our daily routine and use it to really, really broaden our horizons:

1.   Choose diverse books: Instead of only reading books that reflect our own experiences and perspectives, we can choose books that offer different perspectives and viewpoints. We can seek out books by authors from different backgrounds and cultures and read books about different topics and issues.

2.   Take notes and reflect on what we read: Taking notes and reflecting on what we read can help us internalize the information and insights we gain from books. We can write down our thoughts

and reactions as we read and take time to reflect on what we've learned.

3.   Discuss what we've read with others: Discussing what we've read with others can help us gain new insights and perspectives and deepen our understanding of what we've read. We can join a book club, discuss what we've read with friends or family members, or participate in online forums or social media groups.

4.   Set reading goals: Setting reading goals can help us stay motivated and on track with our reading. We can set goals for the number of books we want to read in a year or set goals to read books on certain topics or by certain authors. Hell, you are reading one of the best books in the world right now in this very moment. But still, read other books.

5.   Make reading a habit: Making reading a habit can help us incorporate it into our daily routine and make it a regular part of our lives. We can set aside a specific time each day for reading or incorporate reading into our daily commute or other parts of our day. By making reading a habit, we can continue to broaden our horizons and learn new things throughout our lives.

Focus on nutrient-dense foods:

Good nutrition is about more than just counting calories or following a strict diet plan. It's about nourishing our bodies with nutrient-dense foods that provide the vitamins, minerals, and other nutrients we need to stay healthy. Here are some ways to incorporate nutrient-dense foods into our daily routine:

1.   Eat a variety of fruits and vegetables: Fruits and vegetables are packed with vitamins, minerals, and other nutrients that are essential for good health. Eating a variety of fruits and vegetables can help ensure that we get the nutrients we need.

2.   Choose whole grains: Whole grains like brown rice, quinoa, and whole wheat bread are rich in fiber and other nutrients that can help keep us feeling full and satisfied. In addition, they are very cheap, no

matter what. Especially oats – and if you can, opt for oats with shell. They may be called by a variety of names, so your extra challenge in this extra step is to find out what they are called in your local market. And, seriously, opt for the cheapest oats you can find. Oats are truly and completely the exact same product among all price-ranges. Believe me.

3.   Include lean protein sources: Lean protein sources like chicken, fish, tofu, and legumes can help provide the protein we need to build and repair muscle, as well as to support our immune system and other bodily functions. Do you like chicken? Dried wood worms? Maybe even oats? Well, there you go – you already have three relatively cheap options available to you.

4.   Limit processed foods: Processed foods like candy, chips, and soda are often high in calories and low in nutrients. Limiting our intake of these foods can help us focus on nutrient-dense options.

Practice mindful eating:

In addition to focusing on nutrient-dense foods, practicing mindful eating can help us make healthier choices and enjoy our food more. Here are some ways to practice mindful eating:

1.   Pay attention to hunger and fullness cues: Rather than eating on autopilot or according to a strict schedule, pay attention to our body's hunger and fullness cues. This can help us avoid overeating or undereating. Seriously.

2.   Eat without distractions: Eating while watching TV or scrolling through social media can distract us from our body's signals and lead to mindless eating. Try to eat without distractions and focus on enjoying our food, gentlemen.

3.   Savor our food: Take time to savor the flavors, textures, and aromas of our food. This can help us feel more satisfied and enjoy our meals more. Especially I had to fight to get this right.

4.   Practice gratitude: Taking a moment to express gratitude for our food can help us cultivate a more positive relationship with food and appreciate the nourishment it provides.

Stay hydrated:

Drinking enough water is essential for good health. Here are some ways to stay hydrated:

1.   Carry a water bottle with us: Carrying a water bottle with us can help us stay hydrated throughout the day, even if we do not feel thirsty whatsoever. Wherever I go, I carry a military canteen on my belt.

2.   Drink water before meals: Drinking water before meals can help us feel fuller and satisfied, and can also help support digestion. I used to drink only sugary beverages. Now I drink 4-5 liters of water a day.

3.   Flavor water with fresh fruit: Adding fresh fruit like lemon or cucumber to our water can make it more flavorful and enjoyable to drink. Try berries if you can, enjoy.

By focusing on nutrient-dense foods, practicing truly mindful eating, and staying hydrated, we can nourish our bodies and support our overall health and well-being.
Finding a Hobby:

Finding a hobby that we enjoy can bring us joy and relaxation, as well as provide an opportunity for us to learn new skills and challenge ourselves. Here are some ways to incorporate hobbies into our lives:

1.   Experiment with different activities: Trying out different activities and hobbies can help us find what we enjoy the most. Some possible options would include painting, woodworking, cooking, gardening, and writing.

2.   Set aside some, but not too much dedicated time: Setting aside dedicated time for our hobbies can deeply help us make them a regular part of our routine.

3.   Join a community: Joining a community of likeminded people who share our interests can help us stay motivated and learn from others.

Embracing Craftsmanship:

Craftsmanship is actually about taking pride in our work and focusing on the process of creation rather than just the end result. Here are some ways to embrace craftsmanship:

1.   Focus on quality over quantity: Rather than frantically rushing to finish a project, focus on taking our time and doing our best work.

2.   Embrace imperfection: Accepting that mistakes and imperfections are a natural part of the creative process can help us avoid getting discouraged easily.

3.   Celebrate our accomplishments: Celebrating our accomplishments, no matter how small, can help us stay motivated and feel proud of our work and maintain motivation.

4.   Learn from others: Learning from other craftsmen and women can help us improve our skills and gain new perspectives.

The Benefits of Hobbies and Craftsmanship:

In addition to being quite fun and strongly fulfilling, hobbies and craftsmanship can provide a number of mental health benefits. Such as:

1.   Reducing stress: Engaging in a hobby or crafting activity can actively help reduce stress and improve relaxation.

2.   Building confidence: Learning new skills and creating something from scratch can boost our confidence and self-esteem by as much as 3 times, as a study found.

3.   Fostering creativity: Hobbies and craftsmanship provide an effective outlet for creativity and self-expression.

By finding a hobby we enjoy, embracing craftsmanship, and reaping the mental health benefits, we can enhance our overall well-being and lead a more fulfilling life, gentlemen.
It is important to note that not all hobbies and activities are attractive to all people. You should dedicate a good amount of time to discover what you actually like, and what you can do that does not really feel like work. And most importantly: don't stop when faced with difficulties, no matter how large or seemingly inescapable.

CHAPTER TWENTY-EIGHT
HOW VIDEOGAMES, ALCOHOL, DRUGS & MEDIA CONSUMPTION RAPIDLY DEVELOP AN EXTREMELY WEAK AND DETRIMENTAL MINDSET FOR MEN

Face your own flaws and conquer them, even if that means sacrificing pleasure.

Indeed, the truth that many people never understand, until it is too late, is that the more you try to avoid suffering, the more you will suffer, because smaller and more insignificant things begin to torture you, in proportion to your fear of being hurt. The one who does most to avoid suffering is, in the end, the one who suffers the most. It is his own existence, his own being, that is at once the subject and the source of his pain, and his very existence and consciousness is his greatest torture.

- THOMAS MERTON

Escapism & sedation from the pain of real life. One of the main reasons why as men, we are growing weaker than ever is because we make bad decisions for ourselves. No longer are we facing physical and mental battles with courage & determination, instead we run away and hide from challenges, trials & tribulations. We fear getting hurt, we fear pain, we fear suffering, we fear hardships, we fear agony. TRUE, they are instinctually avoided by us because in order to survive, we must avoid things that are hard and painful, but ironically, because we avoid them, we do not grow, we become just an empty shell of a man, and we wonder why our lives are not going anywhere. Pain makes us grow, way more than pleasure will ever do. In life you need pain to grow, and in order to get anywhere significant in your life, you must face pain.

Life is painful. In fact, pain is one of the necessary components in life alongside pleasure for a healthy life. To reject or the other is, in essence, to reject life. Yet, in our day of age, we relish in pleasure and are willing to pursue it until the very end of time itself, while completely and utterly rejecting and avoiding pain. So much so, in fact, that we do not want to experience even the slightest bit of pain, because it is not in our nature to treat pain enthusiastically and relish it. Yet, that is the position where all of us are at right now with life, we have no choice but to experience pain. But because we do not desire pain, we try our absolute best to engineer and create illusions to separate ourselves to the best of our ability from any pain whatsoever - whether it involves manipulating the reception of pain in the body, diverting our attention, or completely ignoring it. Effectively revolutionizing our mindset and character into someone that is fragile, sensitive, clueless, sluggish, and downright meritless, is simply a byproduct of such behavior. The modern world has brought about a plethora of distractions that we can use to divert our attention from the pain and struggles of everyday life. One of the most popular methods of avoiding pain is through alcohol consumption. Alcohol is a popular choice for people who want to forget about their problems and enjoy themselves for a while. While it might provide a temporary escape from pain, alcohol consumption is a dangerous path to follow. It can lead to addiction, dependency, and other health problems.

Another popular way people use to avoid pain is through videogames. Videogames offer a virtual world that allows us to escape our reality and immerse ourselves in a fantasy world where we can control our destiny. While videogames may seem harmless, excessive use can lead to addiction, social isolation, and the development of a weak mindset. When someone spends hours playing videogames, they are avoiding the real world and its challenges. They are essentially running away from their problems, and this can lead to a lack of resilience and coping skills in the face of adversity. Media consumption is another way that people avoid pain. The media provides a constant stream of entertainment and distraction, allowing us to avoid the reality of life. While media consumption can be a great source of entertainment, excessive use can lead to addiction, and it can also prevent us from developing a strong mindset. When we spend all our time-consuming media, we are not engaging in the real world and developing the necessary skills to deal with pain and adversity.

All these behaviors, whether it's alcohol consumption, videogame addiction, or excessive media consumption, ultimately lead to a weak mindset. A weak mindset is characterized by a lack of resilience, an inability to cope with adversity, and a general sense of helplessness. When we avoid pain, we miss out on the opportunity to learn and grow from our struggles. We miss out on the chance to develop the mental toughness that is required to succeed in life. So, what can we do to avoid developing a weak mindset? Firstly, we need to recognize the importance of pain and struggles in life. Pain is a necessary component of life, and we need to learn to embrace it. Instead of avoiding pain, we need to face it head-on and learn from it. Secondly, we need to engage in activities that challenge us and push us outside of our comfort zone. Activities such as exercise, sports, and hobbies are great ways to develop mental toughness and resilience. Lastly, we need to limit our consumption of alcohol and media, and we need to be mindful of how we use videogames. Life is painful, but it is also full of opportunities for growth and development. We need to embrace and develop resilience. By avoiding pain and seeking pleasure at all costs, we are only hindering our growth and potential. It's important to remember that pain is a natural part of life and that it can teach us valuable lessons about ourselves and the world around us. By learning to face pain with a positive mindset and an open heart, we can develop the mental toughness and resilience needed to succeed in life. To develop a strong mindset, we must also learn to practice self-care. Self-care involves taking care of our physical, emotional, and mental well-being. By taking care of ourselves, we can better handle the challenges and stresses that life throws our way. It's also essential to cultivate healthy relationships with others and to seek support when we need it. We don't have to face life's challenges alone, and seeking help is a sign of strength, not weakness.

In conclusion, avoiding pain and seeking pleasure at all costs may provide temporary relief, but it can ultimately lead to a weak mindset. To develop a strong mindset, we must learn to embrace pain and use it as an opportunity for growth and development. We must engage in activities that challenge us and push us outside of our comfort zone, limit our consumption of alcohol and media, and practice self-care. By doing so, we can develop the mental toughness and resilience needed to succeed in life, and become a better, superior, modern man.

CHAPTER TWENTY-NINE
THE IMPORTANCE OF A MAN IN YOUR LIFE

The relationship between a father and a son is nearly identical to that of a master and a student. Where the master will showcase and teach him everything he knows, and the student will carry on his guidance and legacy into the next generations. A great master will influence and produce a great student, and a great student will demonstrate and produce great outcomes.

A father's presence is very important in a man's life, our perception and eventual portrayal of our masculinity will mostly depends on how our father exemplifies his own masculinity throughout our lives. That is why today we have men who are lost, emotional, aimless and purposeless because of the dire consequences of absent fathers or fatherlessness, couple that with the current social order that tries so hard to shut down masculinity. We have no mentors & guidance to help us prepare for life and all the stuff that it will throw at us. This chapter is a message to all fathers and would be fathers in the world of how profound the effect of your presence is to your son's life in terms of his outlook on life, attitudes, and mental wellbeing.

A father should be the captain of the ship, the one who sets the course and drive the ship, not to let his wife or his children navigate and take the wheel instead. Putting your wife and your children first means you are abandoning their future and their safety, and therefore their lives, prosperity, and finally they themselves, which is not what they both instinctually and intuitively want from you and for the family. That is why it is important that as fathers, you must have a strong masculine frame, a strong foundation of your own world or space in every important aspect and circumstance of life, so that you will be confident in leading your family into a more prosperous place. A strong, dominant and authoritative frame will lay the crucial foundations of how your son will take examples from you and evolve his own masculinity. When we are still kids, our minds are not fully developed for critical and abstract thinking, and the only way we could learn is through pure observation, sensation and mimicking - so it is stupid to try ask and guess what we like, because we will like just about anything we get our hands on. This is the formative phase, so this early phase of your son's life to introduce him to your own masculine world, your hobbies, passions, work and interests. Take him fishing alongside you, take him to watch you practice wrestling, take him to the garage and watch you work on the car, even take him to the gym to watch you exercise and light some weights. This will establish the first stage of the father and son bond.

As he watches you perform all those activities, he will inevitably get interested in those things, and develop the desire to also engage in them.

When this happens, get excited for your son, be proud of him, and encourage him. This will make him feel more involved in the male space and eventually develop a sense of male tribalism. And who knows, maybe you can notice his early talents and inclinations, too. However, do not restrict his time-spending only to yourself. Let your wife spend enough time with him too. However, as we move on to our teenage years, or the learning phase, the connection and bond that your son has developed with you over his youth, will greatly strengthen and will make him feel even closer to you, now that our minds are more capable of making judgements and critical thinking. As your son becomes a teenager, he will probably also cause stupid mistakes and cause a lot of trouble, and often ignore your orders. When your son enters the adult years, this is the individual phase. This is the phase where he will face real world and life problems. At this stage, you need to cut your son off from your support, give him a head start, and let him fall and fail until he forms into a man, learns to solve his own problems, conquer his life, and control it.
This is the stage where your son needs to become his own person, develop his own beliefs, values, and identity. It is essential that he understands that he is responsible for his own life and decisions, and that he can only rely on himself to overcome any obstacles. As a father, your role now is to guide him towards self-sufficiency and independence, while still being there for him as a source of support and guidance.

It is important to note that the relationship between a father and son is not always easy or straightforward. There will be moments of conflict and disagreement, but it is crucial to handle them in a constructive and respectful manner. Always listen to your son's perspective and encourage open communication. While you may have a dominant and authoritative frame, it is important to show empathy and understanding towards your son's struggles and challenges.
In conclusion, being a father is not just about providing for your family financially, but also about being a strong and positive role

model for your children. By establishing a strong masculine frame and bonding with your son through shared interests and activities, you can guide him towards becoming a confident, independent, and successful individual. Remember that while you may have ultimate power over the family, it is important to use this power in a responsible and constructive manner, always keeping your son's best interests in mind.

In the end, being a father is a great responsibility, but it is also a privilege and an opportunity to make a positive impact on the lives of your children. By embodying the qualities of a strong and positive role model, and by using a moderatively strong hand, when necessary, you can guide your son towards a successful and fulfilling life, and create a happy and healthy family environment for all.

CHAPTER THIRTY
THE ULTIMATE MEASURE OF MENTAL HEALTH AND PERSONALITY IN A MAN

Excellence is an art won by training and habituation. We do not act rightly because we have virtue of excellence, but we rather have those because we have acted rightly. We are what we repeatedly do. Excellence then, is not an act but a habit.

- ARISTOTLE

We are what we do, not what we say we'll do or what we think we want to do. A man's actions speaks everything about him, it translates and showcases his values, character and state of mind. We often wonder how a person is doing, are they happy or are they in misery? Are they really okay, or are they actually suffering? Are they on the right path or are they lost? And we try to somehow penetrate their mind in order to find out, or negotiate empathy with them to get them to reveal themselves. But all the answer we are looking for can be simply observed keenly from a distance. A person's collection of habits are the real life translation and manifestation of their own their cognitive and emotional world. A simple observation of their crude/major habits that they do daily can allow us to have a glimpse on their current character and the state of their mental health. What are the nature of good habits and bad habits? How can we break free from the shackles of bad habits that had imprisoned us for years?

Good habits are actions that are beneficial to us, leading to personal growth, health, and success. They can be small actions such as making our bed every morning, exercising regularly, or reading a book before bed. Good habits are developed over time through consistent effort, discipline, and motivation. On the other hand, bad habits are actions that are detrimental to us, hindering our personal growth, health, and success. They can be small actions such as procrastination, nail-biting, or negative self-talk. Bad habits are often developed through indulgence, lack of self-awareness, and avoidance of discomfort. Breaking free from bad habits requires a combination of self-awareness, discipline, and motivation. The first step is to recognize and acknowledge the habit and its negative effects on our life. Then, we need to understand the triggers and reasons behind the habit and develop a plan to replace the bad habit with a good one. This requires consistency and patience, as breaking a bad habit takes time and effort. To cultivate good habits, we can start small by choosing one habit to focus on at a time and creating a plan to integrate it into our daily routine. We can also seek support from friends, family, or a coach to keep us accountable and motivated. Ultimately, the habits we cultivate shape our character and determine the trajectory of our lives. By consistently choosing and practicing good habits, we can create a life of excellence and fulfillment. In order to break free from the shackles of bad habits, it is important to understand the nature of habits themselves. Habits are essentially a loop of behavior that our brain creates in response to a cue, which triggers a routine or action, leading to a reward or outcome. Over time, this loop becomes automatic, and the behavior becomes a habit that is difficult to break. To change a habit, it is necessary to identify the cue, routine, and reward that make up the loop, and then replace the routine with a new, healthier behavior that still satisfies the same cue and leads to a similar reward. This process is known as habit reversal training and is a powerful tool for breaking bad habits and establishing good ones.

Another important factor in breaking bad habits is to cultivate self-awareness and mindfulness. By being more present and aware of our actions and thoughts, we can catch ourselves before we engage in a bad habit and make a conscious decision to do something else. It is also important to set clear goals and intentions for the new habit we want to establish and hold ourselves accountable through tracking our progress and rewarding ourselves for positive behavior. In addition, it can be helpful to seek support from others, whether that be through joining a support group or enlisting the help of a coach or mentor. By sharing our goals and struggles with others, we can gain valuable insights and support that can help us stay on track and overcome challenges. Breaking free from bad habits takes time, effort, and persistence, but by understanding the nature of habits and utilizing effective strategies and support, we can make lasting positive changes in our lives and become the best versions of ourselves.

Habits are a collection of endeavors both major and minor that are implemented int our regular daily routines. They are formed through being provoked by a cue or a catalyst that turned to a committed routine exposure or practice that eventually lead to the collection and sensation of rewards through those routines. As we all know, actions always speak louder than words, because our actions are more closely associated with our instincts, desires and impulses, and are far more of a handful to be controlled, manipulated and concealed than words. The body does not lie. That is why the old saying is that, if you want to really know the truth about a person, don't waste your time trying to talk to them to get them to reveal themselves, simply observe and find out about their behaviors.
Everything happens for a reason, right? Similarly, all actions are done for a reason or a set of reasons, and it is actually no different with habits - they are done by us for two reasons, either to fulfill

certain cognitive and emotional voids or to release certain cognitive and emotional expressions, or both. Here are a set of examples:

A person may read lots of books in order to fulfil a cognitive and emotional void in terms of acquiring knowledge and understanding of a certain circumstance, such as learning human nature, or they may read lots of books just to express their passion in a certain circumstance.

A person might go to the boxing gym in order to release certain emotional expressions such as anger and frustration, or they may go there to fulfill a certain cognitive void, such as the desire to acquire skills in the sweet science of boxing.

A person may watch pornography in order to fulfill his sexual fantasies and dreams, but also express his passions within the sexual act because of the absence of sexual interactions.

A person may consume drugs and alcohol in order to fulfil a certain emotional sensation that they are so desperate to experience a certain emotional sensation that they are so desperate to experience, or do it just so that they can force themselves reliably to express certain emotions that they are uncomfortable in expressing when they are conscious and sober.

So, how can a person's selection and collection of habits determine that particular persons character?

Once again, we simply look at the bare, primal nature of the habits themselves. Healthy and constructive habits are done to keenly pursue meaningful end goals. Unhealthy and destructive habits are done to pretend quench the seemingly unachievable end goals, basically only simulating the desired effect. Healthy habits involve delayed gratifications, whereas unhealthy habits involve instant gratifications. That is also why healthy habits are so much harder to form but are so much easier to break than bad habits, because the rewards take way longer to manifest themselves. And that is exactly how we can tell the state of a person's character by differentiating people who look for quick fixes and people who actually look for the diamond in the mud, and are willing to go all the way, all in. Scarcity impulsive driven mindset vs abundance objective driven mindset, greedy vs calculative, reckless vs prudent, lazy vs active, aimless vs purposeful, undetermined vs ambitious, irresolute vs persistent. Determining and understanding a person's character through their habits will also inevitably reveal the state of their mental health as well. Remember, gentlemen, where the mind goes, the body follows - an unhealthy mind will always direct its focus on looking for quick, easy, and validating fixes for a variety of reasons, because, instinctually, its main priority is to get rid of the harmful, unpleasant, and detrimental sensations that a person is experiencing. Now, gentlemen, do not be quick and hasty to generalize things and conclude that, "Oh if a person takes up and internalizes good habits that means that they have a healthy mind, free from any bad habits that can disrupt that state of mind." This could not be further from reality. Most people, while they have good habits and routines, can also form and have certain bad habits that they internalize, that naturally constantly disrupt, and even cease the flow of a healthy mind. Because, as I have said prior, bad habits are more easily formed and good habits are more easily broken because of their respective nature. A person who regularly goes to the gym is not immune to being addicted to pornography. Likewise, a person who regularly reads books is not immune from suffering addiction to drugs, alcohol, and other things. Bad habits can and will distract you time and time again, and should you gentlemen do nothing about that, they will never stop. So, how can you actually, truly break free from bad habits that have been imprisoning and enslaving you? Or, if not that, how can you try to control yourself in order to prevent yourself from falling into the deep pit of seemingly apparently endless mental mystery?

Well, in essence, you only have two options - the first one is to replace the bad habits through finding new, profound, and healthy fixations that can occupy your mind enough to slowly but surely disregard your thoughts of the bad habits, learn and gain the ability to control them, and finally conquer them, never to see them ever again in your new life. Ideally, this takes form in a collection of activities, and that means a lot to a person on a very personal level. A common misconception is that no one can simply say "Just replace the bad habits with good habits". While this is technically the idea behind habit replacements, it is simply not quite that simple. This is because, if the person does not have any profound interest, curiosity, or dare I say it, obsession of a particular activity with regards to its routines, exercises, and rewards, it is very, very unlikely that he would ever commit on his own accord to it routinely and reliably, in order to eventually turn it into a proper, solidified, internalized habit of his. Even in my case, if I did not have any profound interests in fitness and lifting weights, I would not have broken away from my unhealthy addiction to sugar and caffeine.

The second option is simply instilling a constant state of fear, through making the dire consequences of bad habits far more plausible. In essence, because we are more attracted to the rewards of an activity, and because that is how bad habits constantly seduce you into doing them in the first place, such as presenting you with artificial, yet instant rewards, we instead focus on the bare consequences of what those bad habits can and inevitably will eventually do to us and our lives, in the short term and long term. Naturally, this involves constantly reminding yourself of them through tangible representations of those consequences. Maybe a collection of words on the front page of your little diary that you open every day, or maybe even a wallpaper on your phone, on which you will have no choice but to stare at every single day, every single time whenever you use your phone. Or, alternatively, maybe just downloading an online documentation of someone suffering the dire consequences of those bad habits in an audio podcast session. Anything can work here, gentlemen.

Similarly, the choice is yours. Option one, or option two? Blue pill, or red pill? No rush, please.

Finally, a man's collection of habits can serve as a reliable indicator of his personality and mental state. While negative habits impede personal development, health, and success, good habits promote these things. It takes self-awareness, self-control, and drive to break poor habits, but habit reversal training and mindfulness can help. Habits naturally develop through a cycle of behavior sparked by a cue that culminates in a routine or action that yields a reward.

We may replace negative habits with good ones and lead lives of excellence and fulfillment by comprehending this process. Our habits create our personalities and influence the course of our lives, so it's critical to develop positive habits and eliminate bad ones.

CHAPTER THIRTY-ONE
THE MEANING OF RESPECT AND HOW TO EARN IT FROM OTHERS

It has to be earned

Because men really respect only that which was founded of old and has developed slowly, he who wants to live on after his death must take care not only of his posterity but even more of his past.

- FRIEDRICH NIETZSCHE

Everyone wants to be respected, but today's society, again, blinds you all into thinking that respect is freely given, that your mere existence as a human being is worthy of respect. Well guess what? Respect is never given unless they are earned and deservingly given, you must be someone of value and someone who demonstrates & enforces value, integrity and competence consistently through a significant amount of time. The brutal truth of this world is, people only respect those who can add value to them and those who are socially proven and perceived to be of value. So your delusion of "Respecting everyone" is an absolute lie. People who respect everyone are people who does not stand for anything, and whose worth is meaningless even to themselves. People who give respect so easily diminishes other's respect for them, and eventually their own respect for themselves, as their approval becomes too common and too effortlessly acquired. Everything begins with you, to earn respect from others, you must respect yourself. Everyone loves and yearns to be respected. The feeling of being acknowledged, appreciated and commended for your very own existence and actions is without a doubt an impeccable encouragement and enforcement to our sense of self-worth and a fulfilling sensation that we are someone of true, actual value, that can contribute meaningfully and significantly to society and all of mankind.

As the title of the chapter clearly said, respect is not something that is obtained just because you are a human being and that you exist in this world - it has to be earned. This is because, once again, the world is cruel, murderous, and unforgiving. With any relationship, everything starts with respect. Without respect, there will be no further investment from an individual into another individual. Respect is always and must be earned, and it is not earned in a lump sum or in a bucket full of commendations either, it is simply developed and accumulated through a significant amount of time of continuous demonstration of strength and trust. That is why when it comes to inheritance, it is very difficult for one to truly earn respect from that, because it often clouds the persons mind with presumption, preconception, delusion, and self-made lies that he is automatically, by nature, owed any form of respect whatsoever. While in reality, the respect that he thinks he deserves are actually tremendously doubted, questioned, and contemplated unless proven time and time again until mutual trust has been built. Therefore, gentlemen, to earn respect as a man, you must learn, possess, implement, and internalize these three qualities:

Core values

Integrity

Competence

Core values are the life principles and ethics associated with the reality that you live by with regards to various circumstances and aspects of life. They are formed, modified, and enforced through time and life experiences as you grow up and mature into a full-grown man.

Integrity is simply your capability and courage to implement those core values into real life objectives regardless of outside influence and temptations. And it may sound easy, but integrity is what almost all men lack in our day of age - they think, preach, theorize, engage in philosophy, and say what they believe, but when it comes to practice and taking actions, they either cower in fear of being judged and criticized, make excuses in fear of uncertainty of failure, or attack the person telling them to take action in an attempt to heal their now-wounded ego. I do not need to tell you gentlemen how pathetic that is, and that you are better than this.

Competence is your sense and proof of mastery with regards to many important and crucial activities needed in life with regards to your crafts and arts, your physical and emotional strength, resilience, resistance, endurance, your ability to handle times of distress, your ability to acquire resources, your ability to adapt to build and maintain social connections, and adapt to anything that comes your way. And to add icing on the cake, social connections, or your very own social proof can tremendously boost your respect in society as well. For example, like the great pioneers and inventors of our time, Heinrich Göbel who invented the Light Bulb, only to have Thomas Edison patent it, and Albert Einstein, whom you all know, all spent their early lives developing their own core values, integrity, and competence - only then could they go down in history forever.
A lot of people say that you should respect everyone, regardless of who they are. And, once again, I have to disagree because of that one word, "Everyone". What? So you should also respect those who haven't deservingly earned your respect? The more free and unconditional respect you to people, or "Everyone". the more you will diminish and depreciate your own respect for yourself, and other people's respect for you, not to mention anyone you give your respect to. Why? Because it implies that you do not stand for anything in life and will never do so - it will ultimately leave you vulnerable to deceptions and other people to enslave you, because you are willing to substantially invest yourself in anybody with such ease and disregard for any deeper thought. This is about as smart as a

drug-fueled junkie on the streets. So, gentlemen, treat everyone with decent mannerisms but only give your respect to those who have earned it, or those who have proven themselves time and time again to be deserving of your trust, to eventually gain some of your respect. You can and will judge a book by its cover, but obviously, you do not judge a book by its cover alone. especially with regard to your respect for women. After all, women should be treated with respect. Speaking of judging a book by its cover, one can also give fake respect to you and this one does not really take a genius or an analyst to spot. People who give fake respect are basically people pleasers. Remember, when someone is trying to extensively justify their intentions, this is actually a simple concealment of their true intentions. They will pretend to rightfully submit to you, only to backstab you later on. You may not initially be able to comprehensively make sense of, and feasibly understand it, but you can and will sense the lies and inconsistencies. Now, of course, having certain core values and displaying integrity and competence does not always translate to respect. Like with everything, there are always going to be opposing forces trying to bring you down for cognitive dissonance and hurting their fragile little ego that comes with being a pathetic, weak, and downtrodden people-pleaser. And the only way to disrespect is, again, to associate your core values as much as possible with the objective truth, because whether they like it or not, the objective truth will eventually become conducive by itself.

It is simply a question of them willing to endure the emotional outbursts and the pain of realization long enough for them to accept the truth fully. But let us be honest here, gentlemen - feasibly, most disrespect comes from envious and hateful individuals who couldn't provide any rational, and meaningful arguments about what we stand for, and just emotionally bully us to abandon our own values in order to make them feel better about themselves through a false, weak, temporary sensation of superiority because they felt and are incapable of earning genuine respect from anyone, including their very own family if they have not abandoned them altogether yet. In this case, it is not even worth your time to pay any attention whatsoever, gentlemen. Believe me.

Now, of course, respect does not only come from and given to friends, acquaintances and also colleagues, it can also come from and given to enemies as well. There are two types of enemies: Rivals and Mortals. Rivals share the same or the absolute majority of the same interests, goals, and core values - however, their method of approaching things is different than yours. That is the only difference between them.

For example, two sports teams competing against each other or two businesses vying for the same market share. Despite being rivals, there is still mutual respect because they both understand and appreciate the hard work, dedication, and passion required to achieve major, major success in their respective fields. And to add to that note significantly, I can confidently say that you can trust your rivals a lot more than your friends, as they, time and time again, prove their respectability through their actions. This is simply not the case with friends, you just do not know what they are up to. You do not see their actions; you see what they tell you.

Now, mortal enemies are the complete opposite. They have nothing in common, standing for different values, goals, methods, you name it. Their objectives are at the far end of both sides of the scale respectively, and the byproduct of their objectives is destroying and demolishing the other. The only respect that is given, is the respect for having the courage to stand up for what they believe - nothing else, ever. The rest is ultimately solely the effort of nullifying each other's progress. In the end, if you want to be truly respected by others, you must have the confidence to look at yourself and comfortably have the strength that you are worthy of respect without hesitation, apprehension, timidity, and any thoughts of trying to demand or beg for respect from others. And the only way to develop that confidence is through demanding more from yourself and eventually proving to yourself your worthiness time and time again. All the qualities you wish to have as a man must begin from within yourself. You must cultivate them like fine cheese, gradually maturing. This is what our enemies never learn, gentlemen. And this is why you are already that much superior to them – but there is still a long way to go.

CHAPTER THIRTY-TWO
WHY YOU SHOULD STOP COMPLAINING AND BLAMING AS A MAN

Most of us have been that insufferable crybaby back in the day.

It's your own bad strategies, not the unfair opponent, that are to blame for your failures. You are responsible for the good and the bad in your life.

- ROBERT GREENE

I believe that a lot of you gentlemen have been in that situation or have been a man who just complains a lot over a lot of stuff, even small and insignificant things, to the point where if we can't get the solution to our problems, we start to point fingers to other people or entities that we assume might have some association or correlation to our problems. Even though in reality, most of the time they have absolutely nothing to do with any of our problems whatsoever. Just makes us look like a complete man-child doesn't it when we look at it from other people's perspective, or the outside looking in? Complaining and Blaming are extremely detrimental, unattractive, and abysmal qualities to have as a man, especially today where masculinity is being abolished and untaught, these qualities are ever more present in more men than we could've ever imagined since the manly age of raiders, hunters, scavengers and soldiers. And we are going to discuss why that is.

I used to be one of those men who complained and blamed others for my problems. I would point fingers at everything and everyone around me, thinking that it was their fault that my life was not going the way I decided to take control of my life and turn it around. I started reading self-help books, attending personal development seminars, and working with a life coach. Through these experiences, I learned the importance of taking responsibility for my life and the power of a positive mindset. As I actively continued my personal development journey, I noticed that many other men were actually deeply struggling with the same issues that I had faced in the past. They were complaining, blaming others, and feeling just utterly and completely powerless in their lives. That's when I realized that I had a unique perspective and story to share that could help others.

Just remember, if something isn't going your way if you are pushing to go your way, someone down the road is stopping you. Someone is stopping your progress. If that happens, disconnect from that person. With that out of the way, let us get properly into this chapter, gentlemen. Now before I carry on, I want to remind you gentlemen that the scenarios and contexts that I am implying with regard to this particular topic is outside of both legal and vice circumstances.
We complain and blame because our expectations do not meet the reality that presents itself in front of us, and we felt that we are seemingly unable to handle the weight of that gap and the personal pain and irritation caused by those "Unfortunate Circumstances" that befall us throughout our lives. And even if we do know how to actually handle them, we are either too lazy, too afraid, or too mindlessly and furiously ignorant to get our own hands dirty to clean up the mess and patch our own wounds. So, we desperately try to be relatable to others by venting our own feelings in order to get some sort of sympathy, along with the utmost hope of receiving some form of assistance. At the same time, however, should we fail to get the sympathy and assistance that we hoped for so deeply, we search for a seemingly correlated scapegoat to condemn in order to get their hands dirty for us instead so that we can therefore restore our disillusioned sense of contentment and tranquility, otherwise known as inner peace among more spiritual circles. The environments that we are raised and brought up in can also determine the likelihood of us being chronic complainers, believe it or not, gentlemen. People who often complain can also emerge from an environment that is either too spoiled, too protected, too conservative, or all of them. This is because they are naturally far too accustomed to getting things, even minor things, done for them, and

having circumstances manipulated and engineered to go their way for long periods of time to the point where the massive weight of their expectations on a lot of circumstances becomes their own, slim, and sensitive threshold for discontentment and dissonance in any form whatsoever. And should those circumstances go south on them, even something as small as hitting their toe with a step could send them into a drug-induced-like frenzy, whining, complaining, blaming, and complaining. Now, to complain occasionally and rationally is not necessarily a bad thing - in fact, it can actually work as a decent tool for us to discover our own set of problems, or another set of problems and figure out a way to fix it eventually. But if it eventually turns chronic and frequent, and if it also becomes just a degrading, stupid, ridiculous, and just utterly furious self-constructed sense of annoyance or misery, then it is without a doubt, an insufferable disease that brings absolutely nothing but the contagious spread of ones very own sense of indignation that one is carrying to the table. Therefore, gentlemen, continuously complaining and blaming others for your own misfortunes are extremely repulsive and self-damaging qualities to have, especially as a man where emotional strength, being able to handle stressful situations, and being able to harmoniously solve problems are within our own burden to perform and fulfill. And yes, harassment is just complaining and blaming. Think before you attack someone, or especially me - it could be the last straw that decides whether you will have success in life and become a better, superior, modern man - or die alone, never having children, broke, naturally betrayed by your own only partner you ever got, and of course, bitter and senile. So, of course, these dreadful habits are extremely detrimental to a man's well-being and their own potential, so much so that they can spell doom for your entire life, turning your entire a self-produced torture chamber that you cannot ever even hope to escape. Why? Firstly, because it is an utterly and absolute waste of time - the time that you spent complaining and blaming the unfair world and other people for your own failures, misery, torture, failures, misfortune, accidents, and setbacks could be used to work extremely intricately on them instead, eventually being able to turn them into your very own arsenal of strong advantages.

Nothing can change the nexuses that this world will bring to us. Unfortunate and undesirable circumstances will eventually happen, and most of the time, no one will come to save you from them. People will turn their backs on you. You have to dig your own holes, learn how they work, and then dig yourself out of them, to understand them and allow you to conquer and control them. Yelling and screaming at the heavens or the ceiling of your own one-room apartment, dear gentlemen, will not summon some holy savior that will swoop you off your feet. Far from it, in fact. You need to have the mind and will to withstand the strain to succeed and acquire eternal tranquility and prosperity in your own mind and life. That is why relying on hope or faith alone will never be enough to get you where you want to be, as it is an extremely delusional way to solve your problems. Pointing fingers at everyone around you will only cause them to make it one of their life goals to destroy or enslave you, possibly even taking your female partner with them. Naturally so, you have to do things yourself if you want them done right.

Secondly, complaining and blaming is a way of self-sabotaging yourself of your own potential as a man to give you enough confidence in yourself to give you the necessary moral support in order to find your purpose in life, setting yourself up for guaranteed failure before your journey even begins. You are deliberately removing yourself from your own authority and running away from your own responsibilities, undoing all the teachings that even your mother already gave you, when you were still a child. And really, they are, in essence, simply silly excuses out of fear of taking action and experiencing failures. There is simply no such thing as "The perfect moment". In reality, if you actually want to truly find out the answers to all of your problems, the best single way is to go out there and seek the answers for yourself, no matter what may come your way. Complaining and blaming other entities for your purposeless life will only rob you of the extent and magnitude of your very own potential as a man, especially so if you are still a young man, and will both hinder and obstruct your slow and incremental progress toward real competence and real independence, both of which we naturally attribute a lot of value to, especially in our younger years.

Thirdly, complaining and blaming may lead to you developing an unwanted level of resentment which is a completely unnecessary sense of pain to be left lingering within every single sense you have. And you may not even notice this manifesting. For example, if someone is responsible for your misery, maybe your ex-partner, who put you to an extremely low point physically and mentally during the relationship, and still refused to take accountability for her actions no matter how much you call her out. Well, gentlemen, what would you do then? Would you be a pathetic excuse of a man and carry on protesting only she would do such a thing to you and hoping the universe will give you an answer? Would you keep condemning her and pray to karma to give her a good beatdown to make you feel good about yourself? And if you are keen to do such things, is that state of mind you would like to have to go to the future? I certainly hope not. I would not want to see you gentlemen get horrifically fixated on someone or something treacherous from your past.

Fourth, complaining and blaming will also lead you to eventual disappointment in yourself and the people around you. There is simply nothing more detrimental to a man than to see himself in the mirror and realize that he had become the person he told and promised himself to never be. The damage you will inflict upon yourself will be self-evident when you finally reach the point of fatigue in trying to get others to do your own dirty work and claiming them to be responsible for your own mess, without getting any meaningful and satisfying results in the end. In fact, coupled with the complete opposite and even worse results manifesting the people around you will get tired of your own half-wittedness. And finally, gentlemen, through complaining and blaming you are intentionally confirming and demonstrating your own weak mentality, as you are merely projecting your own incompetence and unreliableness in dealing with stressful situations. Complaining and blaming is the most definitive characteristics of a man-child. Nothing good will ever come out of people who are chronically complaining and blaming, gentlemen - in fact, they will only add more problems to their own lives, simply by ignorantly refusing to take the initiative to solve it yourself. People who similarly often complain and blame are also people who rarely identify, admit, and analyze their own flaws, mistakes, setbacks, broken dreams, and

149

failures, because they are afraid of experiencing any dissonance in their ego investments. So, they masquerade themselves as the sufferers of another entities or individuals conducts. They are simply completely and utterly insane. Do not expect any logic from them whatsoever, and I personally would not believe a word that they say. Now, this certainly does work for women in todays feminized social order, as women, by default, are treated a whole lot more sympathetically than men. But for us, do not ever play the victim game, gentlemen - you are literally trying to play reverse damsel in distress, which will not work and does not exist in reality. You will only turn yourself into a disposable, pathetic, and objective laughing stock should you decide to do so.

CHAPTER THIRTY-THREE
THE POWER OF A MANS WILL IN DARK TIMES

What do you have to lose?

Everything can be taken from a man but one thing: the last of the human freedoms - to choose one's attitude in any given set of circumstances, to choose one's way.

- JAN RUDAT

A lot of us have to face our lowest points in life. Times of dire desperation and absolute despair will bring us to the point where we will question our own existence. With everything & everyone taken away from us, we are left to wonder why we even want to continue living if all that we ever know was loss & pain. We are slowly drowning in our own sorrows and hoping for a light of hope to come and save us. Unfortunately, there is no light/hope that will come to you, the light/hope that will save you is from your own change in attitude and to discover and re-discover your will to live from your own distinct & innermost cause. When you have actually nothing left, all that you have is your character. This is the point where a man will have the chance to fully know & understand himself, what kind of man he actually is, and what kind of man he wants to be, and through the thorough recognition or re-recognition of himself, there he will naturally re-claim his upmost will to live. The will only himself as a true man can fully understand. As humans, we are all too familiar with the depths of despair that can accompany life's trials and tribulations. We may find ourselves stripped of everything we hold dear, left to wonder if there is even a reason to go on living. It is in these moments, when hope seems so distant, that we are forced to confront the most difficult questions of all - what is our purpose? Why are we here as men?

It is often said that a man who has nothing to lose is the most powerful and dangerous man you will ever witness in your entire life, and I agree. Because a man who has nothing to lose, has absolutely no fear, and a man who has seen it all, is a man who is completely free to exercise and unleash his utmost will. On the other hand, a man who has a lot to lose, must be a lot more considerate in his approach, because he has a lot to protect and to preserve, such as his reputation, people and resources. And while the wealth of a man can most certainly enforces his will, it is not what sparks and creates it. We all have desires in this life, some desires are more common and simple, such as the desire to have sex and have social interactions, and the desire to achieve independence and admiration. And behind every desire there is a reason or a collection of reasons governing our intentions and actions towards them but often the reasons that came to mind, and the ones that we and other people tend to understand to a great extent are very shallow and customary reasons which have been stated and explained many times before. However, there are some specific desires that are a lot deeper and darker than what it initially seems, one that is uniquely and exclusively personal, and this can only be noticed, understood, and determined by the individual himself. It can be a lifelong hidden ambition, or a state of accomplishment one is dreaming of experiencing, but what ties them together is the deep-rooted connections and significance with one's character. And just like every other desire, there is a reason or a collection of surface-level reasons governing it, but unlike every other desire, there is another, more complex yet blunt layers of rationales and motives behind them that are all combined to produce a reason or a cause that is so personally engraved within a man's cognition and emotions that he would deliver soul-bound and defiant conduct to fulfill it, even if it means facing death.

This very particular and distinct reason is a man's utmost will. And again, when I said it is particular and distinct, I mean only the individual himself and no one else, can identify and fully understand it. This is the case with every man respectively. To truly understand the state of "Nothing to lose" and to truly unlock that soul-bound reason and desire to live, a man must experience the lowest lows in his life - Events that are so traumatic, dire, and desperate that they can bring a man to his knees and start questioning his very own existence. Major heartbreak from a very long relationship, divorce, sudden loss of loved ones, many years of loneliness, abandonment, and constant bullying can slowly induce this. When everything is taken away from you, when life snatches all the important entities, a man can never fully discover himself, as he is left only with himself for company, reliance, and social contact. That is why some people, whose life is going perfectly well for them so far, will never know and understand the meaning of a man's will. They will never be able to identify that deep-rooted, soul-bound reason to live because they don't need to since they never face the dire circumstances of life turning upside down on them. That being said though, there, unfortunately, are a lot of men who went through the lowest lows of their lives and are unable to discover their will to live, until they eventually succumb and commit suicide, only to experience it all over again less than a second later. The reason for this is very simple and straightforward, really. a man who lost his will to live is a man who is desperately trying to associate his will with everyone and everything other than themselves.

"I must be able to live up society's demands and expectations, otherwise I am nothing. My wife and kids hate me now, I must do everything in my power to prove them wrong"

Well, looking away from such stupid comments many people make, the problem with trying to associate your will with other things and other people but yourself, is that you are trying to control the outcome through controlling their state, decisions and actions, which is utterly and completely impossible. And that you are depending on your very own sense of worth, through their perspective of you, which is extremely unreliable. Your very own soul bound reason to live must be exclusive to your own personal cause that are independent of anything and anyone Selfish? Self-absorbed? Ego-centric? Absolutely, gentlemen. When you have nothing left, and when you have to depend solely on your very own being to survive, you must be purposely selfish, because you are the only tool you have left and must make full use of yourself - no matter what, you simply have no other choice. But with all that being said here, there are, of course, always exceptions. For those of you gentlemen who are at the lowest point in your life, and are currently wondering or are struggling to work out and identify that soul bound reason to live, try to take the trip down memory lane - When you were kids all the way till you grew up, you would have encountered lots of people in person, or seen them in TV shows, movies and videogames. Identify those who stand out the most to you, both in a positive and a negative way respectively. In other words, the people that you deeply admire, and the people that you deeply despise. Identify them and pick out the qualities that stood out from them, both the good qualities that you want to develop and possess, and the bad qualities that you never want to even embody. Merge them together and resonate them with yourself and your inner most desires. That man whom you visualize is the man who you want to become, and through that visualization, ask yourself in the most truthful and vulnerable way:

"Why do you want to be that man?"

and do not answer this question lightly, answer this question with your most transparent and most visceral intent, and you may have to vent out your emotions in order to fully answer this question. However you answer it, that answer is your soul bound reason that you are looking for.

The lowest point in a man's life is the ultimate testament of his character and attitude that will define his future, it is only a matter of making that crucial and critical choice. You simply have to choose to make up a valiant defense for yourself, and to never stop, no matter what.

CHAPTER THIRTY-FOUR
THE CRITICAL MISTAKES OF YOUNG MEN IN OUR DAY OF AGE

Cultivate these, then, for they are wholly within your power: sincerity and dignity, industriousness, and sobriety. Avoid grumbling, be frugal, considerate, and frank; be temperate in manner and speech; carry yourself with authority

- MARCUS AURELIUS

Society has all the tricks up its sleeves to try and make us men involuntarily submit into their malicious agendas. There are specific reasons why we see things that are presented and depicted in the media today, things that are being advertised to us, and endlessly shoved onto all of our senses, to get us conditioned into mindlessly spending our precious resources and convince us all that every expenditure is completely worth any sacrifice, as long as it makes the entity offering the expenditure profit in some way. Streaming services, online shops, social media, and movement groups are all designed for various specific reasons that seemed to lead us all to a very simple and enlightening purpose, but underneath all of that, lies a very dark and grim place of deception and manipulation in order to exhaust every single drop of masculine being within us, starting with our precious money and time. I have always had this sneaking tingle in my mind from years ago and I am very sure that you gentlemen do too, that society is trying to bring us all to its knees. And indeed, over time, it has been nothing but confirmed by government data, and recently, it had been taken to a new level according to a recent scientific study. For example: I was browsing a well-known online shop one day, and just could not help but notice in all its radiance that there is now an option to pay in installments - no matter what you are wanting to buy. Usually, the option to pay on installments is an option to pay for excessively expensive items, such as computers, phones, and other such hardware. But now, a pair of socks that costs a meager 15 bucks can be paid in installments. Now, the first thing that came to my mind in that moment was "Why?" - but logically, and literally, if you do not really have a spare 20 bucks to spend on something as necessary as basic socks, why would you even considering buying something that you feasibly cannot afford to begin with? I am sure you have seen and experienced this yourself, gentlemen. This tells us two things - the first being that we, especially as the new generation, are becoming more and more financially incompetent, stupid, and anti-frugal to the point that we are actually starting to deeply struggle to afford the most basic needs in our daily life, without accounting for any luxuries whatsoever and only opting for the cheapest available options.

And secondly, that big corporations are, in fact, intentionally exhausting our resources by manipulating and pressuring us through endless offers that are ever so tempting advertising whatever goods the respective corporation in question is selling. For me, dear gentlemen, installments are simply band aids in order to deceive you into thinking that you are spending only a tiny amount of your budget, through relieving you of some of that financial burden and embedding into your mind that you have almost nothing to worry about in terms of your purchases, because you are given a lot of time to fulfil your payments, therefore making you feel a lot more comfortable and safe in making more purchases of items that you equally are unable to feasibly afford, no matter how you view the matter. This is especially so with cheaper items that you usually do not give much thought. However, as you all should know, even the smallest of things will, over time, accumulate to greater and greater masses, and this is equally true with expenses. If you spend 10 bucks 10 times, you still spent 100 bucks, and you do not need a doctorate to understand this, but how many times did you forget this, gentlemen? It is important to always remember when making a purchase, and to steadily keep track of your finances, no matter how little you seemingly spend. Recent studies have backed much of this up.

Now, I fully understand that for some of you older gentlemen, this might be nothing new - but for most young men who are just starting out in life and learning how to get by, perhaps just having landed a job a few months ago, this can be the teaching that decides between having a roof over your head, being warm and never going hungry - and being homeless, cold, and starving, eventually ending in miserable death. And naturally, this is only the beginning of the ever-growing list of problems that society thrown into our faces, in protest of our rightful, strong, modern, and superior masculinity. They simply do not appreciate us as their leaders, who can lead us all to great lives.

The next one is in regard to the global, social consequence of social media. More and more people are suffering from deep, crippling competition anxiety. The fear of missing out, isolation and personal inadequacy are all slowly but steadily corrupting them and inevitably, for those unable to cope with the seemingly unbearable pressure, pushes them into suicide or taking out their wrath on society in violence, such as stabbings or shootings. This is especially dangerous for us men, where our respect and credibility, as well as chance of getting a female partner almost purely depend on our ability to acquire resources and our competence in difficult life circumstances. More and more young men who are still working numerous mundane jobs, still trying to figure out their purpose and directions in life, will inevitably get misdirected and plunged into the wormhole of debt and later depression through mortgages, failures, endless loans, and credit card bills, without the help of this very book you are currently reading, gentlemen. I mean, in the United Kingdom alone in 2021, the average amount of debt per adult is more than the average earnings per adult, per the government. Additionally, the government found that almost 8% of British people do not have any savings whatsoever, and similarly, nearly 29% of British people had less than 1000 British pounds saved up in total. Needless to say, this is more than just a bit worrying. Buying a house, buying a car, or a new phone through mortgages, even though your living conditions are still perfectly acceptable, have become almost completely unrealistic for almost every single person in our day of age. I mean, realistically, how are you going to pay for something, that you cannot feasibly afford in the first place? Exactly, gentlemen - you wouldn't. You are simply literally being emotionally misled and manipulated into setting yourself up for your own life to fail and face inevitable catastrophe.

But gentlemen, by all means, I am not telling you that you should not enjoy the fine things in life, not at all, in fact. I simply want to make sure that you actually understand that it is necessary to put your own life first, no matter what - so that you are eventually able to afford and enjoy those fine things in life. Having to paying in installments for something is not being able to afford something. And gentlemen, if it means to live like a homeless person for one or two years to actually set up your own life for good, then that is simply what it takes. And to add to this, you may as well do it when you are young and strong, at the peak of your bodily and mental health in comparison to later life. And finally, the most important and arguably the most overlooked thing that society is trying to hide from us. Emasculation through music and movies on streaming platforms - peer pressure to get us responsible for every woman's livelihood due to their own actions and according to their own terms, resulting in the eventual complete removal of the authority of men. This is the most detrimental to us all, the endless pressure to get married and have children raised solely by our female partner as soon as possible or be labelled as a "pathetic excuse for a man", even though you are not physically, mentally, socially, financially prepared and authoritarian enough to be married. And then, when you do finally get married, you are almost completely removed from your very own authority as soon as the marriage ceremony is over.

Naturally, this also applies to the family. And eventually, you are the one who has to risk losing all of your heard earned money, livelihood, friends, connections, and job, if you are even slightly temporarily unable to please your wife as she leaves you. All this because you have not been given the time to choose a real woman for a real marriage. Ask any old man, and they will tell you the same. Simply put, this is an intricate recipe for inevitable, cataclysmic disaster of your own life, gentlemen. Let us be honest here gentlemen, a lot of men are continuously seduced, persuaded, and eventually pressured by their partner and own family to get married to women even when they are genuinely not ready for it in any capacity whatsoever. And sadly, most men eventually collapse under the pressure, and lose their will, eventually getting roped into marriages only to suck them dry bit by bit. Why? Because many people, given the opportunity, are simply looking to easily cash out in life, by any means necessary - otherwise, we would not have bank robberies, scams, and similar occurrences. Now, with all the financial burden you already have on your sore shoulders, adding the load of marriage, a wife, and to feed and clothe your kids, and maybe even put them through college, is simply put utterly and completely unsustainable to most men today. And this problem will only worsen and worsen. Therefore, if you are not fully prepared, you will most likely be driven to metaphorical and mental insanity as financial stress, marriage problems, kids to entertain and care for, in addition to your multitude of pre-existing problems when you have not even properly set up your life, your chances of suicidal attempts will rise by about 12 times, according to a scientific study. Now, gentlemen, you can truly imagine how bad your life will be if your wife decides to leave you, because you are simply unable to continuously provide for her and the kids. Now, if any woman is reading this and says "Are you engaging in hate speech? Are you trying to discourage marriage?" No, not at all. I am simply promoting the freedom and authority of men and warning them that they need to get their life in order for good before getting into marriage, or it will end very, very poorly for both individuals involved. I believe that humanity will only prosper if men and women are together, in a properly evolved and set-up life. However, in this day of age of the feminized order, this is often not the case, as men are pressured to quickly marry a woman, and completely fumble their marriage and their life in the process, potentially scarring them and their wife in the process, only ending in divorce. If you are against that, then you are against the success and freedom of humanity, and your very own freedom provided by your own husband.

So, you see gentlemen, you are literally one single major decision away from putting yourself into an eventual position of inescapable, inevitable, and ultimate demise. Society will stop at nothing to try and force you to sabotage your own life - always remember that gentlemen.

CHAPTER THIRTY-FIVE
HOW MEN SUFFER FROM MODERN MUSIC

Embrace the Classics

Music possesses much richer means of expression, and it is a more subtle medium for translating the thousands shifting moments of the feelings of the soul

- PETER ILYICH TCHAIKOVSKY

Music has become a very, very significant part of our daily lives. In fact, so much so to the point where it has become a part of us, what we stand for, influencing our very own mindset and even as far as embedding into us a belief system. In moments of emotional vulnerability we often let music guide us because we are able to profoundly relate to them in a cognitive and emotional way, and while it can be a good thing should the music takes you into a much better place afterwards, it is often not the case when it comes to modern music, where they instead take us into a place of misery, grief, uncertainty, hopelessness and emotional turmoil, also known as mental health problems. Especially for men, this results in our eventual emasculation in terms of our mindset because how the destructive pop culture, society, and social conventions re-programming masculinity into the thing that it initially refuses to be.

Music is a very powerful tool of expression. it is a medium that can help us better understand the state of our own thoughts and emotions. A lot of times it is hard for us to make sense and comprehensively make the contents and context of our thoughts and emotions plausible enough for us to properly grasp, because we humans prefer things that are tangible things that can be easily picked up and perceived by our five senses, in order to better comprehend and eventually interpret them. And since our thoughts and emotions are more inclined towards a set of mystical, enigmatic, and ethereal presence within us, we humans will eventually try to find ways to decode them in order to properly decipher them and eventually relate to them. That is why we often write, draw, act, play, build and, of course, sing - in order to express our emotions by channeling, constructing, and structuring them through tangible mediums. And music is one of those very powerful mediums for us to relate our thoughts and emotions to, and better understand them intuitively through the tangible expressions within a collection of properly structured tunes and words. In today's age, music has become extremely vast and dare I say it, almost necessary in our daily lives as they become a huge part of our culture - so much so that they can effectively affect and dictate our moods, determine our mindset, and even goes as far as implementing a set of belief system into our values. This is exactly where both the gifts and dangers of music lies, gentlemen. You see, when we are able to profoundly relate to our thoughts and emotions to the music we listened to, we are inevitably tied onto an invisible string or a leash by the music while being escorted through their narratives in order to witness where the music takes us. In other words, the music becomes our guide that we put our trust to follow in order to understand the state of our own thoughts and emotions and eventually would reveal to us a state of salvation and redemption. Naturally, the same thing happens when we watch movies that we can relate a lot with our own life circumstances, we want to see where the movie takes us, we invest more of our trust into them, and let the narrative of the movie guide us to eventually and hopefully take us to a much better place of realization and understanding. And really, the same dynamic happens when you read this book, or watch a video. The more emotionally vulnerable and lost you are, the greater the likelihood and magnitude of your investment and trust will be. Now, this can indeed be a very powerful and positive tool of influence should the medium guides us into a world of objective and realistic revelations, but it can be a very dangerous and crippling tool should the medium guide us into a world of delusional, dysfunctional, and ignorant fantasies. This is, I'm afraid, happening this very moment in today's world.

Most of today's music constantly tell us to wallow in our emotions, to never move on from the past, trying to relive the past, to not give up on the hope of reliving the wonderful past, to focus on love, that love will prevail, that you are deserving of love, that without a special someone, you are living a completely pointless, desperate, horrible and hopeless life, to humiliate those who hurt us, to be angry and complain about the unfairness of the world, to glorify drugs and promiscuity, to blame everyone and everything else but yourself for your failures, to ignore all criticisms including the constructive ones, to feel entitled to the best the world has to offer no matter who you are, and to make the whole world know that they owe every single bit of appreciation to you, no matter what. In simpler words, today's music tells us that the solution to our miserable life is to run away from our problems, escape reality, lie to ourselves, completely deceive ourselves, and live with the upmost hope that the best times will come by itself without any effort whatsoever. Even one of the artists that make the music themselves confirmed this in an interview with me, who wishes to remain anonymous. Obviously, I have nothing against such artists, they obviously made great music that allows us all to deeply relate to our very own thoughts and often elusive emotions in a never-before-seen way, connecting us to other human beings. It is simply that I wish they could make more music that have real life constructive messages for our mental wellbeing, rather than leading us into an uncertain state of grief, regret, delusion, lies, manipulation, hopelessness, and hate. Truly bygone are the music that reflects and enforces reality, encouraging us to keep on surviving and face our problems, conquering them in the process. Such music used to teach us how to constructively use our emotions, how to actually reveal the truth among countless conmen and cults in this world, that you cannot turn back time, and embedding us to the grueling journey on what it takes to truly become successful, adding immense value to ourselves in the process. Now, by all means, this music is still around today, it simply is not reproduced and consumed enough by any stretch of the imagination, they simply do not receive a lot of attention anymore. They do not deserve as much credit, attention, consumption, and marketability as they rightfully deserve until the end of time. The reason for this is because, as we all understand, painful realities are simply much, much harder to adopt and internalize than hopeful, fun, and satisfying illusions available at the ready, no matter where we go. Even if they were popular and had a huge followership once again as they did in the past, they would inevitably be drowned out by the sheer mass and frequency of today's dysfunctional and personally harmful music. And, of course, many of you dear gentlemen would like to have this kind of music to continuously exist and evolve into all coming generations so that they can positive influence and motivate even your children and later grandchildren - and so do I. But unfortunately, we are still fighting a losing battle until in my guess when the inevitability of the calamities and disorder of today's society becomes too self-evident and too apparent to ignore. Because, after all, we are living in the age of emotionalism, especially as men we are endlessly told to be more in touch with our emotions, to become one with our emotions, to prioritize emotions over reasons when it comes to critically important decision-making, to follow your heart instead of your head. And eventually, what happens then when we do exactly that? The humiliation, degradation, dishonor, condemnation and eventual emasculation of men, because they acted on emotions instead of logic, therefore spiraling their partner and possibly even their entire family in financial difficulties, accidents, and eventually doom, causing the man of the family to be abandoned, to fend for himself with nothing but the clothes on the body. Of course, nobody wins in this scenario. This is why this chapter is so important.

CHAPTER THIRTY-SIX

WHAT GENUINE SEXUAL DESIRE IS & ITS IMPORTANCE IN RELATIONSHIPS

The demonstration of sexual desire can be the most unpretentious, transparent, and obvious force of human nature. Yet, for some reason, they can also be the most seemingly and unnecessarily complicated convoluted and unfathomable transcendence of emotions for those who have a very hard time in distinguishing and recognizing the behavior and experience of someone who actually possesses a genuine burning desire for them and those who do not. Almost none of you gentlemen know that sexual desire is the very potent display of raw, visceral, feral, and unprecedented salaciousness to breed and procreate with the opposite sex. It is full of tension, chemistry, passion, and anxiety. it is immediate, and physical. That is why the best sexual experience you will ever have, is not something that is organized, anticipated, or planned. It is the short and exact moment of pure lustful yearning to engage in your ideal and ultimate sexual experience that you will ever experience in your entire life. The dreadful uneasiness of you missing out the chance to engage in that sexual experience that you want the most is of course the part where the anxiety comes in. You do not need a lot of time or interaction to experience this set of visceral emotions - in fact, most of the time, you do not need them at all. In the small window of time that you glance at and notice this person, you just instinctively and innately make the immediate, subconscious decision that you want this specific person. If you were ever curious what the true meaning of love at first sight is, this is it. Where genuine desire comes from, is from your own innate and distinct mating preference, with regards to ap person's skin tone body shape, vocal tone, hair color, eye color, facial form, and personality. Every single one of us has our very own mating presence within us, it is simply a matter of discovering it, gentlemen. Most men give in to the idea that sexual desire can be forced, discussed, reasoned, and negotiated with. They try to make sacrifices, do the unthinkable, arrange surprises, and showering their woman with lots of gifts. in

163

order to hopefully receive the ultimate reward of being given their woman's sexual access. Now gentlemen, while this may indeed work on some few occasions, most of the time, you will be both surprised and disappointed, and possibly left to sleep on the couch. I do not need to tell you gentlemen about how this makes you feel in detail - we all know that by now. Therefore, what you are trying to do is, you are trying to turn genuine sexual desire into a transaction.

"I've done all these things for you my eternal love, and now you must fillet my banana, there is simply no other way, I will die if you do not do this, you must keep your part of the deal"

And again, while it may occasionally work in a few cases, the chances of sexual experience are far off from the word "realistic" or "feasible". It is not the raw, passionate, deep, and feral experience that all of us men want to experience with women who have the utmost intention to lose herself with us during intercourse - Any sexual experience without genuine desire is just an empty, sympathetic compensation for a deep and lasting lack of arousal designed to prevent insult to the other persons already deeply fragile and pathetic ego. The simplest and most important thing to remember is that arousal is simply not a choice, no matter what the respective person may do, think, or feel. So, do not try so hard, wasting your precious time to reason and discuss genuine sexual desire, because you cannot and will not be able to. Simply sit down, read this chapter to the end, and accept my teachings. If you do not, you will be very disappointed in yourself, and so will be your current or future potential partner of yours. This is why when we are dating, it is so critically important to notice signs and cues, to decipher signals, in order to identify if a woman has genuine desire for you and whether she is a woman deserving of you as a man.

CHAPTER THIRTY-SIX

WHY PEOPLE TAKE ADVANTAGE OF YOU AND HOW TO SPOT THEM

Ever been taken advantage of by someone? Ever been asked to do favors by someone only to have him turn his back on you without any form of gratitude? Someone who just leaves and never acknowledge your generosity by returning the favor or trying to deepen the bond of your friendship/relationship with them. Seems like a stab in the back, doesn't it? Or rather feels like you've been treated as a mere steppingstone to help him achieve/get closer to what he wants. Why do they want to take advantage of you in the first place? Or rather, how could you not spot or notice that they are just trying to capitalize on you to propel them closer to their desires? Let's face it together, gentlemen - being taken advantage of by someone is a hurtful experience that can leave you feeling used and manipulated. It's even more frustrating when the person who used you never shows any gratitude or interest in deepening the relationship you share with them. You may or may not feel like you've been stabbed in the back or used as nothing more than a tool to help them get what they want. It's natural to wonder why anyone would want to take advantage of you in the first place, or how you could have missed the warning signs that they were only interested in using you for their very own gain. But the hard truth is, these types of people are out there, and it's important to know how to spot them so that you can protect yourself from being used and hurt in the future. So, how can you recognize when someone is trying to capitalize on your kindness or generosity? Let's explore this question together, gentlemen.

Have you gentlemen ever been in a situation where you've done someone a significant favor or several significant favors over some time, and that person simply completely disappears into thin air? Not a trace, no calls, and no invitations, and absolutely no gesture nor service of gratitude whatsoever. Either that, or they are completely unfazed by your existence, escalating to the point of trying to avoid you, even in a situation where you are noticeably present? Well, congratulations are in order- you have just been turned into a stepping stone or a free step on a ladder by someone whom you once were too naive to give meaningful and prosperous assistance to. So, why do people want to use you as their own stepping stone? Simply put, it is because you possess, and have good access to something that someone wants to have or wants to achieve. And really, you are merely the blunt instrument of opportunity for them to capitalize in order to fulfil or get closer to their own desires. Most commonly in today's world, it is about professional positions, social connections, and resource abundance, but it can be as simple as emotional availability. How many times during your college years that you've heard rumors surrounding a person taking advantage of another person because of their network of influential people, or access to wealth? Exactly, gentlemen. Now, contextually, people being utilized as steppingstones ever so slightly different from people pleasers utilized as free door mats by others. While people pleasers are taken advantage of because of their lack of value and good attitude, people who are utilized as stepping stones are taken advantage of because of their presence of value and their naive attitude. So, they do indeed possess the majority of the characteristics of each other. In detail, first is a lack of both awareness and confidence. This trait screams one thing: vulnerability.

When you lack self-assurance, especially in social situations you are automatically prone to being indecisive and fearful to causing mishaps and embarrassing yourself, which leaves you nakedly exposed and default into submission to other people narrative, appeal, and intentions. And those willing to prey on your vulnerability, will notice this very early and their initial act of empathy and understanding for you will hastily but naively encourage you to plant the seed of trust between your relationship with them. The more cognitive and emotionally vulnerable you are, the much easier you will be convinced of anything. The second one is giving too much free respect. I have mentioned this in a previous chapter in this wonderful book, that you should never, no matter the circumstances, give anyone too much respect, unless they have time and time again demonstrated their integrity. Of course, this does not mean that you should treat everyone like an asshole, but rather that you should limit the respect you give to people who have not earned it. Find a healthy balance, and then stick with it and adjust it as you go, bit by bit. Naturally, giving too much free respect too quickly only signifies that you are carelessly willing to trust people, and that you are easy to mislead and/or exploit. Thirdly is being too generous. Yes, this one is probably the one trait that can coherently and unanimously relate both people pleasers and steppingstones. This naive and delusional way of thinking or being overly fixated on the "Good things come to those who do good" kind of narrative and/or attitude will, truthfully, only disappoint you in the end. And this is what I fell into believing back in the days myself, so, you are not alone in this regard, gentlemen. Idealistically and morally, it is what we all want, but in the real world, it will never always turn out that way - you will inevitably be pricked by the sharp needle of humanities mischief one way or another. Doing favors for others without question, is an ethical and righteous thing to do and by no means am I telling you to stop doing so. It is just that if you become overly giving for more than necessary, or even if it uncalled for whatever your attentions are, genuine or not, people will eventually be taking you for granted, and your "kindness" will become disposable and lose its value, devaluing you as a man in the process, being no better than a pathetic and weak people please, especially in the eyes of people observing you. Therefore, do not be too captivated on the feelings of others or wondering how your decisions would hurt their feelings, especially in a situation where you are the one who has the most to lose. Having strong boundaries is not a sign of insecurities, but a sign of great care to your own dignity and integrity as a man. This is also why you must be able to identify or at least have some awareness of the types of people who have the potential to take advantage of you, especially while pretending to be your friend, or someone you can trust and/or rely on, even in the most desperate times of need for yourself or your family.

Having strong boundaries is absolutely necessary, gentlemen.

CHAPTER THIRTY-SEVEN

HOW TO DEVELOP SELF-BELIEF AND PERSEVERANCE THROUGH ADVERSITIES

Willpower, grit, persistence, endurance. Those qualities are without question, one of the most desired by every man in this world. All men have desires. All men have some measure of motivation. All men have some measure of goals. The only thing that most men of today are lacking, is the capability to be unstoppably unyielding with regards to any challenges and soul crushing defeats that they will encounter and experience along their way to success. Mostly because of their lack of understanding of how achievement works. Since the dawn of social media, the narrative of success has been identified as this Overnight, catapulting phenomenon, and I'm not surprised because social media only showcased the highlights of one's life, most of them are manufactured and manipulated. But the reality is, success takes time, sacrifice, focus, consistency, and GRIT. The road to success is never a linear graph or a straight line, it is always full of ups and downs, just like life itself. The problem today for men is, we are not taught how to be persistent or encouraged to be resilient, to the point that we never really had the chance to get a glimpse of our goals and desires manifesting. This chapter is finally here to change that. It is here to equip you with the knowledge, tools and techniques necessary to cultivate and develop your own unrelenting willpower and grit. It will teach you how to overcome obstacles and setbacks, how to maintain focus and momentum, and how to stay committed to your goals even when the going gets tough. Really tough, gentlemen.

Like with every personally profound and meaningful journey, whether it is acquiring a skill, building a strong body, or establishing a business, there is always an end goal in mind. Our incentive to start a journey depends on the desired state and rewards that we will relish along the journey, and once we get to the final destination. As many leaders would say, always begin and plan with an end in mind. That vision you have, will always play an important role along and within your unique journey and they will serve as your ultimatum when the going gets tough, and will reveal the answer of the extent in which you are willing to go through those obstacles and keep soldiering on. However, what most people tend to strongly underestimate is the sheer magnitude of the obstacles that they will be going through. After all, gentlemen, what many people would assume and expect of the obstacles that they are going to face are only the usual technical mishaps, setbacks, and failures, that we all can learn from, improvise, adapt, and apply to our next efforts. But in addition to those obstacles, there are also obstacles that come from those technical defeats which are far more "enigmatic" than they may or may not initially seem to be to us - and these types of obstacles will be the only ones that will brutally test your levels of dedication and trust in yourself, especially in the beginning. Yes, in contrary to the typical stereotype that we are all so accustomed to, most people actually quit on their journey right at the very beginning, because of the overwhelming sense of incompetence, lack of progress, stagnation, fears, doubts, failure, setback, impatience, comparisons, harassment, and discouragement from others that quickly extinguish the primal flame of motivation and actively destroy confidence, preventing that person to gain any knowledge, practice, and experience. Naturally, these emotional whirlwinds of thoughts that you inevitably face in the beginning will most likely cause you to deeply question your own choices and decisions if you are not fully prepared for them. This is also why you can often notice and predict people's actions through their demeanor, and whether they have already quit before they even started. Because, in essence, these are the essential trials before the actual storm that sort the wheat from the chaff. You will experience your most soul crushing defeats in the very early beginning of your journey, perhaps only hours into it. We all hate failing and losing, do we not? Especially as men, we all hate that sense that everybody is winning and making it in life, except us, in our pit of despair and misery gradually creeping up on us. Yet, here you are, still bleeding emotionally, trying to figure out your place in this world, but at the start of your journey, like every big journey, it is perfectly normal and acceptable to go through these experiences - in fact, you absolutely must experience all of them, because they are the sole emotional testament of your authenticity towards both your commitment and your sense of responsibility, which are essential to building a stable and even foundation for you to stand on in life. Truly, getting your ass kicked is the best teacher, this is what you must understand first, gentlemen. Acquiring great and valuable skills or knowledge takes intense effort, focus and time. Solving a puzzle starts with you rummaging around, picking up the pieces and understanding where those pieces fit into the whole, complete picture, moving onto initially fitting a lot of pieces in the most wrong places, and only slowly and gradually, piece by piece, fitting them together to eventually finish the whole puzzle. Building a strong and aesthetically beautiful, attractive, and widely desired physique starts with you identifying and understanding your current physical limits, slowly internalizing and mastering your specific selection of exercises, and eventually gaining and adopting that will to serve your goals to the very end, and to stick to your workout routine as you gradually increase your own limit and that of your aesthetic physique as you make strides through failing many lifts, messing up your techniques, identifying your mistakes, and cultivating those areas that fail in a respective situation, until you one day look like Arnold Schwarzenegger himself with your aesthetic physique, and the ladies will be all over you.

As you overcome those early adversities, you will naturally gradually develop that sense of strong, practical, competence. And as you start to notice small results emitting from your work for the first time, so does the increase in your confidence. With every small victory, you grow more and more confident. Some people mistake self-belief as something that is inherited, or as a natural gift that only the truly strong-willed people have, but this could not be further from the truth - self-belief is not a force of nature, but a slow and gradual growth in our sense of self-assurance that is slowly cultivated through achieving minor successes repeatedly, and eventually progress faster and faster. And as you gentlemen will experience those sensations, you will slowly uncover and realize the true capability and capacity of your potential that you have been doubting your whole, entire, life - of whether you should even begin this journey. All of these will result in building momentum and naturally accelerate your progress, because as your confidence grows, so do your incentives and commitment to test the limits of your capabilities. However, the challenges do not stop then and there. Along your journey and as you have established your base level of competence, practice, and experience, the outcome of your work and mental perseverance will be further tested through the criticisms of others and also through the identification and realization of the extent of your own limitations. This is where most people will again be highly tempted to simply quit and leave, abandon the whole journey because of the pressure to please others due to their inexperience in handling harsh criticisms or choosing between what is right and wrong and also realizing that their limitations are not at the level that they expect themselves to be in. So, as they test their limits, they will occasionally slip, make mistakes, and experience a slight or a significant fall from grace in the quality of their work, onto which they tend to further self-deprecate themselves. And if you add in unfortunate circumstances that are out of your control, affecting your performance and progress, the lack of understanding and acceptance can lead to their own eventual self-sabotage. However, the good news is that even though you will be highly tempted to quit, you will not find it easy at all to just let go of everything. In fact, it will be very hard to do so. All the work you have done, all the time and resources you have spent, all the sacrifices you have made, all the people you have lost, all the things you have lost, all the mistakes you made, all the knowledge you have gained, all the wisdom and confidence you have gained, all of your being that you committed to the journey and developed so far, will deeply resonate within you and will most likely completely prevent you from ever walking away because your journey has already become a significant part of your life, something that you hold onto so strongly that if you were to remove yourself from it, a massive chunk of yourself and your life would simply be missing, gone and never to be seen ever again. It has just become a huge part of our sense of routine, lifestyle, personality, interests, dreams, wishes, livelihood, competence, strength, self-esteem, confidence, and self-worth in addition to your very own life. It is only natural that the more time, resources, and emotions that we invest into something, or someone for that matter, the harder it is for us to let go of them, despite the circumstances going ever so bad for us. But, of course, it is only advisable and far, far more reliable for you to invest more of yourself and your time into things that you can profoundly benefit from and full control to the best of your own ability, at any time, in any situation. And even if you gentlemen do eventually experience a significant fall from grace in your journey, all the considerable and important work you have done before will ensure that you will have the complete ability and confidence over your ability to return to your prime state of being, so that nothing was lost in the process. Take my personal example, and I do believe with all my confidence that most, if not all of you gentlemen, can in one way or another relate to this yourselves: I have been in the fitness scene for almost five years now, and in those five years, I have gone through two instances of dislocation of my left shoulder, tearing multiple muscle groups in my shoulders, and having two complete knee-reconstruction surgeries, a broken arm, surviving a trip-mine during a humanitarian mission in Ukraine, and two concussions, all combined of which left me in hospital for several years. Now, gentlemen - did I contemplate about quitting fitness rather than further damaging my body? Yes, I did. But did I ever expect that I will quit? Absolutely not, not in a trillion years. Fitness has simply become such a huge part of my life, and I have invested so much into it that, if I would ever quit on it, almost nothing of my life would be left. Even if it means losing a significant amount of strength and aesthetics, I have had all the skills, confidence, experience, and most importantly the necessary willpower to build back my body, despite the dozens of problems both mental and physical with it that simply cannot be resolved with current technology. And so, I did, eventually once again exceeding my own limits, returning to full-time self-development work. Very importantly, the only thing that can eventually indeed make you walk away completely, for good, is if the journey itself and the end goal does not mean anything to you whatsoever. This is why a man's willpower will not exist without the will itself. It is the deep-rooted, primal personal cause behind the choices and decisions you have made throughout your entire life. To embark on a journey in the first place, your desire and obsession to succeed no matter the circumstances must be greater than your fear of ultimate failure. Because then, no matter how many obstacles you encounter, no matter what happens to you, your body, or your mind, no matter how many setbacks you have to experience, no matter how many crippling defeats and injuries you have to experience, you will always, no matter what, possess that unstoppable craving and tenacity to try to find your way around them or through them. It is all about winning the psychological warfare that you will subject yourself to - the battle between the fight or flight mode inside your own mind, and the constant, everlasting contemplation of "Which is the right choice?" occupying your every thought, leaving you no proper or real rest. The question of how much willpower and perseverance a man possess relies on the answer to that single question, gentlemen - What does this journey personally mean to me?" It is not about how much you can take, but if you can get back up until the day you die, that makes perseverance what it is.

As you embark on a journey to overcome adversities, you will develop a sense of strong competence. With small successes, your confidence will increase gradually. Self-belief is not something that is inherited, but rather a slow and gradual growth in your sense of self-assurance that is slowly cultivated through achieving minor successes repeatedly. You will uncover the true capability and capacity of your potential that you have been doubting your whole life. Challenges will test your mental perseverance through criticisms of others and the realization of your own limitations. It may be tempting to quit, but the work you have done, the time and resources you have spent, and the sacrifices you have made will deeply resonate within you and prevent you from ever walking away. Even if you experience a significant fall from grace in your journey, all the considerable work you have done before will ensure that you will have complete ability and confidence in your ability to return to your prime state of being. The only thing that can make you walk away completely is if the journey and the end goal do not mean anything to you whatsoever. Your willpower is the deep-rooted, primal personal cause behind the choices and decisions you have made throughout your entire life.

Never quit, gentlemen. Always continue. Always improve. Always adapt. Always grow.

CHAPTER THIRTY-EIGHT
HOW THE WRONG PEOPLE TEACH US THE RIGHT LESSONS

It Is Not the Strongest of the Species that Survives but the Most Adaptable

Comfort is a drug. Once you get used to it, it becomes addicting. Give a man consistent stimulation, tasty food, cheap entertainment, and they will throw all of their ambitions right out of the window. The comfort zone is where dreams go to die.

- JAN RUDAT

The Narrative is everywhere. If you cannot break out of your comfort zone, you will never achieve any of your goals & dreams, or even get close to anything that resembles your goals and dreams, let alone experience the taste of your own ambitions. You will only unbearably & despairingly watch that fire be slowly quenched by your fears & gluttony. As much as I tend to stay away from mainstream narrative, it is undeniably THE TRUTH. Another truth is, if you already have achieved your goals & dreams, or are already halfway there while reaping the rewards and enjoying the fruits of your hard labor, there is another trap of comfort, and that is, being too complacent with what you have achieved and accumulated that you become afraid to take further risks because you fear of losing them all. The world continues to evolve and so must you, if you become too content with your state of satisfaction, especially early on, and be seduced by the gluttony that comes with reaping your rewards, you will eventually fall from grace and be robbed from your own potential that got you to where you want in the beginning.

It is a deeply pleasant and calming and/or sensation to simply be wrapped in your very own metaphorical bubble of comfort from which you derive pleasures such as joy, peace, and relaxation, is it not, gentlemen? The pure lack of worries, anxiety, and troubles in a given moment, not having to picture and worry about our own future as men. Naturally, this is an experience that we all wish to exist permanently in any given moment in life. However, as much as we wish to stay ever-so comfortable in this bubble of ours, and as much as we want to avoid pain and adversities in our lives, to never rise to any greatness and to enjoy this one single, fleeting moment, this moment will quickly fade away, and comfort itself will become the very pain you so deeply wish to avoid - as like anything, too much of the good will result in taking it for granted, and only poison us. So if we let comfort consume us for too long, it will inevitably quickly drag us down into a deep pit of misery, and keep us there for possibly our entire lives. No matter how long we stay in this pit, we will begin to mentally rot away in despair and misery, when we could be innovating life itself. Comfort keeps you so dependent on it because it makes you feel safe, impeccable, and invincible, as it staves off your perception of every fear, worry, and problem you may have. But it also staves off your own potential and life possibilities. Fortunately, we humans naturally gravitate towards seeking adventure and change, and that is why we feel agitated when we are not growing for an extended period of time, in certain aspects of life that we engage in. That is why we travel to different countries, that is why we seek new mountains to climb, that is why we try new hobbies, new foods, topics, and subjects to learn and understand, and just new, creative things to simply do. In simpler terms, we humans constantly bound to experience discontent in our life stemming from things like too long or too many repetitions of things such as routines, or simply being unable to explore things and go on even the smallest of adventures - this will quickly cause a sense of tediousness and stress that, if left unsatiated in its full capacity, will impulsively cause us to actively seek chaos to try and break up the monotony of our seemingly soulless and ultimately boring life. Like going straight from a mundane office workplace to a theme part for a huge and extreme roller coaster ride. This chapter covers the consequences of being too comfortable in two stages and focuses on your main priorities and pursuits in life on which you gentlemen hopefully can largely relate to the situations of your other personal endeavors.

Stage One

Now, as much as we enthusiastically want to get outside of our comfort zone, a lot of us also greatly fear to venture outside of it even in the smallest possible capacities. We deeply love novelty, and yet, we fear unfamiliarity because unfamiliarity initially erodes our confidence and makes us feel extremely vulnerable. The first stage begins with you trying to initially venture out of your comfort zone because you are increasingly unable to cope with the mundaneness of your everyday life, how you feel that your potential is slowly rotting away, and your own realization of society's programming and attempts to manipulate you to get you to just sit on your ass and do nothing in your whole life but continually consume its manipulative so-called teachings. To try something that you have always wanted to try, even if you did not know that - such as quitting your job and becoming self-employed, asking the crush of your life out for dinner, learning a new skill from scratch, getting into a field of study, going on an adventure around the world, creating a side-business, or simply apply for that job you always wanted. That overwhelming fear of pain and failure and the endless amount of self-questioning and doubt of whether you will be making the right decision in a given moment will haunt you constantly, and it is even more daunting to consider that mostly, you will be on your own, as most of the people around you that are also fearful to venture outside of their comfort zone, will either strongly try to discourage you to the point of quitting, or force you to remain where you are while leaving you to handle your own struggles all for yourself, without any outside help whatsoever. Part of you just wants to simply let go of everything and go for it, while part of you is still talking yourself into staying within your comfort zone, to routinely do everything to avoid pain and hardship. Depending on the circumstances of your environment, this will most of the time escalate up to a breaking point of where eventually, you become extremely fatigued of your own mental warfare between your desires, fears, anxiety, problems, and the amount of time that you have wasted contemplating that you finally bring yourself to stop thinking and take that decisive leap of faith to break your comfortable but unexciting routine. Either that, or you end up further succumbing yourself back into your wearisome, boring, and ultimately pathetic life that can be shattered by a single major incident, because you simply cannot handle the fear, peer pressure, anxiety, lack of support, harassment, problems, and frustration any further. And gentlemen, to take that leap of faith is actually a lot simpler than most would think, especially when you initially have very little, or even really nothing to lose. The first stage is all about overcoming that dangerous fear of pain, failure, and the doubts of your own capacity and ability - to handle them on your own. Just to encourage you gentlemen, in a new world of unfamiliarity, it is inevitable for us to experience failures and setbacks, and the only question that remains is whether you are willing to learn from them and keep pushing on, no matter what.

Stage Two

The second stage comes as you start to accumulate successes and achievements from your work - the fruit and byproducts of your labor will be evident, and it is only natural foe us to want to reap those rewards and enjoy them to the fullest. However, with success and wealth comes a great deal of comfort beyond what you could have possibly experienced before, financially, personally, socially, circumstantially, and even sexually. And, of course, these forms of comfort and temptation are what can seduce you out of your own way because they can give you a sensation that you have already made it, and that there is nothing more to pursue or to get out of bed early for, even if the successes are still far from what you have envisioned. And as most of us know, pleasure always has a price - and the more pleasure you consume and experience, the more you are dragged away from your original path, as your judgements are clouded by satisfaction which effectively kills your ambitions and purpose almost instantly. Therefore, your successes and achievements are only temporary, and the world constantly moves forward and evolves, so you must adapt to suit its demands in order to survive. Being too captivated and content on the initial successful work you have done in the past, can sabotage yourself from exploring the extent of your limitations, and it is only natural for us to have a great fear not to want to take any further risks whatsoever - to possibly lose all that we have achieved, because now we have a huge status and reputation to protect, credibility to maintain, and resources and possibly a partner and a family to protect. In other words, you have a lot more to lose now. However, to neglect the need to change and evolve constantly, and often daily, is refusing to grow in any capacity. Why? For the simple reason that you are complacent at where you are. This is, in essence, the same as voluntarily accepting your own eventual offer of downfall from grace, and permanently so. And naturally, you will eventually experience discontent with what you have as time passes and you will strongly gravitate towards contemplating to seek further novelties and adventures. In fact, the only reason why you would actually want to stay where you are, and remain complacent with where you are at, is because of your great fear in losing what you already have, and what you have already accumulated. Therefore, gentlemen, you must always look to evolve further in terms of your work, desires, dreams, wishes, and pursuits. Do not be afraid to try out new ideas and concepts, ever. Ideas and concepts are what gets you to eventually exceed your own limits and enter a whole new metaphorical dimension of understanding and expertise in life. As I have already mentioned earlier, human beings are naturally bound to experience discontent continuously and inevitably throughout their entire life. Contrary to what most people think and perceive, discontentment is quite a healthy thing to experience - it is what led to great inventions in the past, it is what leads us in this day of age to attempt to break records and, in fact, eventually succeed at doing so, and leads us to take that fateful initial leap of faith to burst our own bubble of mundaneness that allows all great things to happen and be achieved by us. Without discontent, we just will not have the drive to achieve anything, because our desires and goals come from our own discontentment. Discontent is the enabler and drive for all great things we ever achieved and will achieve in the future. It is important to say that I am not, in any way, saying that you should constantly or endlessly seek discontentment, or to avoid feeling content. Absolutely not. By all means, gentlemen, do enjoy your successes and celebrate them - cherish them to the full extent, by all means. The message of this chapter is to not over-indulge in the gratifications that your initial sense of satisfaction provides you. This had to explained in so much detail as people tend to oversimplify things out of their own laziness which inevitably only leads to more trouble than good. Never get high on your own supply, too much indulgence of the good will do bad. Too much indulgence in the bad will utterly and completely ruin you. Find and internalize the perfect balance, gentlemen.

CHAPTER THIRTY-NINE
BE A RUTHLESS MAN

Selfish people win. Men who relentlessly add value to themselves will win. Because that's what will eventually serves them and allows them to perform on a high level. Men must perform in this world, otherwise they are disposed of mankind's ever so evolving nature. In a world full of distractions & temptations, very few men have the ruthless mindset to discard everything to go after the goal or the life that they want for themselves. Doesn't matter what their friends or parents think. Doesn't matter what their girlfriends or lovers think. His decisions & actions comes from his very own, clear, and precise mental point of view FIRST & ALWAYS. What does it mean to be a man who is ruthless in life? Objectively speaking, to be a ruthless man in one's own life, is to be a man who is brutally absolute and firm in his desires. A man who is uncompromising in his attitude towards building his life to the state and prestige that he desires. A man who makes his priorities extremely clear to himself and, if necessary, to others. A man who does not question or be fickle and uncertain the crucial decisions, sacrifices, and actions that he had made previously. And a man who has an unstoppable will to achieve the things he wishes and that, regardless of if the circumstances surrounding him continuously oppose him and try to make him fail, will always and find and create a way to get the job done to his desires and make him one step closer to get what he wants. A ruthless man is a man with an impeccable level of commitment, obsession, and dedication over a chosen activity. His daily actions are mostly done completely and absolutely in pursuit of his personal objectively, arduously honing his chosen activity to build value in order to be of service to the world and mankind - He is a man on a mission, and a man with a clear purpose. He understands that he should play to his strengths and focus relentlessly on something he is good at and loves doing. But before that, he must think very hard about whether it will be valuable in the future. He understands that life does not reward the undeserving, and that success does not come naturally, especially for those who are even in the slightest way unprepared for it. The bigger his dreams and plans are, the harder it is for him to reach them. A combination of fierce desire and an unwavering "Kill or be killed" attitude fuels his unrelenting pursuit of excellence and his determination to truly prosper in life. Your very own ability to be successful, gentlemen, is your ability to never take your eyes off of the end goal, and to stick and follow a well laid plan, making the necessary and critical adjustments along the way, as appropriate - Just like a tiger, stalking his prey. He just never takes his eyes off the prey, being the goal, until he has it exactly where he wants it to be - within reach of being accomplished once and for all. He has an unrelenting level of focus and determination to persist and to achieve, regardless of the circumstances. One of the hardest things to do in being ruthless, is initially getting rid of everything and everyone that does not align and complement your priorities. This involves removing habits and routines that do nothing constructive but waste your time and resources, and also robs you of your potential. This also involves refusing and removing people who have different priorities than you – now, this is especially hard for most of us initially at first, as we often feel uncomfortable and afraid to hurt people's feelings in saying "No". Our sympathy often gets in the way of our objectivity, and we unnecessarily compromise our integrity in order to avoid confrontations and conflicts. This is detrimental. Especially so if you are not able to overcome or shift your mindset in regard to that needless sense of pity and compassion - you are not wrong. I repeat, you are not wrong. Simply because you do not intend to hurt them by refusing their offers or prioritizing your own objectives before them. In fact, it is what they would, without question, also do if the circumstance is reversed. Any person worthy of respect would undoubtedly understand your decisions, instead taking them personally and getting emotionally hurt, because like all the great stoics said, it is your own choice and decision to feel hurt.

Excellence does not care about your feelings; it only cares about your results. The other hard things about being a ruthless man, is being highly tolerant in handling the vast amounts of disapproval and seduction from the people around you. Aggression, captivation, and ambition towards a desired life circumstance are both condemned, yet also praised bewitchingly by society. On one hand, a lot of people will discredit, disdain, and downplay both your mindset and your plans, telling you that you are delusional, and that your plans are unrealistically dumb because they are uncommon and rarely materialized. And truthfully, most people do this because they are afraid of your potential in becoming better than them. That is also why they try to break your spirit through a barrage of defeatist criticisms before you build any real momentum. A relentless outlook can make those around you feel uncomfortable and lead them to examine their own character and mentality. That is why they impose their own shortcomings onto you - to make peace with their own lack of drive. So, it is important that you weigh in other people's opinions carefully without allowing this to hinder your plans. On the other hand, other people will frequently praise you for your boldness, confidence, and courage, and would be willing to be a part of your slice of life, especially so if you already displayed at least some results. Gentlemen, this is where you must be very careful, as with every human being, they are attracted to even the slightest hints of prosperity and will inevitably endlessly seduce you with offerings of temptations in order to win your approval. They do this through constantly showering you with various validations and offers of distractions to get you to spend more time and money with them, thereby dragging your focus away from your plans, which you will not even notice. This inevitably causes you to delay or even completely avoid getting anything done in any capacity. It is the simple human nature to increase the chances of survival to do so, so take great caution mingling with resourceless and incapable people. Even when you have a dream, you must be responsible in protecting it wherever necessary, and however necessary. Enjoy yourself, but do not get carried away in any way or capacity, gentlemen.

Being a ruthless man is about being objective driven, to the point where nothing else matters more than that. And it is not just about being ruthless with the circumstances and the people around you, it is also about being ruthless to yourself. Most men today are not honest to themselves, or not honest enough to themselves. Honest with what they want, and honest about where they are, as most men today are afraid of even scratching their own egos. Deathly afraid. A ruthless man brutally identifies his own strengths and weaknesses - he knows when his results are not good enough, deeply analyzes his mistakes, and never lets his own emotions get the better of him in the face of hardships, cognitive dissonances, lack of progress, setbacks, and failures. He never sees defeats as enemies, he only sees them as instruments of learning. He does not waste any time to feel sorry for himself or seek sympathy in the low points of his life, he simply accepts his circumstances for what they are, and then makes the decision to be simply better. He is very self-critical and competitive to the point that he is completely willing to do beyond what normal people would even consider in the first place, simply in order to gain just that little, tiny bit of edge over them. Being ruthless and relentless is far from a perfect life, you are essentially going to war with yourself and everyone and everything around you - all in the pursuit of executive results and sheer excellence in order to set up your life the way you want it to be. It is also a very painful life, giving up majority of your youth in order to build a better future, constantly seeking ways to evolve further in all aspects of yourself and your life, and constantly cultivating character for years that is very rarely relatable to many people. So, gentlemen, why would go to this extent to do all of this? Because he simply wants what he wants really, really badly. And because a man has no choice in this world but to perform, otherwise he will eventually be disposed of and forgotten because he was regarded as nothing in his life. Because he wants to go down in history as the legends like Alexander the Great, the Greek god Zeus, and Albert Einstein. Because he wants to be, and will be legendary, to be remembered by everyone in the world for their entire lives, and for all future generations to see and look up to. To become immortal, and aid mankind in its constant evolution.

If you choose to be that man, to follow this book, is your choice, gentlemen.

CHAPTER FORTY
THE DARK AND BRUTAL SIDE ABOUT LIFE

Life. War. Battles. Conflicts. Pain. Suffering. They all are inevitable. Love, compassion, & empathy are without question very much desirable for all of us, in fact it is an ideal that we all fixated upon with regards to our life to the point where we start to promote them to the extreme. But this is reality, and reality does not blend itself to our ideals, it simply as it is. Human beings love to admit their capacity for love & compassion, but never when it comes to their capacity for hate & violence, even though they have displayed and commit such traits in the past, they try to dismiss and bury it as if nothing happened or those traits didn't exists Every human being has a dark side, and this chapter will reveal the part of us that we reject & subdue because they do not represent the ideals of society. Life is war. Everyone loves the idea of peace and tranquility. Everyone loves an ideal world where there is only love and compassion. Everyone loves the illusion of living an easy and a pain free life. Humanity in its nature, is not capable of handing the entirety of truth. That is why develop subjectivism around everything that they could not handle and accept. That is why they resist and reject everything that causes pain and suffering, even those that are truly inevitable. This life and this world have a side that most of us would not rather relish in. The side that we rarely portray and showcase in order to preserve our ideals. The side that is evident in everyday circumstances, but we choose not to pay any attention to. The side that is much darker and sinister that we could even question our own sanity over. Most of us, especially in the modern era, want to believe that both this world and human beings are only and must only be capable of love, compassion, support, help, positivity, and empathy. And truthfully, we all want to subdue and reject the reality that this world and human beings are also capable and have a great capacity for hate, negativity, mischief, damage, and violence. The painful truth is, all of us who believe that ideal are also hypocrites to our very own beliefs. All of us possess that dark and sinister side as well, and we rarely ever want to admit that it is a part of us, a huge part of us, in fact. Even though we have committed such acts over the course of our lives, we still do not want to admit that and truly face it. If we are not capable of violence and destruction, there will be absolutely no laws imposed on us whatsoever no matter where we go.

The Battle of Supremacy

Behind closed doors, every single one of us would genuinely admit to ourselves that we all love to be the one in control. We all deeply love to feel superior and be better than everyone else in this small world. We all love to exercise our pure will and have it manifest into sheer reality on the very spot. We all have a great capacity to be selfish, ruthless, and destructive for circumstances to go our way, even escalating to the point where we are willing to do it at the wellbeing and even lives of others. We just don't mention them because they are both considered politically incorrect and socially unacceptable. These conflicts always exist ever so slightly to the point where we barely notice them occurring. Within friendships, relationships, partnerships, collaborations, and business-ventures, this subtle physical and psychological warfare and power dynamics are tall taking place in order to place ourselves above all others in the pursuit of control and dominance. Deception, corruption, manipulation, accusations, peer pressure, abuse, bullying, blackmail, harassment, lies, betrayal and even murder are utilized by people in fear and desperation for financial or social gains and embed constructivism. People naturally manufacture false rumors in order to subdue one's credibility and entirely remove them from relevancy. People naturally stab each other's in the back for the sake of clout and short-term gratifications and rewards. People naturally gravitate towards declaring, imposing, and following up on threats to watch one crumble emotionally in a conflict, and exit themselves from this world. People also often take others' lives to satiate cravings, do good in the world for personal gain, rise up the social hierarchy, get a promotion or a raise, eliminate competitions and competitors, and future threats. So, the extent on which we are willing to go in order for circumstances to be on our sides are beyond what we initially want to believe. People are selfish, and their priorities come first. The scale and magnitude of conduct one is willing to do depends on

The Battle of Desires

We human beings have our own most basic needs of survivability and reproduction, and we must fulfil them somehow. In the case of men, both financial wealth and access to options for sex are the two most desired commodities, because not only do they allow us to fulfil those basic needs, but they also allow us to prosper much further in them as well. That is why both money and sex always sell. We, men, are competing against one another in terms of physical appearance, acquiring resources, acquiring a life partner and even a family, mental toughness, resilience, strength, competencies, skills, and lifestyle setup - and as a byproduct, we will gain access to options of physically attractive women and the potential of unlimited sexual access. And unlike what most of us would want to believe, and what most gurus would love to tell you, is that all of us can achieve this desired state and be real, tangible, and true winners. The reality is that life at the top is not a place for everyone, and in today's age of high expectations and even higher standards, it will never be a place for everyone. There is and will be more of an uneven distribution of wealth and sex. Those men who will acquire vast amounts of wealth and sexual access are those men who are insanely willing and driven to get there, those who are risking everything and wanting to do what most men would not even contemplate in doing. Whenever there is a concept of winners, there will always be losers - the men at the very top are physically attractive, financially wealthy, and living an adventurous and deeply exciting life, and are therefore extremely attractive to even more attractive women.

The men who are not at the top, who are physically inferior, living through debts, lazy, sedentary, and plain boring will be scraping the leftovers from the floor of the men who are living at the top, or worse, will not even receive those leftovers of what remains of the pie. That is why those men are willing to settle for less.

Desires also highly involve dominance. The battle for desire will also inevitably involve the battle for supremacy, as men who are able to position themselves, whether genuinely or manufactured, over others, are automatically far more desirable to women, because they are perceived to be in command of respect, competence, power, security, wealth, and reliability. Superiority is what women are looking for in men. As they say it, women want to be with men that other men aspire to become. After all, reproduction is also virtually treated as a marketplace in the end, as we all are trying to get the best of what we can have. Those who are both of high value and rare are simply inevitably more desirable, just like high-end diamonds.

The Battle of Choices

All of us are born with our own unique set of cards. Some of us are fortunate, and some of us are not fortunate. Some of us are blessed, and some of us are cursed. Unfair as it is, I have said time and time again, you have to deal with it and make the best out of it, because it is your only available option apart from suicide. This is all about what you choose to do with the circumstances that are given and presented to you. As much as people so often say, "The sky is the limit", in reality, all of us have our own set of limitations with regards to our abilities, possibilities, and opportunities. Our days in the world are numbered and our chances to explore and maximize our potential are also numbered. Time is both our biggest ally and also enemy. We will never know when our due date is to leave this world. There is only so much time you can spend in exploring the choices that you have up the point where you realize that you just do not have the capacity to do that anymore. The last major choice that you made to attempt to steer your life in the right direction can always be your last chance you may ever have. Most people completely and utterly waste their youth - wander aimlessly, make stupid decisions, give half-assed efforts in their activities and desires, and give in to wishful hoping and thinking to direct them to a bright, flourishing, meaningful, and successful future, and start to believe that age is simply nothing but a number, and that possibilities, chances, and opportunities are in endless supply to them, believing that the circumstances will always be on their side, and that things will always eventually turn out in their favor, no matter how dark things may seem, with absolutely no effort whatsoever on their part. As I have taught you gentlemen, possibilities and opportunities are always in favor to those who have the skills and resources, and not everyone is born with a silver spoon in their mouth. After all, we all have to cultivate our own potential and capabilities first slowly and gradually, in order to eventually develop and be exposed to more choices. And similarly, we have to cultivate our own potential, skills, and capabilities first in order to eventually develop and be exposed to more choices - and that itself takes a huge amount time and energy from us. Now add to that the fact that we only have one head, 2 arms and 2 legs - we just cannot be in more than one place at once. Therefore, we have to be very, very careful when we make those crucial and fateful choices in life, that we would want to eventually be willing to fully, all out, commit to - especially in our fateful youth.

We just have to both accept the rewards and the consequences for our every decision we ever make, as they both come with every choice that we ever make. This is also what we very often tend to ignore and underestimate. We all become too drunk in the youthful energy to the point where we feel that we can fully indulge in the freedom and pleasure of aimlessness and irresponsibility for years, until we get to the point where we suddenly realize that time moves very, very quickly and we have wasted the precious time we had during our youth that we could have actually used to fully explore and maximize our then current potential, and this is exactly where extreme regret comes in.

The Battle of Self-Mastery

Gentlemen, this is arguably the most important battle of them all - the battle with yourself is the most crucial and impactful one of them all. Your complete, realistic understanding and ownership of yourself will make or break the trajectory of where your life will be going - because, with everything, it begins in the mind. Your own mind, your own perspective towards yourself, must be as brutally honest and reflective of reality as much as possible. Furthermore, you must be completely able to see things in the outside world as how they are and not how they seem to you. If you consider yourself poor, and it reflects the reality of your own circumstances, admit it. That is in no way, shape, or form self-deprecation, this is self-reflection. It is being brutally honest with yourself so that you can assess the situation you are in and where you currently stand. Self-deprecation is where you emotionally escalate your seemingly dire and harsh circumstances to the point of relinquishing your self-respect, honor, dignity, and self-worth. Every day you are in constant battle with yourself, facing your own weaknesses, problems, emotions, tendencies, trauma, deficiencies, compulsions, urges, and plain bad habits. Your own vulnerability towards distractions and temptations, how you react to comparisons, and your own dark side, that you most likely have shunned away at the back of your head for years and possibly even decades, may also join the mix, depending on the type of person that you are. Understanding yourself to a very deep, high extent, being able to play to your strengths, compensate for your weaknesses, and being able to harness and be in control of yourself will not only bring clarity to the current circumstances of your life, and the path that you are willing to take, but also inevitably put you in a very good position to greatly understand other people and what lies underneath their skin, which you could utilize and even exploit to your own decisive set of advantages, because we humans are not so different in terms of generalizations of our biology and psychology. We constantly have a battle of judgements in our own minds of what is right and what is wrong, and often times, we completely reject the objective truth in favor of subjectivism and individualism because it caters to our emotions and makes us feel sure and comfortable in our own right. All up to the decisive point where we are awakened by reality - then our expectations are suddenly shattered, and we are exposed to the bar mechanics of how things and circumstances actually operate. And that is the one moment where your mindset shift will either take place towards objectivity, or you will stay in subjectivity and individualism and condemn reality for what it actually is. Life is a constant back and forth battle for all of us, whether it is with ourselves, or whether it is against others. Everyone wants peace, but peace can only be achieved through some form of conflict. If you want to live the life you want, you have no choice but to fight for it.

In conclusion, life is not a fairy tale. It is a brutal, dark, and unforgiving reality. There are aspects of ourselves and our world that we don't want to acknowledge, but we must face them if we want to understand our place in this world. We are all capable of both good and evil, and we must acknowledge and accept this duality if we want to become better human beings. We must also understand that not everyone will be able to achieve their desires, and that can lead to negative emotions and actions. We must strive for empathy, compassion, and understanding, but we must also accept and understand the dark side of life. Only then can we truly become better human beings and create a better world for ourselves and future generations, gentlemen.

CHAPTER FORTY-ONE
THE LONE WOLF - THE GOOD AND BAD OF ISOLATION

What a person is for himself, what abides with him in his loneliness and isolation, and what nobody can give or take away from him, this is obviously more essential for him than everything that he possesses or what he may be in the eyes of others

- ARTHUR SHOPENHAUER

All of you lone wolves probably have a reason why you decide to go your own way and forge your own path. Whatever they may be, the reason always has to do with not being able to conform to the norms. Rejections, ridicules & being ignored, all of these factors in to why we eventually decide to bring ourselves to become self-reliant to take on life. The thing that is really circulating the lone wolf sphere of men, is that they are adamant to hardwiring themselves to be alone for the rest of their lives, and in this chapter, I'm going to explain why doing pursuing such a life will lead to further frustrations. We went into isolation because of either, the world rejects both us and our chosen path, and we are therefore unable to conform to normality, and refuse to take the paths society told us to take because we are different, or if we have a great personal mess to clean up and nobody wants to help us, such as if we are in a crippled state in terms of our physical and mental health, and our own grim circumstance of a lack or purpose and an unstable financial situation got us into a position where society wants no part in it and left us to fend for ourselves. Now, because of these initial roots of causation, the path of solitude is often accompanied with hatred and resentment towards everything and everyone that denies and ridicules your proposed attempts at conformity to be part of the norms, and their reluctance to assist you at times of darkness and despair. They reject you because your path is unusual and does not align with their agendas, so it is your responsibility to prove them wrong, to provide value and claim your distinct place within it. And some of you bitter lone wolves might be thinking "I do not want to be used by society! They are plain evil!". Do not be stupidly ignorant, you have to be somehow useful to mankind so that you will be rewarded eventually, otherwise you will have no place in this world, and are genuinely on your own. They are reluctant to assist you in hard times because, you are responsible for both the good and the bad in your own life. Remember?

So, to hate the world for being unfair to you, is like hating the lion for eating your own dog - it is their own respective nature to be both unfair and ruthless. You either play the game the way it is supposed to be played, create new and creative ways to play the game that most don't realize, or you simply exit the game and quit, by suicide.

Good

Now let us discuss what makes isolation beneficial should you utilize it properly, and what makes it detrimental should you go overboard with it, gentlemen. Isolation is only beneficial if you have a clear and set purpose behind it or if you are working to get your own shit together. Purely to isolate yourself because of the resentment due to you not fitting in, or that society does not reward and/or assist you for being who you are in your current circumstances is a sure path to an insignificant and valueless existence that not even the wise would care about. Isolation is a true gift for you if you utilize it in order to cultivate value in yourself in all important aspects of life, whether it is about your physical appearance, mental strength, financial situation, range of skills, and knowledge, whatever they may be. It is not a place where you pathetically wallow in bitterness, hoping that one-day society will realize your worth, purely as a living, human being, starting to treat you right - absolutely not, gentlemen. Society will absolutely leave you for dead and would wish you to be dead if you have nothing to offer because you are nothing but an inconvenience in this ever so in power-evolving world that rewards power and value. This world that we all live in is a power-evolving, gentlemen - weakness does not thrive and will not thrive. In order for isolation to work in y, therefore, it therefore demands purpose. Now, because you have a clear purpose or when you have a clear purpose, isolation allows you to focus and get rid of unnecessary and unrelated distractions It brings you clarity of your own priorities, because what Isolation does, is that it allows you to narrow down your judgments and identify the things that are important and not so important to you at that given circumstance or stage of your life. In a world full of seductive temptations and distractions that we live in, your mind becomes a clusterfuck and dumpster tier of choices none of which align whatsoever with your actual priorities, that you will not fully realize until you get rid of most of those completely irrelevant choices. Isolation will help you develop the capability to filter out all the things that are unnecessarily interfering with your peace of mind in order to get you closer to your objectives, because more often than not, in our daily lives, we cluelessly allow things outside of our control to influence our decisions and actions. The reason for that is that in the outside modern world, we are conditioned to care far too much about the opinions of others any wrong move could potentially damage our reputation and social acceptability. That is also why a lot of the time, we are unconsciously ourselves compromise in order to maintain our status quo in the community.

Being in isolation will get rid of that needless sense of conformity to people who cannot even see or understand the world from your perspective. Isolation forces you to self-reflect, and because you do not have anyone to confine and share your thoughts with, you talk to yourself, confronting your own weaknesses that you would not pay any attention to whatsoever when you are clouded by distractions. Choosing a side between your ego and conscience, battling your own thoughts and emotions, and trying to make further sense of them, you slowly yet surely become more honest and direct with yourself, and eventually, will have a much better understanding of your own character both cognitively and emotionally, ultimately leading you to realize what you truly want from your life from a viscerally personal point of view. The reality is, the most significant decisions that we made in our lives are made alone, in the reassurance of our own point of view, because no one can truly understand them but yourself.

You will inevitably develop self-sufficiency, awareness, and reliance in isolation which ultimately, will make you less affected and dependent on other people's judgements. During COVID in 2020, most people cannot even accept living in isolation for a long period of time, so they reject the idea and confine their emotions to social media to receive online sympathy and attention, thereby removing their position and opportunity to understand themselves better through isolation.

Bad

Now let us talk about the bad of isolation. However, before I start, I am going to talk about the bad from a context of someone who has been literally isolating themselves, no online presence and little to no human contact for months or even years. Years of isolation can be detrimental in terms of being aware and staying updated on a new world information and circumstances. Remember, it is not only the strong that survive, but also the ones who can adapt to any situations. Isolating yourself for years and just being too stubborn to further learn something new, without keeping an eye on society will put you at a massive disadvantage, because what you used to know and believe will be much less or no longer relevant and applicable in the future. Remember, the most dangerous men are the ones continuously listens, thinks, and observe - the ones who always seek knowledge and information. Don to ever underestimate the value and power of information, gentlemen. We can certainly develop the capabilities to survive on our own, however, we are social creatures by nature, we experience tremendous relief when we find others who think the same way as we do. Our state and feelings of authenticity is further amplified when we conform to people with the same values as us, and as much as individual lone wolves would like to think of themselves as the sole outlier among the herds of sheep in society, there are many outliers in this world that share the same values as you do, so do not shun yourself further deep into the darkness and waste the opportunity to get to find like-minded people, especially in this day of the digital age where we can connect with people from the opposite ends of the world, and share ideas together to form a purposeful tribe and help to cultivate one another in terms of knowledge and skills. We all have our limits, gentlemen, and as much as want to be the jack of all trades, there are people out there who are better than us at certain things, and through their assistance, we then can explore new dimensions of our own limitations as would they through your assistance.

Finally, a lack of intimacy. All of us human beings by nature are evolutionary designed to reproduce. Especially as men, we are biologically wired to spread our seeds as much as possible to ensure the survival of our genes in the form of our next of kin. In fact, most of our subconscious motivation in cultivating value for ourselves is to eventually attract a mate and procreate. You build your physique and attract women that you want, and you earn money to women what you want. As much as you want to deny it, as I did previously, it is simply the truth that will become self-evident as time passes. Now I know, some of you lone wolves have bad experiences with women, that is why you avoid intimacy, that is also why you put such a thick shield on to avoid emotional attachments. However, to live alone for the rest of your lives, especially as you get older, is simply unsustainable, gentlemen, and will even increase the chances of falling into depression. We have to solve our reproductive problems eventually, otherwise we can become sexually frustrated to the point where we find countless methods to sublimate our libidos which can only take us so far. Relentlessly working on yourself and engaging in semen retention are just a few of the tools. This book is all you need, however - that much is crystal-clear.

CHAPTER FORTY-TWO
WHY ARE YOU HOLDING BACK?

A ship is always safe at the shore, but that is not what it is built for

\- ALBERT EINSTEIN

Have you ever constantly told yourself that you're not good enough? You are eager & dying to start an endeavor that you have been dreaming, envisioning, and planning for so long, but for some reason, you just can't bring yourself to do it and just take that leap of faith. You start to make excuses involving not being in the time, not having enough knowledge and information & the discouragement from the environment you surround yourself in. This is what I call the art of self-sabotage. It is much less of what is going on around you, but more towards what your attitude is like towards the reality of the matter. In this chapter we discuss why you self-sabotage yourself and why you should stop unnecessarily waiting to start doing what you've always wanted to do.

"Maybe later... maybe one day when everything is in order"

"I just don't know man... it's tough bro... I just don't think I can do it"

"I can't do this I am not good enough man"

"In a couple of years will start doing it"

"This is too hard... I can't bro..."

"But why man?"

Have you ever constantly told yourself that you're not good enough? You are eager & dying to start an endeavor that you have been dreaming, envisioning, and planning for so long, but for some reason, you just can't bring yourself to do it and just take that leap of faith. You start to make excuses involving not being in the time, not having enough knowledge and information & the discouragement from the environment you surround yourself in. This is what I call the art of self-sabotage. It is much less of what is going on around you, but more towards what your attitude is like towards the reality of the matter. In this chapter we discuss why your self-sabotage yourself and why you should stop unnecessarily waiting to start doing what you've always wanted to do. Most of us experience that particular moment of hesitation when it comes to making a bold or daring decision to pursue something that we have always considered pursuing. Hell, even we have those same feelings of hesitation when we are simply trying something completely new to add to our experiences, such as trying a new food that we never even tasted before. But obviously, those are a different caliber of expectations, and naturally, the bigger the risks are, the more hesitant we feel. When it comes to us taking that big first leap to pursue an endeavor, that usually comes with big risks as well as big expectations, because we usually take a lot of time before that to prepare and gather every possible information and knowledge that we could find and take part in, such as endless discussions by overwhelming ourselves with opinions and feedbacks in order to put us in a much better position, to start implementing them when we are in the right state to do so.

But the problem that most people have is that, while they gather all of this necessary information for future implementation, often times, they never actually start implementing things, or even take that fateful big leap in the first place. Why is that? The answer comes back to that particular word of "Expectations". In this current digital world, we are constantly fixated on the word "Success" and its definition. We are fed nearly every day to the narrative of this off-the-scale caliber of success that is portrayed in the media and by society, and those portrayals subconsciously became the measure and the mean standard for our own expectations of ourselves. Your own fear in being unable to meet those standards of success inevitably translates into a fear of your own insufficiency and incapability to produce good results. You froze in place and become emotionally petrified at the magnitude of the tasks that lie ahead. This is also why we hesitate to the point of absurdity, where often times, we always said to ourselves.

"Oh, the timing is just not right"

"Oh, I need more time to prepare"

"Oh dear, I so not experienced enough yet, I really need more time to learn"

"Ah, but I just cannot have enough knowledge about this yet"

It is not so much about your fear of failure, but more towards the unrealistic expectations you have over yourself, because of the content that you consume every single day. The truth is, those portrayals of over-the-top successes are either the eventual results after years of work that you never saw taking place, or they are simply manufactured for the purpose of earning validations in order to satiate an empty self-esteem. Let me tell you something, gentlemen, no one, and I mean no one, is ever fully prepared for anything when they are just starting out. There is no such thing as the time to start to do something. There is no such thing as being 100% or 200% or even 300% sure when you take a leap of faith - never.

You would not know how deep the water truly is until you take a dive into the water yourself. You would not know how to properly run a business, until you actually start running one and learn for yourself. You would not even know how to properly play a simple game, until you actually start playing the game.

The amount of theoretical knowledge that you can have over an endeavor, are peanuts in comparison to the amount of practical knowledge you will accumulate over time by actually being in the midst of the battlefield and really get your hands metaphorically dirty in doing so. You can also watch all the videos you want, read all the books about fitness and self-improvement you want, but if you do not simply implement them to your daily lives, routines, and hobbies, how are you actually supposed to know if those theories truly work for you, gentlemen? Because, if, for example, you read this book and then just leave it at that without acting on my teachings by improving your life and engaging in self-development, this book is literally nothing but a long, easy-to-understand, list of empty words that could help you get into the best shape that you could ever be in that you choose to ignorantly disregard, having effectively wasted your time in learning and not acting on valuable knowledge, gentlemen. There is nothing wrong in being well-prepared before going into battle, in fact, I subscribe to this principle myself. However, it is completely and utterly wrong when you are, or become so fixated on theories to a point so that you simply refuse to implement them to see their results in your very own life with your very own eyes, in practice. That is what theories are all about, gentlemen - do not make this incredibly dangerous mistake. So, here is the brutal reality. No matter how much information, wisdom, knowledge, and intelligence that you can possibly gather, and no matter how matter how prepared you really think you actually are, you can never, in your entire life, come close to being able to fathom the pure unpredictability and the utter chaos that is reality in our own perception as humans. Reality is uncontrollable, we cannot control future events, and it is our job to adapt and adjust along the way, to better facilitate or suit our own circumstances. Knowledge and information are merely metaphorical nutrients for the soil, and in the common heat of the moment where they are indeed applicable, they are ready at our disposal to be implemented. The greatest strategies are not those who have the most knowledge and information, it is those who are able to pick and implement key points of those knowledge and information, in accurate accordance with their present reality, and those whose minds are malleable enough to quickly adapt to the ever changing and rapidly evolving nature of this world, in order to cultivate the new knowledge to apply to their present circumstances. It is important to note that those words have so much meaning than it initially seems - It is more than just about being able to adapt. When something stops moving, they very slowly but surely eventually start to rot and die. This is why the lake water is dirty, and the river water is so clean that you can safely drink out of many rivers in this world. As the old proverb goes: "Who rests rusts". Similarly, the river always keeps going as long as it is a river, and that is why they are able to slowly break barriers of rocks, soil, and plant fibers, to eventually pave new paths for them to further flow through and fertilize new ground by carrying nutrients from one place to another. Whereas the lake just stays there, as algae is slowly amassing and growing until the very end of the lake. Do not get too invested in theories and too dependent on assumptions, only to refuse later completely to even try applying them to your own life, and implementing them into our shared reality, because you are too afraid of making mistakes, thereby facing shame, failure, and possibly social shunning. You simply cannot be, and will never be, 100% sure when you are just starting out - if you are certain that you are sure enough, just go for your dreams and ideas. When you gentlemen do eventually start, everything that you planned and laid out prior, will almost never manifest any way you want them to manifest, and you cannot and will never be able to change that. The absolute majority of your plans, statistically speaking, will turn into chaotic and stressful moments of skilled improvisations, genius adaptions, and new experiments. This is exactly as to why the majority of the learning is done along the way, after you started and took that fateful decision into the unknown. We always learn from discomfort, and not from being uncomfortable. This is the battlefield for yourself, the battlefield where you are made as a man. This is where geniuses are made, and people get their best ideas and inspirations, where legends are born. No matter how much you fail, no matter how your experiments and manifestations of your wishes, dreams, ideas, and desires turn out in their final form, they are goldmines for refinery for future iterations of your remaining wishes, dreams, ideas, and desires. All that matters if that you keep trying, failing, and improving. This Is where you learn to adapt to anything.

So, make it count, gentlemen. Be considerate in your approaches, no matter how small or seemingly insignificant, because you never know what you might learn, and you are never finished with learning in life.

CHAPTER FORTY-THREE
WHY PEOPLE SUFFER FROM ADDICTION

Modern man's difficulties, suffering, and weakness stem from a dangerous delusion about the modern world - a belief that material possessions and external success bring lasting happiness. But true fulfillment can only be found within, by cultivating a deep sense of purpose, meaningful connections, and a rich inner life.

- JAN RUDAT

When they first use a substance, people may perceive what seem to be positive effects. They also may believe they can control their use. But these substances can quickly take over a person's life. Over time, if the addiction continues, other normal activities become less pleasurable, and the person has to encapsulate himself in the addiction just to feel "normal." They have a hard time controlling their need to get off their addictions even though it causes many problems for themselves and their loved ones. Some people may start to feel the need to take/do more of their addictions or take/do it more often, even in the early stages of their addictions. Now, we are going to talk about a very, very important topic for modern men - addictions. We have all been guilty of them in our lives. Especially in this day of age, where distractions are virtually everywhere, never stopping to bring down the rain of temptations in our direct vicinity, testing our emotional strength, integrity, value, principles, and willpower, this corrosion of our very own way of life can make it very tempting to many of us to resort to drugs. Now, when we talk about addictions, we mostly talk about substance abuse, like alcohol, drugs, caffeine, sugar, pornography, videogames, and social media. And unfortunately, in this generation, this has never been more evident. So why do we actually become addicted? What creates this vulnerability within us? Why do we find it extremely hard to resist? And what makes us keep acting on them even though we have the acknowledgement within us that they are extremely bad for us? The answer is plain and simple, gentlemen - addictions occur when you experience a series of constantly amplified sense of emotional distress, caused by the feeling of insufficiency and lacking the desired experiences and sensation in your current life circumstances. Why are you addicted to drugs and alcohol? Because you are lacking or could not experience the rush of excitement and enthusiasm that you crave so much, when you are going about your everyday life that is seemingly ever-so boring, or you are simply trying to escape the painful sensation of your current life circumstances. Why are you addicted to pornography and masturbation? Because you are lacking or unable to experience sexual gratification in real life, so desperately trying to feel that sensation through other people's experience of it online. Why are you addicted to videogames? It is because you lack conquest and strength in real life, and you are therefore greatly afraid of failure, going to great lengths in videogames to gain virtual achievements to try to make up for your lack of it in real life. And because you are always presented with a reset button when you fail, never having to face the consequences. Why are you addicted to social media? It is because you lack novelty in your life, and just like porn, trying to actively live that sensation through other people's experience of novelty, by desperately trying to put yourself in their shoes. That is also why you just can't stop scrolling through social media websites to continuously seek other people's new and profound experiences that you seemingly could only wish for to happen in your own life, unable to do so yourself. Addiction always originates from pain, as addiction is merely the process of ones attempt to escape from one's own pain in the form of insecurities, failures, fears, anxieties, boredom, grief, and aimlessness.

Addictions are merely the tools for you to desperately fill the hole within you that is, in essence, created by these forms of pain. In simpler words, the reason why you are addicted to alcohol and drugs, and possibly other forms of substance abuse, is so that you don't feel the undesired feelings when you are not addicted. The dangers of addiction as we all know it, is that it increases our level of tolerance towards it, meaning the more we use that substance that we are addicted to, the more we become dependent on them, and the more dosage of frequency and quantity are required by us to experience the same threshold of the desired sensations and emotions, all the while we poison ourselves more and more.

All the while failure to fulfill that increasing demand for dosage, will result in withdrawal symptoms and will inevitably amplify our undesired sensations and emotions even under completely normal, stable circumstances. Essentially, the more addicted you become towards something, the deeper the hole and emptiness within you actually becomes. So, it is always a losing battle. Not only do your emotional distress get even more amplified, but now you also have to sacrifice a lot more resources. The same thing I experienced when I was addicted to pornography back in the day, the more pornography that I watched, the more that I felt the urge to consistently watch them in order to keep me feel sane. It is a very, very dangerous path to live on when you are addicted to anything, not to mention the physical, mental, social, and financial damage that you are doing to yourself, while also running the risk of involving and even hurting other people as well as yourself. So, how can we redeem ourselves from this? How should we exactly construct our road of redemption away from addictions? Firstly, you have to make yourself stop fixating and endlessly obsessing over the end goal. Yes, I know, it seems counter-intuitive for the normal narrative of "Keeping your eyes on the prize". Look, it is okay to do that, by no means am I saying that it is wrong, but when you start to obsess over it, it can make you extremely impatient and uneasy. And when you become impatient and uneasy, you are even more vulnerable to temptations of any offerings of shortcuts, such as resorting to your fix for your addiction, and will make more and more unsound and rash decisions and revert back to your old ways in your addiction routine. This is about removing the catalysts that get you to become too eager and hateful to experience the feelings of gratifications of the end results. Secondly, you need to have extreme clarity of your life plans and introduce endeavors that has the same narratives as your emotional distress, that compliments your new lifestyle. Thirdly, you have to keep going - you have to stick to your plan, and never give up. You cannot allow yourself to default to your own addiction.

CHAPTER FORTY-FOUR
THE TOP FIVE WAYS TO BUILD EMOTIONAL STRENGTH

They say that emotional strength is all about being comfortable in expressing your emotions and become vulnerable. SHUT THE F*CK UP. A bunch of nonsense been put on every google search for men to become emotionally vulnerable. There is a reason why it is called "Strength" not "Weakness". Fortitude = Strength. Vulnerable = Weakness. Emotional strength means being able to know & understand the full spectrum of your emotions when they are provoked by real life catalysts and maintain your composure/control so that your cognition still functions well, all despite your very own emotions being continuously and constantly stimulated to be expressed/unleashed. The bread & butter of masculinity is in essence being able to control your emotions, identifying each of their trigger points & finding ways to mitigate their effects to the point where you're not in danger of losing your cognitive & physical control.

Another chapter, another dose of hardships. Welcome back, gentlemen, I hope you are all doing very, very well.

1. See things as they are

The first way to build emotional strength is to see things as they are, not as you want them to be. It's easy to get caught up in wishful thinking and create false expectations about the future. But when reality hits, it can be a painful experience that can cause emotional distress. Emotional strength means being able to see things objectively and accept them for what they are. One way to develop this skill is to practice mindfulness. Mindfulness is the ability to be present in the moment without judgment. People pleasers would stupidly and simply tell you that by practicing mindfulness, you can become more aware of your thoughts and emotions as they arise. This is only particularly true. You have to work hard for multiple days on yourself to practice effective mindfulness. This truly allows you to observe them without getting caught up in them. It also helps you to identify any really unrealistic expectations or negative thought patterns that may be contributing to your emotional distress. Another way to see things as they are is to seek out different perspectives. It's easy to get stuck in our own way of thinking, but this can limit our ability to see the bigger picture. By seeking out different viewpoints, you can gain a better understanding of the situation and broaden your perspective very quickly.

2. Prepare for the worst

The second way to build emotional strength is to prepare for the worst. Life can be a wild ride, full of ups and downs, twists and turns, and unexpected detours. It's like riding a rollercoaster blindfolded - you never know what's coming next.

But instead of just holding on for dear life and hoping for the best, why not prepare for the worst? Think about it - when you're on a rollercoaster, you know that there are going to be drops and loops and turns. You brace yourself for impact and hold on tight.

Preparing for the worst is like bracing yourself for impact. It's about anticipating potential challenges and having a plan in place for how to deal with them. It's about being proactive instead of reactive and taking control of your emotional well-being. For me, preparing for the worst means having a safety net in place. It means having a cushion of savings in case I lose my job or have a medical emergency. It means having a support system of friends and family who I can lean on when things get tough. And it means taking care of myself through exercise, meditation, and therapy so that I can handle whatever comes my way. Because let's face it - life is unpredictable. It can knock you down and leave you feeling bruised and battered. But if you prepare for the worst, you can bounce back faster and come out stronger on the other side. So go ahead, brace yourself for impact. You got this.

3. Minimize emotional attachment

The third way to build emotional strength is to minimize emotional attachment. Now, before you start thinking I'm advocating for becoming a robot devoid of emotions, hear me out.

Emotional attachment can be a double-edged sword. On one hand, it can bring us immense joy and fulfillment. It allows us to form deep connections with others and experience the full spectrum of human emotions. But on the other hand, emotional attachment can also be a source of pain and suffering. When we become too attached to people or things, we can become overly invested in their outcomes. This can lead to disappointment, heartbreak, and a loss of our own sense of self. So how can we minimize emotional attachment? It starts with recognizing when we're becoming too invested in something or someone. It's okay to care deeply, but when we start defining our own self-worth based on external factors, we run the risk of losing ourselves in the process. Focus on the present moment.

Instead of getting caught up in worrying about the future or ruminating on the past, focus on what's happening right now. This can help you stay grounded and avoid getting swept away by emotions. This doesn't mean becoming cold or unfeeling, but rather learning to observe your emotions without getting caught up in them. It's about being able to step back and see the bigger picture, instead of becoming overly invested in any one outcome.

4. Become unreactive

The fourth way to build emotional strength is by developing an unreactive mindset. This doesn't mean you have to suppress your emotions, but rather learning to respond thoughtfully instead of reacting impulsively. Reacting to situations can be harmful, especially when our emotions take over our logic. We can end up making decisions we later regret or engaging in behaviors that don't align with our values. In contrast, responding to situations allows us to take the time to process our emotions and make decisions that serve our best interest.

How do we develop an unreactive mindset? Well, gentlemen, it starts with mindfulness. By being present in the moment and aware of our thoughts and emotions, we can recognize when we're reacting impulsively. This gives us the much-needed space to pause, reflect, and make a deliberate decision that aligns with our values. My personal way to cultivate an unreactive mindset is by practicing emotional regulation. I do this daily through deep breathing, meditation, and physical exercise, all of which help manage emotions in a healthy way. By regulating emotions, I avoid becoming overwhelmed and act in a way that's productive and deeply stable. It's extremely important to remember that we can't control everything. Life is unpredictable, and things don't always go according to plan. Developing an unreactive mindset can help us cope with unexpected challenges and setbacks. By staying calm and collected, we can make better decisions that are in line with our values and goals.

5. Knowing and understanding pain

The fifth and final way to build emotional strength is by getting up close and personal with pain. I'm not talking about just acknowledging it or accepting it, but really getting in there and understanding it.

Pain comes in many forms, and we've all experienced it at some point in our lives. Whether it's the loss of a loved one, a traumatic event, or just the everyday struggles of life, pain is an inevitable part of the human experience. But here's the thing - pain can be a powerful teacher. When we're in the midst of it, it feels like the world is ending. But if we're willing to sit with it, really feel it, and understand it, we can come out the other side stronger and more resilient. To truly understand pain, we have to get rough and personal with it. We have to be willing to face our demons head-on, to confront the things that scare us the most. We have to be willing to sit with our pain, to feel it in our bones, and to let it teach us what we need to learn. It's not easy. In fact, it's downright brutal. But it's necessary if we want to build emotional strength. We have to be willing to get uncomfortable, to push ourselves beyond our limits, and to embrace the discomfort. The thing is pain never really goes away. But if we can simply learn to understand it, to work with it, and to use it as fuel to propel us forward, we can become more resilient than we ever thought possible. Building true, real emotional strength means getting up close and personal with pain. It means facing our demons head-on, feeling the discomfort in our bones, and using it as fuel to propel us forward. It's not easy, but it's worth it. Because when we can understand our pain, we can become more emotionally resilient than we men ever thought possible.

CHAPTER FORTY-FIVE
HOW TO OVERCOME ONES FEAR TOWARDS LIFE

Everyone has fears and feels fear. The nature of fear breeds from unfamiliarity, and that in turn gives way to lack of confidence and assurance. Fear is a tricky little bastard, on one hand we want to avoid them altogether, on the other, we desperately want to see/feel what lies on the other side of that darkness. We want to avoid getting hit, but on the other hand, we also want to be able to take many hits. Many people say that fear is all just a stupid illusion, but I prefer a better term, a natural protection mechanism. You see, gentlemen, fear is our natural, built-in, instinctual response to threatening circumstances based upon the incomplete judgements created by our own initial perception of them, and it can be amplified or dimmed down through the collective perceptions from other people. For example, if we fear depths because we have never been to deep waters before, our sense of fear can be further dimmed by other people's judgements of dept. If a person adds "Be careful of deep waters" it will inevitably amplify our sense of fear, but if a person adds "Never worry, it is so much easier to swim in deep waters", it will dim it. The truth about fear is, that it is not so much about the circumstances that we are dealing with that make us refuse to partake, but more towards the question of our lack of ability and assurance to handle and accept the consequences should the fear manifest itself into reality. Physical pain, emotional pain, damage to self-esteem, mental-pain, demoralization, missed opportunities, failures, losing your job, ruined dreams, ruined reputation, depression, self-deprecation, harassment, bullying, and other negative effects. So, it is really not so much about how deep the water is that gets us pissing our pants, but more towards our incapability to handle the circumstance - if we become helpless in deep waters, or if sharks come for us, and actually bite our legs, that prevents us from going into deep waters. It is not about talking to women that scare us men, but it is more towards getting bombarded by the personal effect of shame and failure if we do get rejected, criticized, or even humiliated by them, that prevents us from making the first move. So how can we get rid of this uneasy feeling when we are trying to break our chains and start taking on new endeavors? I believe that you gentlemen knew or at least have anticipated this one coming, there is no magic pill or shortcuts towards overcoming fear, gentlemen. Additionally, the only way you can get yourself around it, is to eventually familiarize yourself with the circumstance you are dealing with. If you are afraid of failure or falling short of expectations when trying out a certain endeavor, you have to fail a lot to eventually get accustomed to the cause-and-effect relationship and sensation of failing. The very same principle applies when it comes to rejections, criticisms, and humiliations. Only then will your mind develop the capacity to accept the risks that come from the circumstances you will experience, and eventually have the capability to put those fears aside and then concentrate on finding ways to perform better in those endeavors. You can certainly make good preparations to reduce the chances of failure and your fear manifesting itself to reality, and you can certainly change the narrative of fear itself so that you become more eager to approach and undertake them, but if you want to be comfortable in the face of fear, you have to experience fear enough to eventually get used to it. Of course, it is different when the risks involve death - where there are no second chances, you have to accept the consequences from the beginning, no matter what they may be. And trust me, I have experienced this myself. If you can look into the face of death and laugh at it and shake its hand only to walk past it like I can, then you know you succeeded. In terms of familiarizing yourself with fear, it is not always about jumping straight into the fire or taking a huge leap of faith - be smart and methodical about it, introduce ladders of progression here and there along your journey of development in order to baby step your way to more demanding and risky assignments. After all, it is not always wise to go big and take massive risks from the beginning, as the consequences can overwhelm most people in an instant. Don't go from casual, highway street racing to formula 1. You can do this for anything you engage in. Build a system of progressing for yourself, and progress slowly and gradually, but surely and safely. be the wise turtle, gentlemen.

This is also how you conquer and defeat your own fear, as you cannot take it all at once. And always remember that pain leads to growth, and later pleasure. Suddenly, things look a lot nicer, do they not?

CHAPTER FORTY-SIX
WHY YOU HAVE TO LET THE PAST GO

Letting go all else, cling to the following few truths. Remember that man lives only in the present, in this fleeting instant: all the rest of his life is either past and gone, or not yet revealed.

- MARCUS AURELIUS

Stop clinging to the past. Firstly, attaching yourself to the past means you simply refuse to evolve. You can't change the past. Don't waste time trying to relive or recreate the past because circumstances are different and will be different as time goes by. People grow. Personality shifts, circumstances evolve, and priorities change, and even if you can replicate the past, it won't be exactly the same as you envisioned it to be, which only going to massively disappoint you because of your own delusional and unrealistic expectations. We all love reminiscing about the good, the good times in our youth, right? The sense of belonging, excitement, fun, and pleasure. It just seems irreplaceable, especially when you enter the harsh and unforgiving real world of survival where pain and suffering is inevitable to be experienced. That is why you sedate yourself and try so hard to remember the good old days to escape the reality of the circumstances you are in. All the ideal scenarios you want to repeat and all the things you could have done differently to bring those circumstances back into place in the present, all of them are only going to make you feel depressed and regretful at the same time.

We've all seen it recently that the power of nostalgia is extremely effective in getting people deeply invested and attached in something. I'm talking to you, Disney. What nostalgia does, especially through the media, is that it makes you excessively value the past. It does this by retrieving all the key and important moments of the past that you cherish and value to a high extent and present them in a way that it makes you feel that you have something seemingly very important that you can lose. That is why while it certainly makes you feel good, it also makes you afraid in forgetting them gets you to clinging and seduce you to wanting more of them. We see this all the time with music, talking about all the good times with your access all those years ago. I mean, I don't need to mention the artists because they are literally everywhere. Old, new, popular, just hitting puberty, all of them causing millions of people to be depressed in every corner, unable to move on. If this world has the car from back to the future, then fine live in the past as much as you'd like, where you have nothing to worry about. I'm sure everyone would love to do that, but this is reality. Time only takes forward instead of wasting your time, energy and worrying about the good times of the past, being slowly forgotten and fades away from our memories, create better and more impactful new experiences. Instead, I mean all of you gentlemen must be to some degree, have an awareness that the past is a whole different circumstance compared to how you are living currently.

Your priorities are different and so does your responsibilities. Most of the things you're trying to be clinging on in the past won't be relevant or even be of service to what you are currently going through in life. In fact, they can be very detrimental to your own mental fortitude as you are trying to become a fully independent man. Instead of daydreaming about the good memories, utilize impactful lessons from the past as a predisposed blueprint to help you take on future challenges. Don't get me wrong, it's nice to look back once in a while and admire them if you want to, but let's be real here, gentlemen, if they can't contribute to making your presence circumstances better, what use do they have besides been a collection of mental sedatives to lock you in. The second thing is clinging onto the past makes you do things half ass because of artificial safety nets, too much fixating and obsessing over good memories will drown you in an emotional mindset and prevent you from carrying out your objectives and goals, which always requires taking risks and making sacrifices. You know, not just all relationships that you can't forget and let go, but also wealthy friends or relatives that you think you can rely on for help but have completely different paths and outlook in life and you do and old jobs or professions that you are good at, make you a decent living, had great office mates but are extremely unsatisfied in doing. These are what I like to call safety nets because you treat them as contingencies to go back to in case you fail or in circumstances do not go the way you want to because you don't have, don't want or can't create new options for yourself. Your decisions and actions are or will be limited and dictated by the extent or up to a point in which you feel that you are starting to move on from them and forget about them. You will ultimately let others make crucial decisions for you because you can't move on from the past without feeling depressed or regretful. I'll give you examples. One man wanted to go to Cambridge after college. His applications got accepted, but then decided against it because his recent ex said she's going to Miami, and he followed her suit because he had been always hoping for a second win with her. Another example, one man wanted to become a full-time tailor by taking an apprenticeship in Savile Rowe, but then delays committing to it and eventually giving up on us because he doesn't want to miss other yacht parties. That is friends with massive inheritance are hosting and run the risk of being forgotten or replaced by them. You are deliberately setting yourself up in settling for less than what you are capable of. Cut all corners and burn those bridges. Put yourself in a situation where you are backed against the wall and have no choice but to go forward, and there is no better way to do this than deciding to go pack your bags, move to a new area, city, or country even, and start fresh on your own. This will inevitably put you in survival mode and let me tell you why you gentlemen need to experience the sensation. When circumstances turn crucial and desperate, they compel you to waste no time and in turn get you extremely focused only on carrying out your priorities, unnecessary distractions, and anything that does not contribute to your present circumstances will inevitably and instinctually be removed from your mental capacity. Because you are literally fighting for your own life, there are no more safety nets that you can ease yourselves into should things go horribly wrong. No more half-assed decisions or actions taken. You either thrive or you don't, and when the sensation of that circumstance starts to eat on you, you will go to great lengths to increase your chances of survival and will defy your limits of what you think you are initially capable of. Imagine having to tighten up your usual budgets and expenses, cook and ration your own food, wash your own clothes, fix your own broken utensils, find like-minded people to build your own network from the ground up. Taking dead-end jobs to provide extra financial support while you are working on your own endeavor. Those circumstances force you in the hard way to develop necessary survival skills, and with that, you have no time for videogames.

You have no time for binge watching Netflix, and you certainly have no time to cling onto the past because now instead of being afraid of the past, not repeating itself or be forgotten, you are imposed to be afraid of the state of your future circumstances. Burning bridges will put you in an inescapable route where you eventually must not fail, and that is why you won't.

CHAPTER FORTY-SEVEN
MEN ARE NOT BORN, WE ARE BUILT

No man is more unhappy than he who never faces adversity. For he is not permitted to prove himself.

- LUCIUS ANNAEUS SENECA

Men are not born. We are built. Unlike women, we are not valued, respected, aspired, and rewarded purely and simply because of our physical existence. In this world, we are measured through the degree of our performance, accomplishments, and impact. We have to hunt, construct, invent, strategize, compete, conquer, acquire, inspire, and leave a long-lasting legacy in order to be properly classified as a functional, potent, and worthwhile men to exist. The world and life in general are more unforgivingly ruthless to men and all of us know this. We are not privileged and will not be privileged unless we fulfill our burden of performance. And in order for us men to perform, we have to be valuable first. So don't keep on questioning endlessly of why life is unfair for us men. It has always been this way for us since the dawn of civilization. It's just how the feminized world have ignorantly and endlessly conditioned us to think from the perspective of women's natural entitlement to privilege, that we are deserving of everything just by being a walking, breathing human being. Ultimately removing us from our natural instincts as men, to cultivate value for ourselves in order to be capable and confident enough to perform, and instead turning us into generations of incompetent and degenerative weaklings who can't even and are not willing to face all the inevitable and necessary trials to eventually acquire those values and perform to the best of our abilities and potential hardships, tribulations, frustrations, failures as repetitively and cliche edges. They sound because they've been the subject of endless motivational videos. They are the inevitable building blocks or ingredients for us to eventually become someone of true value. We mean included often wine about the agonizing and excruciating sensations that we experienced. When we're going through all those seemingly bleak circumstances, we often constantly question the worthwhileness of going through all of these trials, such as how much longer do we have to endure them?

Whether the light at the end of the tunnel will be like it all cracked up to be or will it just be another needless attempt to make something of ourselves? It is a crisis situation in its own definition, but that is because we always view them as indignations rather than opportunities. Men should treat struggles as necessities rather than excuses. If it turns out to be a worthless effort after all, then at least we know which one is not worth our time to master. A skill or a craft takes tens of thousands of hours of constant practice guidance, intense focus, taking risks, trials and errors, Ted sacrifice and discipline. Someone does not magically become a well-known distinct tailor. Overnight someone does not supernaturally become a great surgeon with no fieldworks. Developing valuable traits like confidence, courage, resilience, reliability, and resourcefulness takes a lot of time to cultivate and they have their own series of trials that we have to go through in order for us to eventually possess and instill those traits. Genuine, valuable traits always have a good or even great backstory to be told. One does not simply acquire these traits and authentically showcase them through mere set proclamations and mindset shifts. You have to put in tremendous practical efforts to understand their components and eventually cultivate them as a part of you. Going through struggles will also inevitably make us greatly appreciate and value the rewards that we acquire through succeeding in conquering them because we basically have invested exhausted and sacrificed a substantial number of resources to eventually get those rewards that we wanted. And I'm not just talking about financial resources, but also time efforts and even emotional resources. The things and circumstances that we acquire and accomplish through great struggles will by default become a significant part of our sense of self-worth.

Whether the light at the end of the tunnel will be like it all cracked up to be or will it just be another needless attempt to make something of ourselves? It is a crisis situation in its own definition, but that is because we always view them as indignations rather than opportunities. Men should treat struggles as necessities rather than excuses. If it turns out to be a worthless effort after all, then at least we know which one is not worth our time to master. A skill or a craft takes tens of thousands of hours of constant practice guidance, intense focus, taking risks, trials and errors, Ted sacrifice and discipline. Someone does not magically become a well-known distinct tailor. Overnight someone does not supernaturally become a great surgeon with no fieldworks. Developing valuable traits like confidence, courage, resilience, reliability, and resourcefulness takes a lot of time to cultivate and they have their own series of trials that we have to go through in order for us to eventually possess and instill those traits. Genuine, valuable traits always have a good or even great backstory to be told. One does not simply acquire these traits and authentically showcase them through mere set proclamations and mindset shifts. You have to put in tremendous practical efforts to understand their components and eventually cultivate them as a part of you. Going through struggles will also inevitably make us greatly appreciate and value the rewards that we acquire through succeeding in conquering them because we basically have invested exhausted and sacrificed a substantial number of resources to eventually get those rewards that we wanted. And I'm not just talking about financial resources, but also time efforts and even emotional resources. The things and circumstances that we acquire and accomplish through great struggles will by default become a significant part of our sense of self-worth. Whether the light at the end of the tunnel will be like it all cracked up to be or will it just be another needless attempt to make something of ourselves? It is a crisis situation in its own definition, but that is because we always view them as indignations rather than opportunities. Men should treat struggles as necessities rather than excuses. If it turns out to be a worthless effort after all, then at least we know which one is not worth our time to master. A skill or a craft takes tens of thousands of hours of constant practice guidance, intense focus, taking risks, trials and errors, Ted sacrifice and discipline. Someone does not magically become a well-known distinct tailor. Overnight someone does not supernaturally become a great surgeon with no fieldworks. Developing valuable traits like confidence, courage, resilience, reliability, and resourcefulness takes a lot of time to cultivate and they have their own series of trials that we have to go through in order for us to eventually possess and instill those traits. Genuine, valuable traits always have a good or even great backstory to be told. One does not simply acquire these traits and authentically showcase them through mere set proclamations and mindset shifts. You have to put in tremendous practical efforts to understand their components and eventually cultivate them as a part of you. Going through struggles will also inevitably make us greatly appreciate and value the rewards that we acquire through succeeding in conquering them because we basically have invested exhausted and sacrificed a substantial number of resources to eventually get those rewards that we wanted. And I'm not just talking about financial resources, but also time efforts and even emotional resources. The things and circumstances that we acquire and accomplish through great struggles will by default become a significant part of our sense of self-worth.

Hardships and struggles are necessary and inevitable, and it is especially way more destined for us men because again, we have no choice but to perform in this world. Otherwise, we will be utterly forgotten. Ridiculed and unappreciated.

CHAPTER FORTY-EIGHT
HOW I OVERCOME MY TRAUMA OF BETRAYAL, ABUSE AND LOSS

If you've experienced an extremely stressful or disturbing event that's left you feeling helpless and emotionally out of control, you may have been traumatized. Psychological trauma can leave you struggling with upsetting emotions, memories, and anxiety that won't go away. It can also leave you feeling numb, disconnected, and unable to trust other people. When bad things happen, it can take a while to get over the pain and feel safe again. Now, when it comes to traumatic experience, it is very different to everyone, and I am pretty sure that I can't speak for every single one of you here because, well, everyone's severity of trauma is different. But nevertheless, I'm going to tell you gentlemen what works for me and how I managed to eventually overcome my traumas. So, it was mid-November of 2019 in Melbourne, Australia. I went there to visit my girlfriend at the time for her birthday, and I was going to stay there for a week and a half. So, it started off pretty normal. We went do the typical relationship thing, you know, eating lunch together, watching movies, this, and that. And then the day of her birthday comes where all of a sudden after we went through our day, she wanted to visit her quote unquote friend's house for a private party. And me being the better cook that I had actually allowed her to go not knowing that that friend was actually a guy. So off she went, and I was left on my own in her apartment like an idiot. Now of course, some of whom might be asking, why don't you just go with her and let her introduce you to her friend? Well, let me tell you why I hated her friends. Bunch of good for nothing degenerates that only eat pizzas and smoke weed on the weekends. Yeah, I don't want to have any associations with them. So, I basically told my girlfriend that she can go on her own and celebrate stupid, right? I know it is stupid. So, I waited for about three hours into the night. It was, I think about one 15 in the morning and I was starting to get suspicious, but then 10 minutes later, her flat friend or apartment mate came back home and then she asked me, why aren't you with your girlfriend in the club? So, I was baffled, obviously. I asked her the club what club she says she was going to her friend's house, and then she replied, well, I just saw your girlfriend queuing up on Ms. Collins, which is one of the nightclubs in Melbourne for those who are wondering. So of course, I was angry and emotional, and without notifying my girlfriend, I immediately take a cab in the middle of the night and went straight to Ms. Collins. I've already had suspicions that she is seeing someone behind my back before I even went to Melbourne to visit her. So, on my way to the club, in my head I was like, I want to see this for myself. I want to see if she is really cheating on my back. I want to see the hard evidence right before my naked eyes. So, I was in this really determined state to find out the truth. So, as I arrived at the club, I had to cue for another like 20 to 30 minutes just to get in the club. So, there I was in the club, prowling the dance floor, prowling the bar, prowling the tables to witness a crime scene in action live. So, the whole time I'm in the club, I was looking for this flash of a peculiarly Shaped blonde hair, and eventually I caught a glimpse of her in one of the corners of the dance floor dancing and making out with another bloke. Yep. Most of you gentlemen who have been cheated on would probably found out through either a friend witnessing the events, or you secretly dig up her phone when she's asleep to find out that she's been sending naked pics to another man. Well, I had to witness everything live right before my eyes. Well, at least I got exactly what I wanted. I've uncovered the crime scene. Shame then that I can't call the police on them, I'm just kidding. But anyways, witnessing that, of course my heart was floored like impulsively, I want to go up to them and punch the guy in the face. But fortunately, my rational brain was still working. Even in the midst of a devastating heartbreak, I realized that I'm a foreigner, and any trouble with the law in Australia would've made the situations a lot worse for myself. So, as I exit the club, I was still processing the whole thing. I was connecting the dots of everything. You know, her strange behaviors during calls, her excuses to go to sleep early and many other things. It all came to make complete sense. In the end, she's been banging this bloke behind my back the whole time for months. So, I decided to move out, pack my things, and move out on my own and spend the rest of my days in Melbourne grieving about what happened. That experience, that betrayal really scarred me more than anything I have ever, ever experienced. But long story short, that traumatic experience made me very bitter, vengeful, verbally abusive, spiteful, and just viewing them as this really, really cruel creatures.

we tend to become very biased and extreme to one end after we experience a traumatic event. And that was me. I became very biased towards women. I just view them as this bunch of evil malicious succubus for quite a while. But I'm a very curious man. So, I needed answers. I started seeking for answers. Why would she cheat on me? I mean, there must be a reason or a collection of reasons why she would do that. Behind every action, there is always a reason behind every effect. There is always a course. So, I started researching and learning about female nature, and that's where I discovered the red pill. And then from there, I started learning and reading about the dark side of human nature, evolutionary psychology, evolutionary biology, learning about human thoughts, learning about human emotions, learning about human behaviors. And through that process, I actually became even angrier, not towards anyone or anything, but at myself for not knowing or discovering all these knowledge and all these information beforehand so that I wouldn't have got through all those troubles and all those shenanigans and get traumatized because of not knowing all this information and also discovering that society has been lying to me all this time through the movies, the music, the books, everything that they have thrown at me ever since I was a kid, has conditioned me into a delusional idealist. I was living in a fantasy all my life and through discovering all this knowledge and information and starting to live realistically through rational and logical judgments, slowly and surely, I was able to free myself of all the pain because now I understand how things work. So basically, what cured me for my traumas was deeply educating myself of how the world works through the principles of cause and effect.

In other words, the truth. And I think that is what all of us needed to do. You know, understanding will lead to acceptance. We may experience cognitive dissonances and frustrations when we try to understand these things at first because of our own ego investments in previous narratives. But eventually, like I always said, the truth will become self-evident to us. And it is a matter of time before we get used to it. No matter how much you try to resist the truth, you will eventually fatigue. So, by knowing and understanding the reasons of **why a woman** would cheat on a man, I was no longer confused. I was no longer perplexed, and I was no longer hopeless because now I have the knowledge. And with knowledge, we gain understanding. With understanding, we become accepting. And with acceptance comes peace. Because there is no longer this void of perplexity that haunts us, that confuses us, that endlessly makes us ask, why did this happen to me? And yes, it applies to my trauma of being abused as a kid by my parents as well. I was always regularly beaten with a belt and locked up in an isolated room for hours. I would always wonder as a little kid, even until then of why mom and dad were such monsters back in the day. And of course, again, after educating myself of how parents can become abusive, I start to understand why they would do such things to me, the reasons behind their anger and violence, and how their own struggles and circumstances contribute to their own behaviors. And I was no longer angry or bitter to them. And the same thing happens to the trauma of loss. If you lost a dear friend, it is an unfortunate circumstance that you have no control over if you lost a family member.

It is basically a natural evolutionary progression. It is an inevitability, and that is it, gentlemen, we can't change the past and all the traumas that we have experienced. There is no way you can turn back time and redo what you have done. Don't go online looking for sympathy and go to those you know stupid Instagram pages where they show quotes like no matter how bad a situation becomes; everything will get better in the end. Shut up. It's just like saying a deep stab wound would heal by itself. Just let yourself bleed out to death. Traumas are deep wounds, and they require time and effort to eventually overcome. And that is why my solution to you, gentlemen, is to educate yourself as much as possible about your bad experiences. Information is free nowadays, and they are just at the tip of our fingertips. All you have to do is look deeper into the wormhole. At first, you will be bitter, and at first you will be angry for knowing the truth.

CHAPTER FORTY-NINE
STOP BEING FAT AND OVERWEIGHT

Now, there's nothing that makes my blood boils more than hearing men's excuses for not getting in shape. Ooh, I don't have time, man. Ooh, I'm too busy, man, shut the hell up. You're not that busy in real life. You're just merely prioritizing unproductive things like your videogames and you're jerk off session and lying down in bed for hours scrolling on social media. In fact, why can't you spare just an hour or two of those useless periods of consumptions to go to the gym and get in shape? Oh, life's too short to exercise, you know? Yeah. Well, life is very short for you to continue down the path of self-sabotage and living the life of a dysfunctional degenerate, which is completely idiotic. What you were doing besides putting effort and time to the gym and eating healthy is merely escaping from the reality that you can't handle. That is why you drown yourself further in misery by playing your videogames and looking at porn hut while simultaneously eating fast food. Just seeing an overweight man walking down the street, it makes me sad genuinely, and the sadness replicates on their faces as well. I mean, just imagine the arrays of physical problems that they have to face and endure just because of their own inept decisions. Diabetes, joint problems, lower back pain, stroke, high blood pressure, heart attack, metabolic disorders, low testosterone, and kidney failures. I mean, I have never experienced being overweight, but I have experienced being massively out shape. I was extremely skinny fat, and that experience alone made me realize that I need to get in shape in order to improve my quality of life to the way I wanted it to be. I was smoking two packs of cigarette a day, eating fast food and other processed foods for supper, and then washing them down with either soda or whiskey while living a sedentary lifestyle, playing videogames, and watching porn all the time, nearly every day. I was weak, depressed, unconfident in social situations, and just the overall demeanor of being out shape makes me feel like a degenerative slop, like a man with no direction in life and only keeping himself alive through ingesting the same substance that is going to accelerate his own demise. I was suicidal for a while and getting in shape was the thing that saved my life because it gave me a sense of direction and purpose. Being physically functional is just as important as being mentally healthy. Gentlemen. It translates to so many other endeavors, even your own work ethic, financial position, and relationship quality. People who are overweight and obese are 55% more likely to experience depression as well as higher chance to experience social discrimination, ridicule, and isolation. Looks do matter, gentlemen. There are scientific and mathematical evidence of human beings' preferences for visual, aesthetic pleasure. Leonardo da Vinci wrote about them in a book called Divina Prop back in the 14 hundreds, and speaking of relationship quality, people who are overweight will inevitably have lower levels of testosterone that people who are in shape, and we all know what that means. Yes, poor performance in the bedroom, which will lead to reduced intimacy and less satisfaction coming out from your partner, which will inevitably increase the chance of separation or infidelity.

Physical health and appearance matter in relationships and other social settings because everything is judged externally. At first. People could care less about your personality if you are someone whom they do not want to interact with in the first place. You don't have to get jacked like giga Chad, nor do you have to get skintight shredded like Bruce Lee. Just being an overall physically functional and relatively strong man is enough. Though the word enough is relative to every man. It is evidence that people are more likely to want to interact or approach physically. Good looking individuals. Having a strong masculine stature brought shoulders and low body fat is an indication not only of good and optimal genetics for reproduction, but also a great sense of self-respect and a valuable mindset that many people want to associate with. I mean, I'm assuming that some of you gentlemen who are reading this chapter are already in shape or at least working towards getting in shape. You gentlemen will be lying to me if you say that Being in shape does not change the circumstance of how people behave towards you, people will take you more seriously and treat you with more respect because your initial impression is higher up on the list of the evolutionary desirable traits and criteria of the male human being. Now, some of you overweight men might say, oh, You're just fat phobic.

Here is the thing about body positivity. It's lying to all of you. It's a delusional and ignorant fantasy claim of pride to once own sin of gluttony and overindulgence. You think you are being loved and valued, but you are secretly being ridiculed, despite stigmatized, and eventually eliminated from any prospects of reproduction, and you will not be cared if you ended up alone and just being overweight or obese due increases the probability of you ending up alone in life. I mean, who the fuck would encourage someone to continue their journey towards type two diabetes and having one of their legs amputated? It's absolutely absurd. If this starts to sound like it's personal, it is because most of my elderly family members died due to heart failures in kidney failures due to living a sedentary lifestyle and being overweight. And these people and organizations are supporting people being unhealthy and overweight while their bodies are slowly rotting their organs from the inside out. Social agendas and social constructs make you feel very rich in your dreams, but very poor in reality because they appeal and empathize to your emotional needs yet ignore the practical cause and effect of your own circumstance. They keep you wrapped in a bubble of delusions until reality pops that bubble and expose your deficiencies and destructions to your own naked eye. If you really value your quality of life, you have to fight for it. If everything comes easy, everyone will be kings and queens. The world does not owe you anything and you only get what you deserve. If you want to know what's on the other side of the storm, stop voluntarily. Position yourself in a situation that only drags you away from the finer things in life because that is exactly what you are doing by continuing to be fat and overweight. And the worst part is most overweight people know how to get themselves out of that situation, but still choose not to.

They make excuses to compensate for their own lack of drive and defeatist mindset. Do not hypothetically hope for all the finer things in life that you want to have, and then blame the world for being unfair because of your own incapability. The only person to blame here is you because you refuse to be responsible to make yourself capable.

CHAPTER FIFTY
THE ONLY REAL WAY TO HAVE REAL CONFIDENCE

Confidence. Confidence. Confidence. Without a doubt, every single person in this world wants it, it is arguably the most attractive & desirable trait that a person could showcase. As they say it, energy is addicting & contagious, when you're confident, everything & everyone around you becomes invigorated, and things just seem to go smoothly, even though it may turn disastrous, the overall demeanor of the group & the atmosphere just renders it irrelevant. Women loves confidence more than anything, as confidence demonstrates the assurance of leadership, which is what they look for most in a man, to be able to lead. To have confidence is not easy, some may luckily have it, but for most, we have to build it from the ground up.

Everyone wants confidence, right? When we are confident, everything in life just seems so easy and it's a very, very attractive trait to have around people as well. We all want confidence like the snap of a finger, like we all want it now, every time and in every situation possible. Being your authentic self is one thing, but wrapping confidence around that authenticity is another. Let me explain. Confidence is simply the feeling or sensation of reassurance of success or prevailing in your own judgments, knowledge, capabilities and experiences towards the situation, environment, and body of work. You exude in showcase mastery of important aspects and circumstances and life, as well as having profound understanding of how to navigate through various stages of life in simpler words for the TLDR generations. Basically, you genuinely know, understand, and can excel in what you are doing, and you know how to handle different, difficult, and essential situations in life over and over again. That is why achieving and possessing high levels of physical strength, mental resilience, financial wealth, vast arrays of skills and intelligence, resourcefulness and social connections will naturally generate unprecedented level of confidence because you know and understand what it takes to have all those crucial and desirable attributes. And if you were to lose all of them, you would know how to get them all back again from start to finish. Essentially, what people notice from you when you are genuinely confident in yourself is the emanation of amused mastery or perceived competence, meaning you gentlemen oozes an aura of profound expertise in every bit of every step that you take in your life. And like I said earlier, people will perceive that you have the capability to handle different, difficult, and essential situations in life. Genuine confidence is only achievable for people who have the courage to go through a lot of challenging situations in life. Again, it's not rocket science. If you want to know, understand, and master different situations and circumstances in life, or you're going to have to go and experience them yourself and cultivate yourself from there to obtain those profound skills, knowledge and understanding. And speaking of cultivation, confidence itself is cultivated in a gradual and progressive manner. You won't get to have massive confidence in one lump sum. It is accumulated through overcoming trials and challenges and eventually having the reassurance that you can overcome those trials and challenges repeatedly should they be presented in front of you once again or numerous times. Now, can confidence be faked? Certainly, it can, but I wouldn't recommend it if I were you.

This whole narrative of faking it till you make it is a very inefficient thing to do. You see, gentlemen, confidence can be faked, but it's only a matter of time before you let your guard down and expose yourself. You see, faking involves lying, and lying as we all know, is extremely tiring when it gets too much for our own good, it gets you to overthink and exaggerate and slowly makes you less believable and sincere in your words, which will eventually lead to inconsistencies between them and your actions. And we human beings are social creatures by nature. We have the inherent capabilities to sense social cues through our intuition, like body language, tone of voice, and even subtle gestures like an eye twitch. People can easily sense if you are lying through the disparity and the incongruency of your words and actions. It's a very, very simple process of our natural intuition when it comes to social interaction, gentlemen, so don't underestimate it. In my case, I would rather admit my incompetence and inexperience in certain situations rather than fake confidence, because eventually you are the one who's going to inevitably lose and lose a lot more than just your dignity and respectability. Even your reputation will be tarnished, especially in today's age where word of mouth can spread to a million people in just a couple of hours. Confidence is seemingly displayed through who you genuinely are as a person, how smooth and articulate you speak your firm and assertive tone. But in reality, it is about what you are capable of that eventually morphed into a part of your character or personality, which is eventually identified as charisma. Yes, there is no charisma without confidence. If you look at Tony Stark and James Bond, they both have their own distinct characteristics and personalities. One is the brash, an outspoken individual. The other is the quiet, mysterious, and reserved individual. But both of them possesses the same set of attributes that lead to those charisma, and that is, once again profound skills, knowledge, and understanding of their own chosen profession and way of life. In other words, they both possesses the same set of attributes that gets them to possess unprecedented levels of confidence. There is no charisma without confidence, and there is no confidence without courage, and there is no courage without commitment.

CHAPTER FIFTY-ONE

WHY MEN HAVE TO STOP SETTLING FOR LESS

The hardships of success, they can be very irritating & atrocious to endure, especially when our mind & body are wired to go after & experience pleasure as quick as possible & wherever they are conveniently placed for us (The path of least resistance). Unfortunately, we all know that the great things in life, the finer things in life, the desired things in life & the worthwhile things in life, doesn't come easy, they always require a significant amount of time & effort for us to have the capacity & capability of handling them. We only get what we deserve in this world, and when we are naturally impatient to the gratifications that are placed in front of us, regardless of your circumstances in life, they can bring you into a state of a pretentious makeshift of the true success that you initially desire for yourself. Especially in today's world where gratifications are shoved into our 5 senses constantly.

Now, at some point in our lives as men, we aspire to become someone more. We put a lot of effort in cultivating ourselves into new heights, which would inevitably strengthen our sense of self-esteem. And with that, of course, our ego would naturally want to demand more out of life. We start to raise our standards and keep visualizing what could possibly be best for us in this world. It is a very, very tingling sensation when you realize that you deserve way more out of life than what you initially thought. But we all know that life isn't always about cleansing glitters, especially when you're still climbing the ladder of success. There is always going to be moments of stagnation, despair, and deprecation, and this is where most of the time the turning point to oblivion will start to happen. Where before you start believing that you deserve everything that this world has to offer, now you decide that you may bit off more than you can chew and start to settle for lesser things in life that you utilize as a pretentious makeshift for the greater things in life that you desire, like masturbating to porn. Instead of having sex with a beautiful real-life woman, you are essentially sabotaging the progress that you have made so far. By deciding to settle for easy and immediate instant gratifications, you can even sabotage selves even when things are going seemingly well. You see, gentlemen, why do I and many other YouTubers promote delayed gratifications? It's because pleasure or gratifications or temptations will always have a price, and when you are still climbing the ladder, especially in your youth, you can't afford to pay the price or make sacrifices that would jeopardize your future setup. Essentially, the price and consequences of pleasure that you will have to pay when you are still young and still lacking resources is much, much more detrimental to your livelihood than when you are an already established and resourceful man where you can better afford to pay the price and consequences without jeopardizing your own livelihood. Of course, by no means that I'm trying to say that you gentlemen should avoid gratifications at all costs.

Absolutely not, because that is impossible. Human beings are intrinsically motivated by rewards and gratifications or something that they can gain out of something that they work on. Essentially what I'm trying to say is that when you are still struggling in climbing the ladder of life, don't make choices that would result in temporary satiation, but would cost you permanent disappointment and regrets, especially in today's age where distractions are fed constantly 24 7, 365 to all your five senses directly through the predisposition and ease of access through our phone. We are literally more equipped to endure delayed gratifications back in the days of Nokia where our phones are purely purpose built for communication and not entertainment. The reason why most modern men are willing to settle for less in life instead of the finer things in life that they've envisioned for themselves initially is because they cannot handle falling for instant gratifications, both when things are going tough and also when things are going well. So how can we have a better angle of approach or attitude towards the instant gratifications that has been presented in front of us nearly every day? Now, I know that those type of contents can be useful for inspiration and motivation, but when we consume too much of it, it can lead us to a compromising state of mind. Let me explain. You see, we human beings are inherently impatient creatures. We find it hard to wait. We want our desires to be satisfied as quickly as possible. And when you are constantly teased of your desires through shots of fast cars, money rains, and hot women, you will be more tempted than ever before to know what it feels like to be in the shoes of those big Guys or ballers that you see in success porn videos. And that is where this type of content could get you to become extremely uneasy and impatient to feel those gratifications, which will make you inevitably vulnerable to impulsive decisions like when you see a hot woman in one of those videos you can't afford. But imagining yourself having sex with that woman. And because you are impatient and agitated to be in those circumstances, you will inevitably settle for less and watch porn instead to fulfill that craving or have sex with a much less attractive woman just because you'll take what you can get or even paying a huge sum of money for a lady companion. Another example could be the sports cars that you see in those type of videos. Similarly, you just can't wait and are so eager and so fixated and desperate to feel those sensations of what it's like to own and drive exotic sports cars, which could tempt you to buy lesser-known sports cars that you can't afford through debt or mortgage, just as satiate the sensation that you crave because of continuously being teased by those success porn videos. Secondly, you need to pay attention when you are rewarding yourselves. Now, like I mentioned previously, we can't afford to negate or neglect gratifications altogether. Rewarding ourselves is necessary in order to keep the momentum going and further solidify our sense of self-esteem and self-actualization. However, this is where things could go south on you, especially when you think things are going very, very well. You see, gentlemen, when we reward ourselves, we rarely pay attention on what could have been or what could have gone wrong. Of course, why would we? Things are going well; we are feeling good. Why would we ruin the moment by questioning them? Well, it's because we tend to reward ourselves way, way more than what we actually deservingly should. A nice dinner could continue into a night full of alcohol parties and drugs. Even something as simple as giving yourselves a day of rest could turn into a full week of rest. And before you know it, over rewarding yourselves will become a habit. And bad habits are much, much easier to form than good habits.

So, you have to be wary of when you start to slip, when you are rewarding yourselves, gentlemen, because when we are feeling good, we rarely question things. We just go with the flow. It is only when we face the consequences of slipping up, then we start to wonder what had gone wrong. Thirdly is to seek command from a place of higher authority. Now, this one is very important, at least to me, to always have a reminder from a person that is of higher authority than myself, whether it is a fellow YouTuber or a role model that I've admired to constantly remind me of what is right and to not slip away from the path that I've chosen. Now, the reminder can be anything. It can be a video, a podcast, an audio book, a quote, whatever they are. You have to find ways to make them plausible enough for you to notice them based on your own preferred and most effective learning style every single day. Like for example, putting quotes as the wallpaper of your phone or your pc, so it serves as a reminder every time you turn them on. What figures of authorities that we genuinely admire do to us is that they implant to us a deep sense of self-awareness. And when we are self-aware, we do not want to disappoint ourselves or take any actions that will take us further from our desire itself. If we are attacked by distractions, temptations, and gratifications every day, we have to bring the fight to them. We have to know how to combat them and win the fight every single day, otherwise they're going to overwhelm us eventually.

Fourth is to identify the rewards and consequences of every gratification that you are tempted to bathe yourselves in. And not just identifying it but make them plausible enough to be instilled within your mind, like writing them down in a notebook or a journal so that every time you are seduced by gratifications, you would have the mental capacity to weigh in your decisions more carefully. I mean, do I even have to explain this? When you jerk after porn, yeah, it feels good for a couple of seconds, that is the reward, but you're going to waste an hour or two finding the perfect video waste even more time getting aroused and getting your dick hard and then feeling like shit and regretful after your nut yourself. Number five, and this is in my opinion, the most important one. Always move forward and look for new challenges within your chosen path in life. Life is a conquest when we're not moving forward because we can't let go of the past or because we fear of what's ahead of us, we will feel stagnate and lacking the excitement that we want out of life. So, when we regress, what happens? What happens when we can't find the excitement out of life through the endeavors that we do? Because we can't move on, and we are too afraid to take risks. We seek for that excitement through synthetic means and lesser beings. That is why when things are going extremely well, don't underestimate it and stay comfortable. Human beings will naturally seek further novelty no matter where they are in life. And if you stagnate in one place for too long, you will inevitably regress and sabotage yourself to your previous self-deprecating state. It's like standing in front or reaching a complete dead end where you have absolutely nowhere to go but backwards because there is nothing left to look forward to. That is why you will become desperate to try and experience that excitement and exhilaration through instant gratifications. Submitting to instant gratifications will eventually make you settle for less in life because what they do is that they make you conform to the rest of society, that you cannot be something more than what society tells you to be and that you could never bring yourself to a state where you deserve more than what you are currently deserving. Now, when things are going tough, don't sedate and self-deprecate. When things are going well, don't underestimate and slip away.

CHAPTER FIFTY-TWO
THE TOP 3 REASONS WHY YOUR LIFE SUCKS

A lot of us experience this sensation. For some reason we feel that our life is so insignificant, unmemorable, pathetic, lacking & just plain depressing, and then to make things worse, we could not figure out why. It's just this feeling of absolute dread, decadence & decay caused by the seemingly insurmountable amount of stagnation within our lives. What causes this feeling? What are those things that make us regress towards a miserable state, where we apparently have very little to no choice but to sedate ourselves to feel alive & worthwhile. Everything involves the environment that you put yourselves in gentlemen.

we're going to discuss the main reasons why our lives are miserable and what changes you could make to turn your seemingly bleak and hopeless existence into something that you can look forward to every day you wake up. Now, as we live and go about within our daily lives, we developed a sense of routine and a sense of perceived attitude towards different circumstances that surround us. Meaning the environment that we put ourselves into will play a very important role with regards to influencing the state of our judgments, point of view and frame of mind towards many different and important aspects of life, such as our attitude towards facing adversities, personal growth and uncontrollable circumstances. Place or direct yourself into a good nurturing and cultivating environment. You will both discover and experience never before realized. Seemingly hidden possibilities, opportunities, potential and state of mind that will propel you towards the significance of flourishing, progressive growth, place or direct yourself into a contempt, lifeless, and deteriorating environment. Then you will undoubtedly face the common feelings of boredom, regression, lethargy, dullness, and neurosis, where the lack of personal growth, excitement, enthusiasm, creativity, and conquest will plunge you into a state of emptiness and decay in which you will try to hopelessly or desperately attempt to counteract with sedations and enslavement involving synthetic beings in simpler words. The reason why your life is miserable is because you are unable to surround yourself with the right environmental attributes or characteristics that can constantly help to elevate your own attributes to new heights. Experiencing ecstatic insights within your own psyche and culminating into a developed sense of genuine fulfillment, pride, maturation, worth, wellness, and accomplishments within you. Basically, you surround yourself with shit that is why you are miserable. So what are these quote unquote shitty environmental attributes that have been critically poisoning and dissolving our attitude or approach towards life in the modern era? All this time, there are three main ones. Number one, shit contents. Now, come on. This is an obvious one and don't try to lie to me or yourselves on this one, gentlemen. Let's be honest here. In today's age, we spend most of our time daily online, in front of the screen, so either our phone or computer. And aside from doing work and engaging in communications with your mates and family, the only other choice you're going to have online is to consume contents. Now, what type of contents you consume is going to dramatically affect your attitude towards your daily routine and the circumstances that surround you. It is very, very important that you consume contents that have actual meaningful effects and practical applications to your real life circumstances. Remember, it's always entertainment versus information when it comes to contents. And of course, most of you are probably expecting me to stay. Stay away from entertainment, stay hard, keep showing information, knowledge, and testimonies every single waking moment of your days until you die. Don't waste even a second on watching movies even with your grandparents because they're not going to get you anywhere and they're ruining your life. Come on, let's be realistic here, shall we? Yes, of course. I will tell you gentlemen, to consume more information than entertainment, like read more eBooks and listen to more self-improvement podcasts instead of watching social media.

I mean, that's what I've been saying in the Death of Modern Men chapter because for us daily, it is a constant mental battle to get consumed in either distraction or knowledge. But let's get even more specific here. The thing that really matters is the quote unquote type of information and entertainment that you consume. Now in terms of informational contents that you consume, it is always a wise decision to consume information that you can relate and apply to your current real-life situations because if you don't, there will be no actual realistic progress that is going to be made and you're only going to feel even more lolly-gagged afterwards. Like if you are currently in financial shambles, don't spend an entire afternoon learning about the first and second world war in terms of entertainment, I'm not going to say that they are completely useless because they aren't. If you consume the right ones, they can actually make your day a lot better. That is why consume those types that uplifts your mood and spirit to take on further tasks within the day or those that nudges you away from procrastinating much more than necessary. Like in my case, watching a simple three-minute UFC promo video wakes me up instantly and gets my day started. Don't consume those types of entertainment that gets you to run away or confine yourself from your real life problems like porn or too much videogames or too much fantasy and idealistic with you TV series or even worse, those type that gets you to emotionally dissolve yourselves within your real life problems instead of finding a way to solve it like those sad and miserable songs about hopelessly clinging to your past relationships that gets you to feel pathetically sorry for yourself for months on end. Come on mate. If you manage to get your ex when you're a bum, imagine where you could fish when you're an established hunk. Number two, shit people.

Now this is probably a subtopic that I would have to make a separate chapter about because I could go on endlessly about understanding the people around us for 10 lifetimes and still would not have figured them out completely, because human beings are both immensely and extremely complex and they will always be gray areas we haven't yet explored. But regardless, we all know how the closest people we hang around and associate ourselves with have a tremendous influence in how we think and feel about ourselves, our choices and decisions in life, our habits and routines, our values and principles and our perspectives regarding everything that is around us. Close people that we trust will always play an important role in shaping our future because we eventually have to conform into their collective common thoughts and fundamentals that we share amongst one another, meaning eventually we will have to showcase our own set of strengths, inclinations, vulnerabilities, and deficiencies. Because developing a genuinely strong and trustworthy social bond often requires us to be transparent and that alone takes a long time and without a doubt, a lot of shared activities, trials and tribulations, actionable assistances, gifts, celebrations, clashes, debates, convincing and proposal to eventually achieve. That is why it is always necessary to carefully select these people, people with great characters, people who are not spoiled or privileged, people who understand how to navigate through life, people who have a lot to bring to the table, people who push or inspire you to take risks and be courageous and people who dare to call you out on your mistakes and get you to introspect so that you could grow on a personal level. And of course, people who truly stick by you through hard times, which is, let's be honest, extremely rare nowadays, oftentimes, especially when we are still socially inexperienced or inept, and if we haven't developed enough sense of confidence, self-worth, and individuality, yet we tend to conform to whoever we find convenient and available for us. We tend to become desperate necessities for social connections or intimacy because we do not want to be alone and because we are afraid to be the odd one out, this could cost us a lot because if we conform to the wrong group of people, we run the risk of feeling forced to conform to social values or fundamentals that we deep down do not agree to and partake in shared activities that we do not enjoy ourselves.

And the longer we keep putting pressure on ourselves to keep going, the more those undesired social fundamentals and activities will be instilled into us until eventually they all become a sense of involuntary normality for us, and we will be in constant war with ourselves mentally between either being criticized or condemned when we retaliate and feeling safe but uncomfortable when we don't. I mean, imagine feeling forced to worship the Kardashians, gossip about dead celebrities, complain about the unfairness of the world, talk about a whole bunch of social dramas and smoke weed by your mates every single weekend when every fiber of your being genuinely wants to do none of that shit. It's extremely miserable, frustrating, and horrifying to be in such smorgasbord of discomfort around fuss and whiz and will only be a complete waste of your time and potential. So yeah, get rid of those people whose attitude towards life. It's not the one that you would want to share with alongside your journey, gentlemen. It's so much better to be alone nonconform for a while and having a clear direction of where you're going than being held back or contained within an impotent and petrified community. Number three, ship mindset.
Wait, what? Our mindset is a part of our environment. Yes, it is. Everything starts in the mind. Gentlemen, when we wake up first thing in the morning, we are immediately placed within the garden confinement of our own psyche and conscious identity. Our mind is the place where judgments are made, perceptions are formed, and attitudes are instilled. Whatever external stimulus went through our five senses, they are imminently digested in order for us to establish a base level of understanding and plausibility. But there are internal stimuluses that are arguably of stronger influence than all external influences we have in our world, namely our conscious and subconscious attributes like the id, the ego and the conscience or superego. Now, the workings of these inner voices are again,

extremely complicated and I'm certainly not car union enough to be the best in explaining it scientifically, but in simple words, how we collectively and internally converse to ourselves altogether with regards to many different and important aspects of life, will eventually have a much more impactful effect on the way we express our demonstrations to the external world and our declarations to our own internal world. A simple example can be when you fail a certain task, your own sentiment towards that failure will be a lot more important and impactful to your own internal welfare and external expressions than the actual affair of the failure itself. For example, one person could fail and still could think and act like nothing happened. On the other hand, one person could fail, and he could bring himself to the brink of taking his own life. It's all a matter of how the mind approaches the different and unique circumstances of life. Now, forgive me, this chapter is getting a bit long and starting to get quite gibberish, but I want to split this category of shit mindset into two extremely crucial forms. Firstly, the mindset of passivity. Now, this mindset is the one I mostly have a problem with because it involves around an idol and idealistic view of the world. This is where you just sit there praying and hoping for great and meaningful things to happen to you without taking any form of action or fighting back against any form of abuse or tyranny. Passivity and conformity breeds contempt, lack of creativity, demise of enthusiasm and cravings for immediate indulgence. And in today's society, there has never been more people willing to be enslaved under a system that favors the high society like accepting your fate in working in your boring, tedious, arduous, bland, and oppressive nine to five job, while at the same time daydreaming about your desire to become a free man and engaging in endeavors that you voluntarily take part with the need for other people's assessments, take control of your life and start living life on your own terms.

And finally, the mindset of self-deprecation. This one you gentlemen are very familiar with as it involves around you, pathetically accepting your fate at the hands of your own involuntary admission with regards to your untapped, unrealized, and uncultivated potential. I'm not good enough. I don't deserve this. I'm hopeless. I can't possibly do this. I'm going to die a loser. Those defeat statements can only come from your own impulsively, shallow judgments, fear of the taxing roe towards significance and an emotional or superstitious attachment to misfortunes. Never underestimate and depreciate yourself when it comes to how the unfairness of life has affected your current seemingly bleak circumstances because all it takes is just a single internal mental decision to completely turn it into your favor. If you gentlemen notice the whole theme of this chapter is all about a single word stagnation and life will only start to get worse if you stopped moving forward. That is why if you ever feel like a miserable bum on any day, make sure to direct yourself to commit to a certain significant, personally meaningful endeavor, to satiate your natural subconscious pursuit for growth, survival, and prosperity. Or in one word, happiness.

CHAPTER FIFTY-THREE
THE MOST IMPORTANT MESSAGE TO FUTURE LEADERS

How power corrupts your mind, it does this by amplifying our deepest & darkest desires, where we eventually lose consciousness of what initially matters, and start to become insatiably obsessed solely with what makes us feel even more satiated/what cultivates our own circumstances/agendas/ego investments to better state without any other consideration outside of that.

We all know human beings are and will never be satisfied, we always pursue novelty regardless of how many we already have possessed & experienced, and power arguably removes the idea of contentment from our mental dictionary completely. With power comes choices, a lot of them, and we always want to exercise/capitalize on those choices to increase our chances for survival & prosperity, to make our lives easier and possibly more exciting/lively.

But as a leader, it is not as simple as acquiring as much power as possible and relishing yourself within it & disregarding everything else around the responsibility of your position without any consequences, it is much more complicated than that, because every choice has rewards & consequences. And human beings always focus on the rewards without paying much attention to the consequences. Power. Everyone wants power. That sensation of ultimate authority, mastery and resourcefulness, it's addicting is what it is. That air of invincibility, rain and finesse just dominates everything. The very notion that you are capable to excel, influence, intimidate, and command everything that is within your vicinity just gives you this insurmountable level of self-belief, confidence and control power gives us the self-induced acknowledgement of pride, of our own capabilities and the vast array of possibilities and opportunities that they can generate or the number of doors that they can open for us to choose accordingly to our own pure desire and will inevitably putting us in a position of further prosperity where we can capitalize and maximize to keep expanding our own ascendancy towards our ideals of perfection or a perfect and undisputed life. Unfortunately, that is the point where power could turn its back on you should you not become aware of its corrupting properties. Human beings ultimate, deepest, and darkest desires involve two things, and that is infinite control and infinite prosperity. We are innately an inherently selfish being. We always prioritize our own needs and wants first before everything else, and through that we always want circumstances to go our own way, even those we have no control over. That is why most of us get angry and complain of why circumstances didn't turn out the way we expect them to be or the way we want them to be. As your power increases, it gradually grants you more resources, status and authority over many things such as the ability to influence people's thoughts and actions, the ability to build entities both physical and nonphysical like buildings and humanity or political movements and the ability to partake in more challenging, tempting, and previously hard to access endeavors that provide more novelties to satiate our cravings as we are given or presented with more control and opportunities, we will always be tempted to exercise them time and time again, and by all means, you should as a leader, you must exercise them to experience growth.

However, this is where they can corrupt you if you let yourself go and indulge yourself by the impulse. As I've said before, we are inherently selfish beings, and we always prioritize ourselves before others and power corrupts us by escalating this natural instinct of ours to an uncontrollable, deceptive, and hallucinatory level. As more doors are opened, as more possibilities and opportunities are presented before you and as more degree of authority is bestowed upon you, you will eventually be spoiled for choice and vast of temptations will start to slowly overwhelm your initial quest and attempt to diverge you to many different often unrelatable and destructive directions. Your selfish nature will naturally want to facilitate your thirst towards covertness, and that is where your own power will start to disintegrate you from the inside out. As the saying goes, the only thing that interests people with power is more power. In reality, a leader's power is not this fantastic and enigmatic force of nature that you can utilize at your immediate will. That is just the illusion that power gives. It is hugely different from when you are still cultivating yourself from the ground up where you have all the power and authority towards yourself. As a leader who has established a reputation, majority of your power comes from serving those in need, giving them what they need the most and earning their support. In other words, most of your power as a leader comes from the people you serve and earning their trust enough for them to support you by sacrificing a part of their time, capital and voice to eventually present you with the authority, resources, and opportunities that you can capitalize on. Whether it is for selfish or selfless means that here, why the most effective indication of power and credibility is the amount of people that are loyal to you and support you with the utmost passion and enthusiasm or in modern language, it's also known as the social proof.

Certainly, when you're a leader, everything starts with you and that gives the conception or assumption that you control everything, but you don't. You certainly control the orchestration of the direction and destination where you and your supporters might want to go and end up, but whether that path and destination can give your supporters the results or the outcome that they want, it is all in their power to judge you and your leadership. That is why no matter how good you think a product, or a project might be for your customers and followers, in the end, the market will determine the reality of its potential. As you become more established, credible and reputable, you will inevitably have a lot more to lose expectations of you will grow and failing or forgetting or dismissing to deliver your promises to your supporters. You will lose your power much, much quicker and easier than you gain it or can attempt to gain it back. That is why you must not let your own selfishness for congress get the better review when you are presented with the number of opportunities, resources, and authority that power can seduce you with. Of course, it does not mean that you can't reward yourself significantly for the promises that you've kept delivering to your people. You should and you must in order to amplify your momentum to keep on delivering. What you can do instead is utilize those opportunities, resources, and authority to cultivate both yourself and your supporters to reach new heights and insights in life. You could be selfish and selfless at the same time. That's where you can establish a deeper, more personal bond with them as you are experiencing growth alongside them because it is not only the direction where you want to go, but it is also a direction where they want to go or have the curiosity to give it a try. Certainly, when you're a leader, everything starts with you and that gives the conception or assumption that you control everything, but you don't. You certainly control the orchestration of the direction and destination where you and your supporters might want to go and end up, but whether that path and destination can give your supporters the results or the outcome that they want, it is all in their power to judge you and your leadership. That is why no matter how good you think a product, or a project might be for your customers and followers, in the end, the market will determine the reality of its potential. As you become more established, credible, and reputable, you will inevitably have a lot more to lose expectations of you will grow and failing or forgetting or dismissing to deliver your promises to your supporters. You will lose your power much, much quicker and easier than you gain it or can attempt to gain it back. That is why you must not let your own selfishness for congress get the better review when you are presented with the number of opportunities, resources, and authority that power can seduce you with. Of course, it does not mean that you can't reward yourself significantly for the promises that you've kept delivering to your people. You should and you must in order to amplify your momentum to keep on delivering. What you can do instead is utilize those opportunities, resources, and authority to cultivate both yourself and your supporters to reach new heights and insights in life. You could be selfish and selfless at the same time. That's where you can establish a deeper, more personal bond with them as you are experiencing growth alongside them because it is not only the direction where you want to go, but it is also a direction where they want to go or have the curiosity to give it a try.

CHAPTER FIFTY-FOUR
BEING AMBITIOUS WILL SAVE YOUR LIFE

A lot of people say that having ambitions will jeopardize your happiness & mental health. The excessive & competitive drive to attain wealth, power & status is too much work & too much mental hassle to sustain for long periods of time - is it really true, though? Or is it just a collection of excuses of one's tremendous mental barriers/vulnerabilities in lack of confidence, fear of criticisms & reluctance due to passivity, to pursue & achieve greater things beyond what they initially thought they are capable of? This chapter will explore on why being ambitious and striving for greater things will do wonders for your psychological wellbeing, especially for those men who are burdened with the rotting properties of passivity for a very long time.

Now for most of us young men, we've all been in that particular situation. We've all experienced or least have tasted the withering and put feeling of not having a place to go and not having a place to belong. We wandered aimlessly and cluelessly for far too much and too long to the point where we start to relinquish our fate to the world and hopefully, they take us somewhere we can find a sense of actual meaning and direction we yearn desperately for both meaning and direction or at least one of them. That is why we often find ourselves unable to stop asking where to go and or what to do when we feel stuck and stagnant in life. And if we can't or unable to find the answers to those questions for a long enough or at least one of them being answered, we will inevitably start to turn those questions point of view onto and against ourselves and eventually engaging in self-destructive inner monologues to degrade and deprecate our very own potential or existence effectively jeopardizing our very own psychological wellbeing because there are apparently no solutions to the sense of insignificance, uselessness, and fruitlessness that we experience when we are caught within the hollow space of passivity. Now, why does having a set of clear and strong goals or ambitions is the undisputed cure or answer to all those questions and problems? Firstly, the bloody obvious one, having ambitions will give you a definitive sense of direction to engage in a determined pursuit. Purpose is the reason behind what you do, whereas ambitions are the directions to undertake to fulfill that purpose or at least your own personal needs with any form of ambitions. They all start with a transparent, definitive, and realistic visualization of where you want to eventually end up in life or at least reach within a given timeframe in terms of character, wealth, achievements, accolades, status, and professions. Then you progress towards identifying what needs to be done to realize that vision, the challenges you'll face, and eventually getting even more micro and specific in how to become competent in all those things that needed to be done from you. Taking the very first step, essentially having ambitions will gradually and subconsciously present you the realization that you have found or carved out a path or a bridge for yourself to walk on or cross to a preferred destination, a place to go remember and that will give you a very powerful sense of relief from the aimlessness and void that you experience in your daily lives. But that's not all. We all know that the world itself is chaotic, unpredictable, and fast evolving, and we human beings want to achieve growth or evolution through a gradual and hopefully a complete understanding and mastery of the world that we live in. However, we only have so much time and capacity to handle all of them at once, so many countless directions to follow. That is why we have to narrow down the scope of our judgments, choices and decisions so that we are able to commit to a few selected directions or parts in order to become proficiently familiar with them in terms of the way in and out, so that eventually we can find, carve out and capitalize on new directions and paths for ourselves to undertake after the old ones become too stale for us to evolve.

This is what having ambitions can and will do to you and for you, giving you directions to commit yourselves to, and at the same time presenting you with the ability, confidence, and opportunities along the way to carve out new parts for yourself after you've mastered the old ones. A snowball effect inevitably satiating our continuous need for growth and novelty as human beings. An example can be someone who chose to be a filmmaker for 10 years and after he succeeded earning the resources, establishing a credible reputation, and meeting new people who undertook different directions, he decides to take his foot off the gas for a little bit and dedicate his time and resources to pursue the art of brewery. The second thing is excitement. With everything that involves great rewards or prosperity, there will always be great risks and a lot of pressure, and inevitably with risks and pressure comes fear. And there is a significant difference between committing and dedicating yourself involuntarily towards directions and endeavors that you are afraid of and are not willing to do because you find the end results personally unappealing or not worth the effort and committing and dedicating yourself voluntarily towards directions and endeavors that you are afraid of, but are willing to do with every fiber of your being because the end results are in perfect alignment with your visions, necessities and desires. When you experience anxieties for future outcomes, it is a vastly different sensation. If you have absolutely no sense or lacking a sense of possibility, comprehension, anticipation, and enthusiasm of the outcome than when you are. When you lack or have absolutely no desire for commitment towards a risky and high-pressure endeavor, you will inevitably become overwhelmed with fear and be reluctant to even take the first step, eventually abandoning it altogether. But when you have those impeccable levels of yearning, longing, and eagerness, regardless of the feelings of fear or hesitancy that surrounds you, they will eventually be overwhelmed by your much stronger sense of excitement to achieve the end results. If you gentlemen ever feel scared or anxious to do something like entering a competition, for example, but your abnormal levels of curiosity and enthusiasm to obtain or relish the end results are so strong that you ended up doing it anyway regardless of all the risks and pressure. That's what having strong ambitions feel like every human being secretly desire something massive to work for, regardless of our natural instinct to pursue the path of least resistance, we all deep down and want the opportunity or opportunities within this finite lifetime to prove ourselves that we are not just here merely to exist. The dedicated pursuit to unlock an unprecedented sense of self-esteem and self-actualization when you finally attain something or at least reach a point of significant threshold of realized potential and capabilities that you have set for yourself initially within a given timeframe is without a doubt, the only way to fulfill the absolute peak within every human being's hierarchy of needs. The hunger for the ultimate sensation of satisfaction, gratification, and triumph. When you reach the end goal that you visualize most of your waking moment is that uneasy but seemingly chronic excitement that incentivizes you and keeps incentivizing you regardless of fear or pressure or occasional setbacks. And finally, having strong and clear ambitions will give you peace. Now, of course, I'm not talking about peace as in relaxing in a mountain lodge, sipping tea with your dog or lying down on a secluded private beach, drinking tequila with absolutely no sense of urgency and absolutely nothing to worry about. No, of course not. What I mean by peace is a sense of alleviation or liberation of a large burden from your shoulders, the sense of big relief. Remember, everything comes back to that clear vision that you have of where you see yourself five years from now or 10 years from now. In essence, you've already predetermined and pre manifest the next chapter of your life. And that very vision unshackled you from the unbearable weight or ordeal of confusion and insignificance that you have been agonizingly enduring all this time. No longer a sense of floating or roaming around aimlessly in this vast universe, no longer a sense of pointless fruitless and stagnant contemplations late at night of what should I do and where should I go, and no longer a sense of dread or apprehension with the amount of time you have wasted and the time you have left to make something out of yourself. And of course, the other important thing regarding peace is being able to identify what matters and getting rid of all the unnecessary and the detrimental elements out from corrupting and wasting away the precious time within your finite lives. And when you have strong and clear ambitions, you will by default have strong and clear priorities. You will know the things that matters most through sheer instinct standards and routine, and that will help you tremendously in keeping you in line within the scope of the direction you've chosen, despite seemingly more glimmering offers and provocations from other sources. Now at this point, some of you might be asking, how can I discover or find my ambitions in life? And if I'm going to be honest, despite the matter of ambitions being a relatively simple or direct matter when it comes to individual assessments, it is actually a lot more complicated than that, and it may take more than one man's perspective to fully encapsulate your needs because everyone has different circumstances in their lives. But if I were going to give you my best assessment in finding ambitions, it will be to aim for a direction or directions that allow you to tap into an extreme level of immersion and captivation because it is not how many hours you put into something that counts towards you fulfilling your endless quest for growth, mastery, and understanding within your chosen directions and endeavors. But it is how long you put quote unquote intense and unmitigated focus towards them that realistically counts. It does not matter if you love the process or not, although it is much preferable that you do. But all that matters is that you keep that vision alive no matter what. You must keep craving the end results badly enough. And another thing to mention is that one person's level of captivation and immersion towards a matter or endeavor is positively correlated with both the level of deep interest and curiosity. One has to thoroughly understand it and the level of trust as a real-life problem that it presents for one to desire in solving.

CHAPTER FIFTY-FIVE
THE MALE AGGRESSION

Want to know the internal reason why you're feeling stuck & frustrated in life? Both what made you afraid to pursue/achieve growth & what made you vulnerable to the problems of world? You lack aggression. Your lack of aggression is what gets you to think too much that caused you to become overwhelmed with fear, that eventually lead you to miss opportunities, remain stagnant & waste a lot of precious time.

Your lack of aggression is what makes you fragile & susceptible to inevitable undesired/painful circumstances from both people & nature, penetrating your mentality and controlling your frame of mind and eventually, your actions.

Aggression is viewed & preached as an undesirable trait for men, they call it "TOXIC", because they always associate it with anger, hate & violence. But they are necessary for our survival & prosperity in this power hungry & extremely competitive world. Society only looks at one side of the coin when it comes to aggression, without taking the other, more important side, into deep consideration. Fair enough, because human beings in general, love to rush into conclusions & generalize things because they hate the feeling of not being able to have a firm grasp/understanding of a particular element of life, but often, they are stubborn & ignorant enough to not see things from different perspectives to further solidify their judgements.

That is why, this chapter will explore that particular side, and explain to you why having, showcasing & imposing aggression is necessary for men. You must not reject it/repress it.

Now, scientifically speaking, all of us men are born with higher levels of testosterone, providing us with much greater capacity and magnitude for aggression. However, when it comes to the male aggression, the first things that come into our mind is all about the undesirable and unattractive qualities with regards to anger, hate, violence, and destruction. In this feminized world, we have been conditioned and programmed from an early age to perceive the male aggression in such a negative way, to the point where men ourselves start to reject, repress, and even feel repulsively disgusted by our own capacity. For audacity, we have been numb to believe that being soft and compassionate is the only way to make it in this world that love will prevail no matter what evil that bestowed itself upon us. That is just plain, ignorant, and stupid. If someone bullies you, would you just sit on the floor and pray that that blow will eventually stop the harassment? Pathetic and cowardly is what you are. Stand your ground and figure out a way to defend yourself.

Aggression is not necessarily destructive at all. It springs from the innate tendency to grow and master life, which seems to be characteristic of all living matter. Only when this life force is obstructed in its development do ingredients of anger, rage, and hate become connected with it. We focus too much on the dirty side of the coin when it comes to aggression. While aggression is strongly correlated to anger, they are not the same. Anger is more of an emotional reaction. While aggression is more of an attitude when a man is aggressive in his approach to circumstances, it does not mean that he is always susceptible or vulnerable to anger, dangerous but not violent, ruthless, but not vicious, formidable, but not terrifying, such as if a man is extremely thorough or detailed in his analysis towards a matter, it is considered as an aggressive trait or tactic or strategy, but that doesn't mean that he's held bound to inevitably experience or showcase anger when he conducts his analysis. In fact, aggression is absolutely necessary in life and in survival, especially for men as if done right. We can properly and constructively utilize the cultivating properties of this particular dark site, quality of our psyche to our advantage in navigating or breaking through the ruthless and competitive challenges of life way more than the nourishing but vulnerable qualities of compassion could ever do for us. These cultivating properties of aggression can be classified into two very important traits, initiation and assertion, offense, and defense. When it comes to initiation, it's all about the ability to take initiative as a man. Most of us all have been sufferers of hesitancy, and this is what happens when you repress your aggression as a man. The feeling that holds us back from taking action to start any conquests and endeavors or because of fear, which upon failure will eventually manifest itself into anger, disappointment, and regret, or because we are unable to push past that hesitancy due to us being afraid of society's punishments in the form of criticisms, condemnations, and repulsion. When we showcase our aggression towards a particular circumstance and in the end, it left us with nothing but being bombarded with, with our own unbearable and shameful frustration because we are unable to eventually unlock and test our potential by putting our desires into practical actions. Aggression, when it comes to taking initiative is all about the conduct of imposing our will to every thought that we fixate and action that we take. The traits of boldness, courage, decisiveness, meticulousness, eccentricity, straightforwardness, resolute, adaptability, resourcefulness and mastery are all cultivated through the aggression of taking initiative and being the leader of every step that you take going forwards in your life. It doesn't have to be all about purposeful endeavors. Even as simple as going out for a date requires the initiative to plan it all out and eventually execute those plans. All of those traits are all about creating and manifesting your own desired circumstances to the best of your abilities, the perfect blend and magnitude of visualizing, planning, and acting. When it comes to assertion, it's all about the ability to display and enforce your boundaries as a man, or in other words, the act of claiming your authority. Like I mentioned earlier, if someone bullies you, takes you too far or push your buttons too hard, what are you going to do about it? Let him keep kicking you in the face as you lay down on the floor, or are you going to assert yourself, acknowledge your worth and defend yourself? Now, of course, when it comes to people we don't know, it is much easier for us to decide to defend ourselves, but what if this person is your best friend whom you've acknowledged and trusted for a long time? In this case, we've all experienced that particular sensation of being afraid to hurt other people's feelings or offending them to the point where they will try to assert themselves as well and potentially escalate the situation into a conflict and eventually fracturing the relationship. Again, this is all because of our conditioned fear to face society's punishments for defending ourselves from unfavorable misconducts and engaging in conflicts which will eventually leave us being taken advantage of by other people and become extremely vulnerable to manipulation, deception, and even physical harm. This is where aggression will assist you tremendously regardless of your status of companionship with anybody who extensively disrespects you. It is your own right and jurisdiction to reclaim your authority when it comes to your very own wellbeing or dignity. Even if it means engaging in conflicts, you will always have enemies. Remember, trades such as being able to call people out on their bullshits, reject undesirable offers, denounce unfavorable, conducts, standing up for your own beliefs or principles. Protect yourself from physical harm and assert your authority are all cultivated through the aggression of enforcing your boundaries. Those traits are all about preserving and displaying your commanding presence and control over yourself and the circumstances that are bestowed upon you. If you allow people to keep disrespecting you, they will continue to do so until they have complete dominance and control over both your thoughts and actions. Aggression for men is absolutely crucial to be unlocked, accepted, embraced, harnessed, and properly utilized. If you gentlemen want to thrive in anything in this highly competitive and power-hungry life, when was the last time any powerful man didn't showcase his near unwavering aggression through either his words or actions or body of work, if you repress and reject it, it will eventually implode on you and spiral out of control with tremendous consequences. This is where the hate, anger, and violence will manifest themselves. Just like any emotion that is bottled up or contained for too long without any attempt to be properly understood and eventually expressed or satiated, we all have dark side qualities that society tell us to get rid of, especially with regards to men, but shutting the mouth from your life and being apologetic for having greater capacity and capability in them is the same thing as feeling sorry for yourselves, for being born with a dick and a pair of balls.

CHAPTER FIFTY-SIX
THE ONE WAY TO NOT CARE

In the modern age, it is very hard to not care about a lot of things, when we are constantly bombarded with distractions, people telling us to give a f*ck on irrelevant & meaningless things, and our own lack of purposeful/determined path in life. In the self-improvement/self-development world, we have to acknowledge the capabilities & limits our own mental capacity/mental bandwidth. And when we are already habituated by thoughts & endeavors that do little/do not contribute positively to our lives, such as checking what people are up to on social media/playing videogames & watching porn for hours on end at any given day, to the point where they start to corrupt our thoughts and make us feel bad about ourselves, and downplay our own existence, we have to come to a realization, discard and realign the things that fill up our mental bandwidth with constructive & immersive thoughts & endeavors instead. Otherwise, we will be spending precious/critical moments of our lives in mindless & irrelevant stagnation. There has never been a time within the history of this world where there are too many excess, irrelevant, redundant, and gratuitous elements that penetrates the world. Our mental bandwidth every day corrupts tranquility and encapsulates it within a degenerative roadmap than the times of the modern life that we are currently living in. So much so that we eventually become overwhelmed, inhabited, and controlled by their simple, effortless, and painless properties to the point where we start to compromise, forget, and even abandon both our desires and conquests to act, grow, achieve, and build a better life for ourselves. Social media stories, videogames, pornography, depressing music, streaming services, people, shallow opinions and conducts random events and noises. The seemingly minuscule and harmless effects of these modern distractions constantly seduce us into their world. Because of our aimlessness and ruthlessness, an attempt to drift is soft into a life of consumption through sacrificing our potential by feeding us irrelevancies coated with in inapplicability. I guess that's why the men back in the days of good old-fashioned letters and expensive grammar phones get to get things done and accomplish more out of life than the modern men of today due to less access forms and quantities of irrelevancies disturbing their daily lives. In simpler words, your lack of solid and committed directions in life is the sole reason why you gave too much fuck about too many things that are completely unnecessary and insignificant, such as checking what people are up to on social media, jerking off the porn, and then proceeding to play videogames. Minding and involving yourself in other people's business, paying too much attention to minuscule unfortunate events and so much more without a clear visual trajectory of where you want your life to go. Every single step of the way and every single moment along the way, you will be easily disturbed and eventually consumed by all forms of obstructions of the modern world. We humans naturally pursue growth and novelty because we instinctually want to achieve a thoroughly complete sense of comprehension and mastery of this ever so fast, evolving world, and if we stop growing or evolving alongside it, we will abolish our chance of surviving and thriving in it. Just like an animal that has to adapt to its surrounding habitat, it has to evolve or die. That is why we always need directions in life to go and keep going constantly all the time. And if we don't have or lacking any, we will naturally march towards whatever it is in front of us with the least resistance, even if they barely or do not contribute to our need for growth. At least we are experiencing some form of sensation to occupy our cravings for novelty, but we all know without resistance there will be no growth, only stagnation and eventually regression. So, the solution is quite simple, gentlemen, and it is everything to do with priorities and not just any priorities, but devoted priorities, priorities that are personally meaningful, properly significant, mentally captivating, circumstantially, constructive or cultivating, and both cognitively and emotionally immersive. You have to live by these priorities' day after day routinely and eventually habitually. These priorities are those that have rippling effects cognitively well after you are done with them for the day. Priorities that incentivize you to explore much further and deeper within their space to the point where they fill out your mental bandwidth completely day after day in such a manner that barely or even know other forms of entity could divert your attention and captivation. In fact, it would irritate and aggravate you when irrelevant things are thrown your way. I'll give you my own example. I treat fitness very seriously. It has become like a religious ritual for me, and I'm sure many of you gentlemen also treat fitness the same way. Every time I work out, I'm in the zone, no other thoughts of anything but to perform and complete the session to the points where I could conduct further research on information and contents relating to fitness to further cultivate my understanding on the endeavor. For hours on end, even long after I had finished my session for the day now, at one point last year, me and me may went to the gym together as he never worked out before in his life and asked me to come and show him the nuts and bolts of things, and during our rest period, as I was recovering and catching my breath for the next set of heavy squats, he suddenly came up to me and said, you maid, haven't you heard there's a big container truck that fell over sideways in front of your complex? That's horrible, dude. It was carrying a truckload of fruits and vegetables. Now they're all complete wastes. It's so sad, bro, and I didn't answer him back. All I did was give him a disappointed look because all I can think of in my mind was, are you serious, mate?

Don't you have time to worry about more personally important stuff than some clumsy or unfortunate event? And I could see the look on his surprised and slightly disgusted face and what he's thinking. How could you be so cold? Don't you know the driver has families and he might not get to see his wife and kids again? I don't care about him, mate. I don't know the guy, nor does he have anything to do with my life or me in his, he got in an accident. Tough luck. That's his problem to solve, not mine. Stop pretending like you care about him because it's the politically correct answer to say, if you really do genuinely care about the driver, do something about it. Visit him in hospital or donate some money to his family instead of feeling sorry for the guy and trying to seek attention or cloud for bringing up an unfortunate event. Selfish, egocentric. Yes, absolutely. Thank you very much. What do you think? The woods, I don't give a fuck means if people have a problem, when you don't give a fuck, just tell 'me to fuck off and mind their own business. Oh, yeah, they can't because they have none. That's why they pay attention to needless any irrelevant things. Anyways. These priorities can literally be anything realistically and circumstantially progressive, that you can thoroughly put your mind into things as simple as fitness, cooking, and meditation, but also can be as complicated as engineering, design and composing. It's all your own choice, gentlemen, and it's only you that can clarify what you want and willing to immerse yourselves in. Now, for a lot of people, identifying these priorities can be relatively easy, but for some whose minds have been engulfed by so many unnecessary and irrelevant things that disturbs their tranquility and composure to the point where they start to jeopardize or damage their mental health, they have to completely disengage, detox, and retreat. When you are in moments of utter perplexity, overwhelmed and bewilderment, it's time to totally remove or discard everything and go into isolation for a while where you can collect your own thoughts and definitively determine the things that you really want out of your own life, and plan out the ways to get there eventually, so that when you come out of isolation, you already possess the mental clarity and the visceral yearning to start taking the actions necessary. If you can live your life daily with your set of determined intentions in every step that you take and in every endeavor that you do, you would most likely maybe indefinitely become unreactive towards things and circumstances that are not related, nor have anything to do with your resolution towards your desired life, to not give a fuck is as simple as asking yourself, are all the things that I'm thinking doing, paying attention to and spending time on will contribute or benefit significantly to my own personal development that will eventually make my circumstances in life better? If yes, keep doing them. If not, throw them away, forget about them, and move on to the next. That's literally it. However, never think of not giving a fuck as an instant hack or a quick fix because it isn't, especially when you are already significantly habituated by a lot of stagnant and degrading things in your daily lives. Just like any mindset shift process, it requires complete realization, determined intention, and daily practice that will eventually be instilled as a habitual response through self-cognitive and behavioral conditioning.

CHAPTER FIFTY-SEVEN
THE TRUTH OF WHY MODERN MEN BECOME QUITTERS

Quitting & being a quitter is literally the worst. Giving up on something meaningful & significant just makes us feel cataclysmically guilty & disappointed on our own potential & existence. Our own incapability to handle failure and come back from adversities are genuinely shocking in today's age. I wonder why? We absolutely envy those people who just never give up, who has an unbreakable level of grit & perseverance, and who take failure like it's a blessing or a gift of some sort, and then they come back even harder from a seemingly pointless & hopeless state. We all want to be like that, but how? And why can't we be like them initially?

we're going to talk about being a quitter. It's a very popular topic that I don't see many people diving into it quite as deep as I anticipated.

Now, I'm guilty of this phenomenon back in the day, and I'm extremely sure that many of you gentlemen are also guilty of this or maybe are suffering from this disease. Yes, I'd like to call it a disease because it literally does nothing but make you feel even more shit than you already are. Now, generally, and generically to avoid or to remove the quitter mindset from eating away, your soul is simply to not give up when you fail, right? To change your perspective of failure from a monumental and irreversible life altering course towards the doomsday of hell to a necessary steppingstone in order to further cultivate ourselves towards a higher level in many aspects of life that we originally gave up in or on the verge of giving up in, everyone has been telling you all the same thing. You've all heard it a million times, never give up. But what they rarely mention is in terms of the nuts and bolts of how or the way to rewire your mental firmware completely to that desirable point of view. Well, I'm going to try my best to deliver it to you gentlemen in this chapter. So first of all, let's look at failure through a rational and logical lens, shall we? Why do we fail? We fail because of a singular or a mixture of these three reasons. Number one, avoidance of responsibilities due to disinterest, fear, and illness. It's simple and obvious. If you're not putting in the time and effort necessary in order to cultivate your level of skill, knowledge, and experience within a craft or situation, or because you lack enthusiasm, being afraid of failure and are too lazy to take on an enormous challenge, or in other words procrastinating way too much to the point of neglecting accountability, then you will by all means, increase your chances of failure or lack of good results.

Number two, insufficient fundamentals, and preparation. Now, as much as you want to put in the time and effort on the right thing, sometimes it may not be enough to yield good results or because you haven't delved deep enough into the complexities and intricacies of the problem within a craft or situation, or in other words, you are too quick to generalize things and didn't pay enough attention and understanding into the details. We can certainly often get too ahead of ourselves and think that we know and understand what needed to be done, but in reality, we are unaware of our own lack of attention to the details due to our inborn haste to make sound judgments as quickly as possible. And number three, an unfocused, unstable, and preoccupied mind. This is what happens to those who choke in high presser situations and those who are slow learners, they are unable to be mentally present enough in the moment to focus on what's in front of them. And instead, their concentration bubble gets gate crash and drifts off into distractions precipitated by things such as anxiety or future circumstances, emotional attachment to past circumstances, and letting other forms of curiosities or temptations interfere with their mental bandwidth. Now, from that logical sense, when we face failure, we basically are aware that there are certain components that we lack that caused us to deliver unsatisfying results or to make major necessary changes so that we fulfill all those components. And all we need to do is to identify the holes in our work and where our weak links are and emphasize more on them so that we can deliver better results the next time we try. However, in the age of emotions of today, we are unable to think this way.

And instead, we took failure and look at them from an intimately personal standpoint and linked them into a mystical and metaphysical narrative where we attach our own default emotional reactions towards it for seemingly being permanently born to be cumbersome and incapable. And there we can do nothing about it besides self-deprecating ourselves through bawling our eyes, out, getting envious from people who are capable and seeking sympathy from people. You see, gentlemen, with the reason why we took failure rather too personally nowadays is because we have developed an unhealthy emotional and superstitious attachment or narrative towards failure. We treat our current incompetence and unreliability as if there are bound to our eventual fate by the spiritual cosmos of the universe and this kind of irrational, mythical, and spiritual thinking all started early in our age within our upbringings, how the environment and the people around us, especially figures of authority that we look up to and their level of control over us embed the idea of failure or anything for that matter, will have a dramatic effect in our attitude towards many aspects of life. I've said these exact same words in an earlier chapter, but it tears without a doubt crucial within our childhood that we are instilled on mental firmware that could assist us in tackling the circumstances that life will throw at us as we grow up during our period of adolescence, especially by our parents as human beings. The teachings and narratives that we grasp during our childhood years will have a huge rippling effect even when we are grown adults well within our years because our profound level of curiosity as children amplifies our sense of passion and enthusiasm, whether it is positive or negative, which will predispose us to develop strong memories and a religious or instinctual responses over them.

That is why we are often able to recall and remember circumstances from our childhood way more clearly and thoroughly than what we experienced during our adulthood. So if our overly controlling parents respond to our failures and instill them to us as a God-given sickness, then of course we will treat our failures as such every time we experience any form of failure, such as if your father repeatedly called you a quote unquote useless, brainless piece of shit who don't deserve anything, and I wish you had never been born every time you got a D in any of your school tests, then you will inevitably reflect that narrative to yourself every time you face failures. But if your empathetic and reassuring father responds to you by saying these words, when you experience failures, where do we force? Then you will inevitably recall that narrative to yourself every time you face failures. Two completely different attitudes towards a similar circumstance. Now, unfortunately, for a lot of us grown men in the modern era, we have been instilled those crippling and defeatist narrative towards failure by our parents and now being nailed into the coffin even more through the disillusioned and depressing emotional contents that we consumed every day of the year, as well as the demoralizing people we surround ourselves with every end of the week. And that made a lot of us gentlemen on suicide watch reminding and defining our lives. There's nothing more than just a pointless and painful existence no matter how much we actually try to be better, even if we are already genuinely trying our very best. And that miserable sensation is all because of what narrative you have exposed yourself to and what narrative you are currently exposing yourself to that eventually contaminate your own mental dialogue with yourselves. Remember gentlemen, the core often unseen and un interpreted objectives of our daily habits or routines will become the blueprints of the manner of approach in which our mentality dictates us. So how can we rewire our mental firmware to have a completely different and constructive view towards failure so that we don't concede into submission through the emotions we experience during failures? Simple, expose yourself thoroughly to the complete opposite narrative, both internally and externally. What you use to conceive and believe can be intricately shifted through the curiosity and deductive reasonings of another belief set and eventually getting the results that you want out of them. Like for example, this chapter exposes you to a new narrative towards failure than what your parents or the people around you may have instilled within you all this time.

And if you apply this narrative into your life and start to notice results and improvements, you will gradually adopt this narrative and abandon the old one. That is why a lot of us turn to motivational or self-improvement contents and figures of authority that are quite tough love. In order for us to break free of our previous mentality and belief set that didn't get us anywhere we want to, it will take time to adopt a new mental firmware and it will be uncomfortable as our mind is like a muscle. It needs to be trained to adapt to a new stimulus and environment. Diverting your mind away from what you are used to routinely or religiously visualize and cogitate will be an uncomfortable process, but it is absolutely necessary to make cognizant changes if you are not getting the results that you want out of your current arsenal. And I don't want to sound like a motivational speaker at all, but it is necessary to say this, quitting is a choice as long as you don't quit living. There is always a chance for you to get somewhere in life. They are both rationally and metaphorically true.

CHAPTER FIFTY-EIGHT
THE SINGLE MOST EFFECTIVE WAY TO HANDLE CRITICIZMS

"Don't give a sh*t about what other people think of you!!!" is what has been fed to us for as long as we can remember that line. That statement can only come from people who once cared too much and paid the price for being vulnerable, naïve & ignorant about how communication between people works & behaves in reality. Opinions & criticisms are inevitable when it comes to communication, and being too enthusiastically & idealistically open about them, makes you prone & unprepared to defend yourselves against the extremes of verbal abuse & bullying, and being too begrudgingly resentful about them, will eventually make you become deluded within your own opinion and sabotaging the opportunity for you to grow. It's all about selecting which of them we should care & which of them we should care, and how do we select them?

we're going to discuss about how we should deal with the opinions, perceptions, and criticisms of other people. This is an extremely important one, as it seems people are still struggling with this particular issue, even though they have been remarked millions of times to not care about them. Eventually, it gets them to become chronically frustrated and inevitably compromising their own mental health through imploding their own mental dialogue with themselves. Now, let me just start by telling you gentlemen, a simple truth. We cannot completely ignore people's opinions and treat them as if they're just some gusts in the wind. We are social creatures for many different reasons, and we are biologically hardwired to engage in social interactions or activities in order to help us further solidify our judgments and make better decisions with regards to many different aspects about life and the world we live in to complement our chances of survival, that here's why we have the natural tendencies to compare and contrast ourselves with other people, that here's why we love to exchange ideas and opinions, to cultivate our level of knowledge and understanding from different perspectives. And before some of you say, oh, you're wrong, we don't naturally seek social interactions. I'm more comfortable on my own. In fact, I feel even more alone when I'm with people. Well, that's because you are hanging around with the wrong people that don't compliment your own values and circumstances. Of course, you wouldn't last. Every loner and lone wharf are secretly hoping and trying to find a pact that they can conform to stop lying to yourself. If we are natural loners, loneliness won't be a problem to human beings. Social media wouldn't even exist, and they wouldn't have become the mecca of the world's operations and activities they are today. However, as much as we like to naturally interact with other people to showcase or exchange ideas, concepts, and opinions, it won't always be a walk in the park. Disagreements, arguments, debates, criticisms, and even verbal abuse are bound to occur when we are dealing with the awakening and collision of multiple cognitive dissonances and ego investments. When we start to care too much or get too invested in them, it can compromise our own mental wellbeing. Because of the complexity and polarity in both the way human beings make judgments and the way they communicate or deliver their judgments; they can throw us off balance. That is why we are constantly fed by the opposite narrative to not give a floating shit about them. However, there is a problem or limitation with this narrative. Caring too little or completely ignoring people's opinions and judgments of us will eventually shield us away from our own potential for further personal development and can escalate to us being diluted with our own incomplete or shallow judgments, especially with regards to our own character, knowledge, and set of attitudes. Now, I will wholeheartedly admit that I was also guilty of being too ignorant and delusional to say that I absolutely and completely don't care about what people think about me, the usual love me or hate me attitude while in reality secretly I still do to an extent even now. You see gentlemen, what made all of us so bewildered, insecure, and frustrated in dealing with other people's opinions of us is with regards to three crucial reasons that must be understood. Number one, we do not know the extent on which of them and how many of them we should care about. Number two, from whose opinions we should care about. And number three, the attitude on how we should perceive opinions from the many ways people can deliver them. In other words, one, we have very little awareness and acknowledgement of our own set of trades that we both should pay more attention and shouldn't pay any attention to when people give us their opinions about them. Two, we want to know from which specific type of individuals we should pay attention to when they give us their opinions. And three, how we should perceive opinions from different types of tonality in which they are delivered with. In essence, it's all about filtering, which we should care about and which we shouldn't care about. Now, in terms of the traits that we need to pay more attention to when people give their opinions on, in this case, it's going to be slightly different from person to person, but it all comes down to these four metrics. One, whether those traits are personally meaningful for you and your wellbeing. Two, whether they are crucial or critical for survival. Three, whether they contribute positively to your very own personal development. And four, whether they are things that are in your control. You want to care on the traits about yourself and people's opinions about them that will quote unquote constructively and realistically contribute to those four metrics. If they do not constructively and realistically contribute to any of those four metrics, do not give a rat sauce about them or people's opinions about them. For example, things such as your personal appearance, lifestyle knowledge, and financial wellbeing are things that you can control, contribute massively to your own personal development, and they are crucial or critical for your survival. And things such as your height, the shape of your nose or your genetics are things that you have absolutely no control over, and they contribute literally nothing to your personal development in terms of from whose opinions, criticisms, and judgements we should care about. It's fairly simple and straightforward. Really identify those people who fulfill at least two, but ideally all of these three criteria. Number one, people of much higher authority and reputation than yourself so that you have more assurance of their credibility or competence in the areas of life that you want to improve on. Number two, people that you can significantly relate to your real-life circumstances, so they actually understand the nuts and bolts of what you're going through both cognitively and emotionally. And number three, people whom you can take significant or full aspirations from so that you can be showcased and have more clarity in the direction you want to go in life and the steps that you have to take. So, it's pretty simple really.

If you gentlemen encounter an online troll or an online bully whom you have absolutely no acquaintance or association with, and who doesn't have any form of credibility, relatability, and positively encouraging reputation, why would you even care of what they have to say? And speaking of online trolls and bullies, now we come to the part on how we should perceive people's opinions from the vast array of tonality and medium that they can deliver them with. Now, this is probably the part where all of us struggle the most. In fact, I think this is the main reason of why we eventually in begrudgingly decide to not care about people's opinions on us. The way people's opinions, criticisms and judgments are delivered are very important to the perspective or the attitude in which we eventually acknowledge them. One, criticism can be delivered in two different ways in tonality, and they can have dramatically different effect on how we grasp them. Of course, all of this depends on the individual's level of familiarity and tolerance. For example, one person can criticize another person's appearance through an empathetic and nurturing tone. Like, this is quite worrying me, mate, your weight gain is making you harder to be taken seriously by others, and it's starting to take a toll on your health as well. You should consider going to the gym and start a weight loss journey. I'll help you out, and another person can criticize through a brutal and straightforward tone like, look at you, you flabby bird. No wonder girls don't want to fuck you because you literally look like a molten mashed potato. You are willing to die a virgin. Go and lift some weight. And many of us struggle to grasp the latter because we are too occupied with the emotional impact of a non-empathetic or non-formal form of communication. But if I'm going to be honest, when it comes to personal criticisms, and your feelings. Really, the only thing that matters is not how the opinion is delivered. It's what's in the opinion itself. Look for the substance behind them, gentlemen, no matter what tonality they are delivered with, if the opinions or criticisms have absolutely no substance reflection to your reality, relatability, congruency, and constructiveness within them, you should absolutely don't give two shits about them all in all though, gentlemen, the most important thing is your own brutal and realistic assessments of yourselves. So many of us are afraid to do that, and we rely on people's opinions to dictate our thoughts and actions no matter how useless and insignificant they are to us, because for some reason, we care more about people's opinions on us than our own assessments of ourselves indefinitely and eventually making us seeking or prioritizing their approval over our own Gentlemen, your own practical and reasonable judgments of yourselves are what will ultimately be the deciding factor of how genuinely satisfied, confident, and proud you are of your own existence. Because that is why you will radiate to everyone that encounters you, regardless of their opinions and criticisms. If you are able to become more level-headed and pragmatic towards yourself and your circumstances than any other person on earth can be to you. All of the things that I've said previously wouldn't matter much. Unfortunately, today that is hardly the case. As we are afraid to even look at ourselves in the mirror and judge ourselves with a level of honesty that causes discomfort yet incentivizes the urge to grow.

CHAPTER FIFTY-NINE
HARD WORK

How is the word hard work defined in the minds of all of you gentlemen? Is it about constantly delivering physical and mental punishments to yourselves while hoping for the best outcome to manifest itself in front of you? Is it about collecting Callister so that you can remind yourselves of what you are actually capable of and that you can push yourselves a lot more? Or is it about utilizing your intuitive wittiness to find and create opportunities that allows you to navigate and maneuver around the pitfalls or dead ends and catapults you higher up on the ladder? For me, hard work is a perfect combination of both dedication and sacrifice, both whose effectiveness are dictated by the most precious commodity or currency of the mall time. We all know time is the most valuable thing in a human life because time represents our own individual limited period of existence. As you can never, ever get it back once you spend it. Unlike money and the extent of our power control or effort to try to prolong and save time is barely minimal or most of the time impossible to make even a noticeable impact. The sole principle or law of time with regards to the human life and human nature is absolute. You will only get more or the most out of anything with the amount of time that you are willing to put in or spend on it. In terms of dedication, it's all about your level of commitment, a measure of devotion towards your obligations within the fields of work or endeavors that you have chosen. And yes, it is straightforwardly measured by the amount of time you are purposefully allocating on a daily basis into fulfilling those obligations and your own willingness to go beyond your call of duty. The value of time in this case is way less about chasing the numerical additions of how long you carry out your work, but it is about how much of those time you spent daily engaged within your utmost concentration to cultivate your capacity of knowledge, understanding, and experience, because those are what will inevitably and effectively contribute to your state or position of progression. I spent 12 hours a day learning how to code, or I go to the gym two hours a day, but what portion of that time do you actually spend concentrating at your hardest to elevate and refine your capabilities through polishing your practice or repetitions? What portion of that time do you actually spend reaching, discovering, and testing your limitations? And what portion of that time or beyond that time do you actually spend analyzing, investigating, and experimenting further to potentially discover new augmentations within the scope of your knowledge and understanding in your fields of work? Those are what truly matters, not the time you spent getting distracted or doing mindless dimwitted and pointless work that does not contribute to anything, but rather get you to store or regress. How I personally picture dedication is living a disciplined, regimented, and scheduled military life, or purposefully constructed for your own development. And yes, let's be honest, it is far from living the perfect life and it is most certainly far from being considered as favorable and pleasurable. They are initially unpleasant, but it is undoubtedly considered as quote unquote absolutely necessary for your own sake with regards to the wellbeing of your present and future circumstances, putting in the time to wholly commit to the essential deeds when you don't feel like it is not a pleasant thing to experience. A lot of the times you will want to punch someone in the face just to relieve yourself from the frustration, boredom, and pain coming from the arduous and the Ted of your regiment, not to mention the bitter taste that will attempt to discourage you coming from the unpredictability of uncontrollable circumstances that will go against you, such as experiencing lack of results despite the efforts and being halted or slumped from your progress because of an injury. This is where you need to remind yourself and keep the vision of your end goals remain as clear as they were when you started because without them, you will eventually and often prematurely yield as you virtually and plausibly have nothing left to hold onto in terms of sacrifice, it's all about identifying and managing your opportunity costs. It's pretty much the measure of the magnitude and frequency of physical translation or demonstration with regards to your principal priorities in comparison to all the others, the value of time in this case is more in the numerical additions. As the amount of time, you spend doing one thing can be allocated additionally or entirely into the time you spent doing another more important thing, it's an innate behavior. What you prioritize most will always be the one you put most of your time, thoughts, and efforts into as they say it. People never lack the time to do something or go somewhere. They just don't prioritize them enough to be willing to sacrifice a significant portion of their time for them.

Your actions will always be more impulsively acquainted with your instincts and desires than your words will ever be because words are much easier to manipulate an action to sacrifice something in order to cultivate and attain. Another thing may sound like an easy feat, but it isn't. Sacrifice isn't merely just a simple choice. It is quite a significant dilemma between all the things that actually are significant in your list of priorities, and you have to give up some of them that you are personally fond of doing or at least are habituated in doing in order for you to attain significance in the other more predominant endeavors. It's all about which eventual circumstances in life do you want more to manifest, and which daily endeavors will bring you ever so closer to that circumstance. And it's not easy, I'm telling you to do much less or completely stop doing the things that have become habituated within you. Like videogames, relationships and social life are definitely not easy just to instantly disregard and neglect because you already have spent a lot of time on them, and they have become a significant part of you. But ultimately, the same question remains, which end destination do you want more, and which collection of endeavors possess the clear set of steps or directions to take you there? If they do not move you any closer to the end destination, then allocate much, much less time on them. Or simply just don't give them any time of the day. Like for example, unless you are still a teenager and really bloody good at videogames and aiming to be a professional gamer one day, what good is there for you playing videogames for 15 hours a day? Why don't you do things that facilitates you towards your goals instead? The same thing with relationships and social life. If they become stagnant, discouraging, and aimless and pretty much turn into roadblocks in front of your ambitions, then let them go or commit way less time on them. It won't be easy, and it certainly will bring some emotional tension between you and them, but there are no feelings involved here. It's simply a personal decision. There is no need, need to feel bad about the petty feelings of someone when it comes to making crucial life decisions that you want because they have no right to tell you how to live your life as they are not responsible, and they don't pay your bills. Be ruthless because you're going to die one day and one of the worst feelings to swallow is regretting the time you waste not exploring your potential or because you're too occupied yet forgotten in the shadows of other people's lives. Now, for those of you who argue that working smart is far absolute to working hard, in an ideal world, yes, because we all want to work the least and achieve maximum results, but in reality, you need both. Hard work alone is not enough because you can't face the world blindly. You have to know what you are doing. You have to know the waters you're going to be venturing deep into. You have to have a firm idea or at least some idea of the scope of every decision you make and every action you take within your chosen fields. Don't spend time committing into an endeavor that has no clear end goal or won't eventually affect the circumstances of your livelihood significantly, because that is when and where despite all the hard work, it won't get you anywhere close to your eventual destination. Smart work alone is not enough because you must be able to sustain circumstances beyond your control that can negatively impact your efforts and results. And without the tenacity, perseverance, and grid that is developed through hard work, you won't make it far down the line. Figuring out more efficient and effective ways to get results is one thing. Sustaining circumstances that will get in the way of your efforts and results is another. That is why many crypto investors who had no idea what they're doing or what world they're in or contemplated suicide and even some did commit suicide when the massive crash happened. And another thing to mention is that to eventually do smart work, you need to cultivate vast amounts of knowledge so that you can possess a profound understanding of the game that you are playing, and that purely comes from hard work.

CHAPTER SIXTY
THE VICTIM MENTALITY

Being caught too often within the receiving end of the unpleasantness that the world has to offer will a lot of the times completely break a man's spirit and turn it for the worst into the opposite extremities. The mountainous accumulation of pain that he experienced in his reality will shatter all of his expectations and ideals that he had been conditioned for years to believe and hang onto. And we all know reality is always a lot darker and way more sinister or unforgiving than the barrage of overly delusional optimism and make beliefs that we are often fed with by those who deny reality and wrap them around their own collection of so cystic subjectivism human beings are inherently incapable of handling the entirety of truth on how the world actually operates in the most transparent and rawest level. And when all of the confidence within their own romantic assumption's assurances, predictions, forecasts, and hopes are utterly demolished by the natural law of the universe and humanity that they refuse to acknowledge and understand the immense magnitude of dissonance, disappointment and disbelief will unleash a seemingly endless string of negative emotions that would cloud their judgments and eventually dictate both their decisions and actions. The profound feelings of anger, despair, hate resentment, bitterness, and lust for vengeance overwhelms his state of mind and transform him into an extremely single-minded anarchist. I mean, being a man who was bullied, betrayed, abused, condemned, banished, abandoned, and forgotten, they will accumulate a collection of painful experiences that will, without a doubt, generates endless questions within him that need desperate answering. Because of course, we all learn significantly better from painful experiences rather than pleasurable experiences. And if he can't find those answers or if he's unable to accept those answers that had been given to him, he will inevitably develop his own selfish answers based on his own shallow and incomplete perspectives that only prioritizes the satisfaction of the immediate reaction of his instincts or ego towards his bleak circumstances. And that is to react impulsively. And yes, innately speaking, forgiveness is a hard thing for human beings to eventually learn and adopt. Vengeance is our natural response. In order to eradicate threats, eliminate competitions and satiate emotional cravings, it's the classic villain mindset to utilize once painful experiences to inflict pain to those who delivered pain to him in the first place. And to those who has an experience, all the pain that he had giving everyone who wronged him a taste of their own medicine to witness their state of agony, suffering, and eventually their unpleasant demise, it's an extremely impulsive decision. That is why being a hero is a lot harder than being the villain because a hero has to withheld and overcome all of those impulsive tendencies. Now, it is not to say that experiencing the victim mentality ourselves isn't a normal thing that occur when we experience pain. It is in fact very normal to feel that way. It's simply an emotional response. But what separates the ones that eventually succeed in controlling those negative emotions and those who let them soar into a cataclysmic force of destruction are those that are able to effectively compromise and disconnect the self-evident reality of the circumstances that they experienced from all of their previously adopted or conditioned ideals, expectations, perspectives, and ego investments. Our lingering hatred and bitterness does not come from experiencing painful or unfair circumstances. No, it's all because our spiritually invested propositions are practically contradicted by the visible, noticeable, and perceptible reality that cause tremendous level of dissonances and disputes in which our sense of self-esteem or self-worth refused to concede and or could not handle. In conceding, for example, a lot of us wholeheartedly believe that human beings are purely creatures of peace, love, compassion, and empathy because we are gifted with those capabilities, and yet we refuse to acknowledge that we are also gifted with destructive and mischievous qualities as well, such as our desire and capacity to physically hurt other people and tell a bunch of lies to fulfill our selfish intentions. When other people start to display these supposedly sinister qualities, they identify them as ridiculously and utterly inhumane, who while also denying their own capacity and capabilities to perform such conduct should the situation cause for them to do so. They refuse to accept that those dark qualities also make up a significant part of being human. Like if they're forced to defend themselves from someone who wants to kill them to the ends of earth, they will have to put him down for good in order to put a stop to his never-ending murderous intent and survive. The victim mentality is actually the initial emotional phase when our optimistic narratives are contradicted with reasonable evidence. Because we are desperately trying to find a way to prove our own claims, and because we are unable to do so, our stubbornness will seek a way out by impulsively trying to find false defects and inconsistencies within those evidence. Kind of like Amber, her trying to desperately justify her claims against all the evidence that has been brought up against her. In the end, though, whether that mentality remains or not, it all depends on your ability to momentarily compromise against incoming reasonable narratives and perspectives in order for you to further evolve your own knowledge and judgments regarding certain circumstances that before you, because if you remain unyielding pigheaded within your own bubble of ideals, while keep getting contradicted with firsthand tangible or plausible evidence, then you will remain resentful and keep pointing fingers at the world for operating within its own nature. The sad thing about the victim mindset is that internally he's also desperately seeking for someone who would sympathizes with him and understands both his circumstances and conducts. But unfortunately, this isn't the movies where one could follow him alongside every step he takes, and also experience the exact same circumstances that he went through to fully understand him. Because in the real world, most people couldn't care less as one's own problem is one's own authority and responsibility to solve. No one wants to be with someone who is a sensitive, miserable, and emotionally nihilistic wreck that hurts other people for pleasure or because he couldn't endure a series of bad days and bad luck, which let's be honest, happens to everyone on this planet. They just refuse to give them any form of highlight for other people to notice. No one will respect he who does not even try his best to change his circumstances for the better, and instead continuously moaning, grumbling, and protesting their problems to desperately look for any forms of concern.

CHAPTER SIXTY-ONE
SELF-HATE AND INSECURITIES

Never let your degenerative thoughts about your own unfortunate & uncontrollable attributes, overcome your desire to strive to experience the finer things in life. No man is born equal, one person's circumstances maybe slightly/significantly worse than another, and that can throw you off balance mentally about your state of worthiness. However, your tenacity to become more despite the disadvantages that you are born with & those of your own doing, will eventually put you in a place where you can be equal/better than those who are initially more fortunate than you. Insecurities are one of the hardest things to deal with on a personal level, and it's made even worse by the presence of social media through the overstimulation of novelty. It's the gutted feeling of inadequacies, insignificance, and incompatibility to keep up or attain to the metrics, benchmarks, standards, and expectations of the world, of which, let's be honest, are significantly unrealistic and overly stigmatized or manufactured or manipulated. Life as we know it is absolutely unfair, and it has always been. So, people are born with different circumstances. Some are fortunate and others are born without limbs or food on their table. This is just the reality of the world we live in, gentlemen, and as I've always said, millions of times we have to get used to that truthful narrative and accept that a lot of us are born with noticeable or significant deficiencies, shortcomings, and disabilities. We all desire to be accepted as social creatures. We all want to be acknowledged and be a significant part of a mutually connected community. However, the bitter reality of our nature as human beings is that we always instinctually want to avoid or exterminate the minority, crippled lonesome, and the unfortunate because they run the risk of jeopardizing the state of our welfare and survival. Like if you are part of a community where protection, resources, fellowships, and reproduction are strongly engraved or established, why would you run the risk of compromising your own state of wellbeing by leaving them to join a lone, crippled and impoverished individual? Of course, your survival instinct will dominate your judgments by showcasing hesitancy, dismissal, and rejection, and it can even go as far as imposing discrimination, underestimation, ridicule, mockery, and even abuse if we feel bothered or threatened. In other words, those of us who are disadvantageous will not be primarily prioritized by others and will eventually get completely ignored by them.

In the case of US men in the modern world, the issue of physical shortcomings, genetical defects, unfavorable history or background, and the state of incompetence and unreliability are the main sources of our insecurities. Short height, lack of hair, lack of resources, small genitals, limited knowledge, shortage of skills, and absence of family. This degrading sensation of pure insubstantiality, inconsiderable, wretchedness, and worthlessness just eats away at us to the point where we desperately wish to be born a completely different person. Unfortunately, that wish is nothing but to complete and utter impossibility and to make things worse, no matter how much we condemn the unreasonable and unrealistic standards of the world, they are already established and will always be imposed on us for as long as we live, and they're more likely to get even more amplified. So how can we overcome this? There is only one way compensation. There are insecurities that are completely out of your control, and you can do nothing about and insecurities that you have significant control over that you can eventually turn into a worthful, or valuable advantages and supremacists cultivate those that you can control so remarkably until they overshadow those that you can't control. For example, you can't control how tall you are, nor can you control the length and girth of your dick, but you certainly can control your body composition and your level of knowledge and skills, which will eventually give you control over the level of resources that you can accumulate. If a man who is short, small, and bold, but is exceptionally built, able to fight humorous and wealthy, he wouldn't be primarily known as the short, small, and bold guy. Sure, they may get mentioned from time to time, but that's not what he will be acknowledged and remembered for because those are not and won't be.

His valuable standout qualities that people are looking for and will be paying more attention and consciousness to. Life is significantly competitive, and for all of us that are unfortunate and disadvantageous, we have no choice but to do more and work much harder in order to eventually become equal in significance to the others or even more significant than them. Another thing that is worth mentioning for the insecurities that you can't control is with regards to the matter of attitude. The amount of attention and consideration people give to your deficiency significantly depends on your own level of attention and consideration towards them. People will give a lot of shit about them only if you give a lot of shit about them. Demeanors are contagious. We all know that, and people can innately sense this through subtle social sub communications like your body language, tone of voice and level of eye contacts. So, if you are internally deprecating and selling yourself short because of your insecurities, people will eventually develop that same attitude towards you. You must be the one who dictates the narrative of your own presentation towards other people because people will ultimately judge your character based on the level of authority you have over yourself. How you think about yourself will ultimately lead to how others think about you because they radiate into plausibility and tangibility through your physical demonstrations. So, control the narrative of your deficiencies and twist them into a positive demeanor. I'll give you an example to make things clearer to you gentlemen. One of me mates have unusually long and lanky legs. They're so anatomically disproportionate in comparison to his torso that even how heavy he squats doesn't significantly impact their size. We occasionally poke fun on his skinny legs as all of us men would do in our friendships, and if he was so insecure of them, he would've said things like, yeah, man, it sucks, bro. I wish I was born a different person in an extremely depressing manner and maybe further escalates his deprecation by endlessly explicating his insecurities. Instead, he said these words, dudes, I deeply apologize that I caused severe discomfort within your eye for aesthetics because fortunately, my families were direct descendants of African giraffes that all of us had to get custom-made pants because no available size pants would fit a soul without exposing our naked ankles. Obviously, he hasn't got the best sense of humor in the world, but he exaggerates the narrative of his deficiency to the point of unreasonableness, and he puts them in a positive limelight with the definitive tone inevitably taking control and dictating the narrative for all of us that is in the room with him, which makes us develop an attitude towards his deficiencies the way he did. And again, we all know that positivity and resolute is contagious or infectious. So, cultivate those insecurities that you can control to turn them into valuable traits and twist the narrative of those you can't into a positive narrative so that people will subconsciously overlook your shortcomings in favor for your quality attributes and upbeat or absolute demeanor. Ensure there are people who will try to constantly pray and capitalize on your deficiencies no matter what. In that case, the best thing you could do is completely dismiss them because predatory people will always try their best to get an emotional reaction from you to establish control, and pretty much they're doing that to divert attention away from their own insecurities. If you are massively insecure, there is absolutely no use in feeling sorry for yourselves, hoping that someone will come and sooth your brows and eventually give you a blowjob because again, the world doesn't care and will ignore all of you who are crippled. How often have you ever heard or seen a homeless disabled beggar on the streets get picked up by wealthy individuals and eventually living the dream life?

Especially if you're a man? I say never depressing and unfair. Yes, but it is undoubtedly possible to eventually thrive if you are willing to do significantly more as a disadvantaged individual in the end. As always, it is your own choice to make.

CHAPTER SIXTY-TWO
THE STATUS GAME

It may pain, some of you gentlemen to hear this, but it really helps out a lot when you know a lot of people and when people like you, opportunities, lessons, assistances, new experiences, favors and connections, all of them play a huge role in determining the eventual circumstances of your life. Like one could be given a job opportunity of a lifetime if he knows the right people and one could get out of a catastrophic life-threatening situation like a prison sentence if he knows the right people. When people like you or want to work with you or are fond of you or like being around you, it will by default entice a positive mental reaction, projection, and judgment from most of other people who haven't known you yet by subconsciously reaffirming or pred declaring to them that you are someone of respectable qualities and value. It's like a restaurant with a long queue up front. Most people will positively wonder what makes this restaurant so special that so many people will want to wait for a long time just to dine in it. Social proof right now, I know I've said this a million times, but a lot of the narrative that is being shoved deep into our throats these days, especially within the self-improvement world, is to absolutely not care whatsoever about what people think about you and how they view you as an individual and are used to believe this wholeheartedly back in the day, and for sure it has its own set of appeals and applications in certain circumstances of life. Like when you are taking your first major risk in life and people are finding it very hard to believe that you can make it, or when a group of shallow minded people are criticizing you without or lacking the presence of any rationality and objectivity whatsoever, then it is appropriate to adopt or utilize that mindset. However, after some further analysis and personal experiences, that mindset actually have some limitations that may end up sabotaging your own growth as an individual along the way when you become overly fixated about it, especially when it comes to wanting to associate yourself with respectable and reputable individuals that can contribute tremendously in a positive way within your life. That limitation being, it can dilute and seclude you within your own bubble of attributes and beliefs that are still in need of much further improvement and evolution, especially when you are still young. You see, gentlemen, no matter how much we like to do things all on our own, eventually we will reach a point where we can't do everything by ourselves. We have our own limitations to what and how many things we can do simultaneously within our given skillset, scope, timeframe, and both physical and mental bandwidth. That is where we need the right group of people around us to help one another grow to new heights in life. And in order to become someone respectable enough for these respectable people to want to associate with, we must develop and establish a reputation for ourselves to eventually earn their attention and consideration. In other words, status bluntly speaking, it's the way you sell yourself to others and how high you are valuing yourself. Now, of course, it doesn't mean that you have to go to the extent of begging hard to be acknowledged by literally prostituting yourself. No. It's just simply building a valuable reputation for your own sake so that circumstances are more likely and have more chances to go your way because you will inevitably develop a reputation as you are climbing the ladder as it is a default after effect of the accumulation and magnitude of your work or deeds, and there is so much on the line when it comes to your own reputation, so you must develop and protect it at all cost because as you become more established, more people will take notice of you and some of them will also be secretly wanting to bring you down and sabotage your ascension because of course not everyone is going to like you and it only takes one word to completely incapacitate one's credibility. But anyway, so how can you elevate your reputation or improve your status as an individual to help you ascend further up the ladder? Number one, having a polarizing and imposing appearance, I mean this is a no-brainer really. It's the most basic and simple way to build notoriety as everything and everyone is judged externally at first. No matter how many delusional cons say that you cannot judge a book by its cover, it's absolute bullshit. Everything is judged and will always be judged externally at first. A book's content wouldn't matter much if someone is not enticed or intrigued enough to pick a top and flip its cover to read what's inside of it. It's the same thing with looks and appearance. How you look determines the way you present or package yourself, your body size, shape, composition, and personal sense of style, they all will project a series of glimpses or snippets in terms of the quality of your character in the minds of other people. Basically, people can and will subconsciously judge what you are and who you are as a person just by the way you present yourself in front of them, and we all know how important first impressions are. No matter how valuable or special you think you are, if people can't or won't take you seriously, they wouldn't bother to make further efforts to get to know you further or even want to be affiliated with you in any way, shape, or form. Like if you want to buy an iPhone and it's packaged in a red plastic bag like the apple that you bought in a supermarket, you would inevitably think that it's a bit anticlimactic for such an expensive item to be presented in such a cheap manner and you will subconsciously start to have doubts in its quality and capability regardless of its actual quality and capability just because it looks so mistreated, unattended and neglected. If you highly respect yourself, you will inevitably take great care of yourself, and it is the first sign of a highly valuable trait and attribute as a person. So, build your body and dress impeccably nice, especially as a man. Better yet, dress differently or superiorly than most people because we all know that commonality eventually brings contempt, so it is much better to be overdressed than normally dressed or underdressed as they say it. There is absolutely no harm in being ahead of schedule and being overdressed as anything in life that is worth doing for your own sake is worth overdoing. Plus, it separates you from the rest because you bring a distinctive stimulus that people will be more intrigued by and inevitably pay more attention to. Number two, being a man of the people. Now of course, it isn't just all about looks, it's also about your attitude towards life and people in general and being a man of the people. It's not all about licking their asses and desperately thirsting to get a blowjob back from them like a pathetic people pleaser, nor is it about trying to always be the center of attention in every social interaction. No, it's all about giving people few or many a good time and worthwhile moments to look back and remember because people may forget your name and they may forget how exactly you look like, but they will never forget how you make them feel. It's about becoming someone people would want to hear more from and someone people would want to be more with, and there are no better ways to do that than cultivating and implementing these three timeless and foolproof methods. The first one is sense of humor. Now, who in their right sane mind does not want to have a good laugh? Everybody wants it. Well, everybody except those who takes everything too personally like a sensitive little push just like the modern blue head walruses humor takes away the repetitive dress and mundaneness of everyday life and it livens the atmosphere to where you can take a momentary break from the stress and seriousness of real-life problems and just look at life from an amusement and entertainment point of view. There is no question that people with a good sense of humor are so magnetically attractive as they are able to turn the negativity of a mood into a positive and enthusiastic demeanor, and who doesn't love to be around with someone who possesses that capability? It's infectious to turn the most reclusive and depressed man in the room into someone who's not afraid to showcase their passion. People love to feel good and love to releases those chemical endorphins from our brain then makes us feel good and let's be on shall we. We all could use a lot of that for as long as we live. Now, for those of you who are wondering how to cultivate a sense of humor, the easiest way is to lightly poke fun over your own weaknesses, escalate circumstances to the point of rational or reasonable absurdity, or just introduce some ambivalent irony into the mix. How do you think the British got the best sense of humor in the world? Sarcasm, baby.

The second one is wisdom. Now, having wisdom is not about being a bottomless emotional tampon for people who can't handle their own problems, nor is it about trying to desperately solve one's problem by any means necessary because I know for a lot of us, especially men, we'd like to go far and beyond our capabilities to try and solve another person's problems, women's own emotional problems, especially that only they themselves are able to solve. Having wisdom is all about giving people a much-needed realization and clarity of their own shortcomings and letting them make their own choice whether to eventually take accountability for their problems or not. Now, I know some of you are going to say, well, won't you take away from the whole giving people a good time and making them feel a good narrative? Yes, it will initially, but eventually what realization will give people is that liberating sense of relief no matter how much dissonance and emotional conflicts they experience initially, eventually they will no longer feel lost about where to go and what to do because wisdom simply points them towards that direction that they needed to go and the matters that are in need to be put to work to eventually make their circumstances better. Of course, it's all their choice whether to make or break to cultivate wisdom is not easy. You have to experience a lot of circumstances in life, especially the unpleasant side of it.

You must be able to relate to the other person both cognitively and emotionally, and you must also be able to see things reasonably from different angles and perspectives, both from a large picture and the intricate details within the connection of the dots of both cause and effect to arrive at a realistic and meaningful conclusion. And the third one is storytelling. Now, this is something not a lot of people emphasize about the ability to tell a good story will do absolute wonders for you because what good storytelling does is that it captivates people's curiosity by letting them project their own fun or horror induced imaginations as you cinematically or dramatically narrate them of your accounts and it can escalate the anticipation in something that they are looking forward to or not looking forward to in trying out or experience. People naturally and innately seek novelty in various forms and by expressively narrating them accounts and experiences that they are in treat or afraid by but may have not gotten the chance to have a firsthand experience themselves. It'll induce the much-needed sense of enthusiasm or dread towards their expectations. It's all about getting people to tap into or run wild with their imaginations, which will both cognitively and emotionally captivate them enough to pay full attention to you. And imaginations are never boring because it represents people's ideals. Plus, it gives you the opportunity to invite and physically introduce them to those experiences firsthand as the point man, the one they're looking forward to. Of course, subconsciously giving them something significant or major to remember you buy. Another thing that storytelling tells people about you is that it gives people an insight into your life, the types of adventure that you seek, and an extent of your character traits as a person to become a good storyteller. Just like someone who has good wisdom, you must experience a lot of stuff in life and that can only come by you willing to take a lot of risks cumulatively because with every adventure there are always risks involved, but that's what's being a man is all about, right, and you must also vividly remember your accounts in a very intricate way so that you can narrate them however intimately and dramatically you want to captivate the person in front of you or the people around you. But the best thing about being a good storyteller is that you most likely will never run out of things to say and again, we could all use a lot of that as well. Number three, skills, accomplishments, and lifestyle. I'm going to combine skills and accomplishments together here because they're pretty much tied together like a mother and a toddler.

Now, in all honesty, nothing subconsciously screams and exudes control, command, confidence, dominance, and leadership than possessing a lot of necessary skills to navigate through life. Whether they are crucial survival skills, the ability to accumulate vast amounts of resources and social skills, all of them radiates a sense of security, guidance, and superiority as they take a considerable amount of time to learn, adopt and polish. Other people will innately be more inclined to want to work with you, learn from you, and lean on you at times of distress as when it comes to important life skills relating to survival and welfare. They are undoubtedly a collection of evergreen worth practicality that people of all generations would want to assimilate, possess, or at least be a big part of. The level of proficiency and competency you have regarding different fields are most of the time. In direct conjunction with the number of resources, accolades, establishments and positions you will accumulate, letting your resume speaks and radiates volume by itself through people's word of mouth without you ever needing to say a word. For me personally, it is the ultimate sign of social hierarchal prominence. Another thing that exudes high status is having a lifestyle that only few people can afford access and consider. Now, of course, it doesn't have to always involve jet skis, yes and private jets just live a unique, distinct, and exciting lifestyle full of novelty that most people rarely witness or hear about because like I've said before, commonality brings contempt. It doesn't generate enough excitement, no curiosity for people to want to be a big part of or even have the notion to give them a worthwhile thought. Number four, authority, and integrity. No matter how good looking, humorous, proficient, and wealthy you are, if you do not have a strong sense of authority over yourself, your life and the circumstances around you, people will capitalize on that weakness and leach off of you until you have nothing left. What I mean by authority in this case is having the frame of mind that patently originates from your own point of view, first and foremost towards everything in your life. For those of you who are still confused in the self-development world, it is defined as the masculine frame. Basically, it's about how you want things to be like and how you want them to operate or behave within your own space with regards to work, people, family, activities, et cetera.

Most people let others decide for them how things and circumstances in their lives should be like subconsciously, letting them take control over their decisions and actions, which is unquestionably both foolish and dangerous for your own sake because you basically allow people under their own free will to repeatedly cross your line of defense and just take advantage of you endlessly. If you want people to notice or acknowledge the level of respect and limitations towards you, you must make it clear to them by implanting a strong sense of dread and imminent consequences within their mind through demonstrating your unmitigated authority over yourself and the circumstances around you because people will constantly poke you or push your buttons to find out whether you are the kind of person who is a spineless cower that can't stand up for himself, or if you're actually someone who has a strong character that put things back in line, if they do go out place. The perfect example of this is the dynamic between Will Smith and his wife Jada. The next one is integrity. Now I'm going to make it short on this one because it is without a doubt one of the most straightforward methods to earn respect, trust, and acknowledgement from others. Just say what you're going to do and then go out and actually do it. Most people underestimate this particular trade because they perceive that saying or declaring something has a similar level of complication as going out on actually doing them. Just declaring that you're going to lose weight and get jacked this year is a completely different game or world than actually losing weight and getting jacked. As most of us have known and experienced, people often try their best to sell themselves too highly in front of others, exaggerating their capabilities and over-inflating they're own assurance of trustworthiness. But in reality, most of them don't even have the capacity to fulfill those promises they've made to us and themselves yet alone make an actual effort to do so. So it is important for you to be a man of your word, to showcase the honesty, significance, and eagerness of your efforts and commitment as people will appreciate that highly because believe it or not, it's actually still quite a rare sight to see even today. And finally, number five, be genuinely invested in others. Yes, it's not all about us, but it's also about them. People are inherently impatient, and they can't wait to talk about themselves and their lives. The trouble is most of them are so occupied with wanting to open their mouth that no one wants to eagerly listen to what one has to say thoroughly before another person interrupts, and that is where you come in. You see gentlemen, being a good listener is also a valuable trait that people are looking for. Just being able to sit there and be totally encapsulated within one person's string of dialogues without interrupting or making any form of judgments until that person has expressed or that he or she needed to express will get them to lower their guard down and open up more to you. People experience wide ranges of emotions through daily events, and oftentimes they either bottle it up to the point where it starts to infect their behavior and demeanor, or they express it online just to get that much needed release or to look for a sympathetic response only to find out that no one actually understand them or give a fuck about their problems. Every single person in this world desires to be accepted and understood, and by being a good listener, by being genuinely or entirely invested in what one person has to say and express, by making an effort to fathom their interpretation, they will slowly open up and instinctually consider you as someone that they could trust as they are in a state of both cognitive and emotional vulnerability, and yet they don't feel anxious nor threatened by you. Of course, don't just open your ears and not endlessly like a good dog. Ask them questions. Ask them to elaborate their statements to further showcase and establish your profound interest in them, making them more comfortable to eventually establish a bond with you. Now, I understand for some of you hardcore, don't give a fuck about other people's perception of you individuals. All of these may be considered as absolute rubbish, but the truth is, when we've built a reputation for ourselves, people's perception of us can significantly impact the trajectory of our lives. And let's be honest, when we want to allow other people to be a big part of our lives, we also want to extensively qualify them if they are someone whom we can trust and rely on, or if there's just a bunch of sneaky snitch bastards, we all care to a certain extent of how people perceive us. The big difference is being someone who wants to be perceived by people based on their own metric of how they ideally want to perceive themselves and those who want to be perceived by people based on how ideally and endlessly people want to perceive them. And I can guarantee that as men, all of the above things that I've mentioned are within your set of ideals on how you want to eventually perceive yourself as a man, which will inevitably lead to how others perceive you as a man.

CHAPTER SIXTY-THREE
THE TRUTH ABOUT LOYALTY

The deeds that we've done to please our significant other, all in the name of love, peace, devotion, loyalty & compassion, turns out to be our own undoing that resulted in our significant other losing their respect & desire in us. They left us wondering within our broken shell of why the more we love someone, the more we spend time on someone, the less they appreciate us.

It can be literally the most suffocating experience both physically and mentally. When you got separated from that special, someone whom you've poured every single ounce of your time, effort, resources, and being into or even worse, that special someone decided to leave you for someone else without saying a word. Despite everything that you've done for her, you will inevitably feel like your whole world had come crumbling down and a huge part of you is missing, seemingly taking away the very core reason for your existence. When we're young and naive, love easily blinds us. We all know that the notion that this special someone is quote unquote destined to be with us for the rest of our lives despite all the hard times that we are mentally and practically unprepared for or because we are convinced that the stars of the zodiac cosmos are perfectly aligned through the Milky Way, connecting the threads of the twin flames and paving the way towards the unbreakable magical aisle of the soulmates, right? Well, until our daily prayers got utterly ignored and our hopes got completely shattered by the natural mechanics of human nature, that is then we wonder Cluelessly like the ignorant idealists that we are of why the spouses of the fairy godmother and the angels of love didn't work. Even though we've done everything right now, the easiest thing to do and what most of us men do initially is that we start to put the entire blame on her for being a corrupt individual that turned her back on the righteous path of loyalty and faithfulness within the God protected realm of unconditional and unmitigated true love. Then we send our hateful prayers to karma, hoping that it will come after her and collect the massive moral depth that she owed us. Either that or we self-deprecate ourselves in utterly pathetic fashion, sedating our misery, we synthetic liquids and hoping that another fair lady would sympathize with our emasculated, sorrow, and rescue us by emptying our balls for the night. Now, I'm not going to beat around the bush any further here, and let's just cut straight to the chase. The word unconditional does not exist in the dictionary of love. Love has always been and will always be conditional. If love were unconditional, A Victoria's Secret model would spread her legs for a fat, smelly and broke man living underneath a bridge with only 20 bucks to his name.

Loving someone is first and foremost will always be about whether that someone has the attributes or most of the attributes that we are looking for from a significant other based on their gender. Is she hot? Is he tall and strong? Is she a virgin? Is he wealthy? It's always about what are you first before who you are, and if those attributes that one is looking for are gone, so will be the so-called love you are going to be receiving and experiencing from that person. Now, apart from the vast differences in life, cultures and priorities and severe mental health issues, turning the relationship toxic and abusive, the most common reason of why relationship fail is because of the failure in fulfilling the respective gender roles that they are expected to deliver within the relationship, and this failure is the eventual result of the cumulative effects with regards to the eventual absence, lack of diminishment and powerlessness surrounding those attributes that one is looking, looking for from their partner within the relationship that eventually culminate into a loss of both respect and desire between each other. If one fails to fulfill their role, the relationship is inevitably bound to fail. A man's default role in the relationship is to lead, protect, and provide. A woman's default role in the relationship is to follow support and nurture. For example, if she was initially hot, feminine, soft, spoken and nurturing when you met her, then over the years she slowly becomes lazy, fat, and smelly, while also revealing to be in an insufferable, nagging, and drummer field. Bitch, would you not eventually lose all respect and attraction that you initially had for her? Would you not be instinctually end biologically enticed to leave her and look for a better woman that can make your life a better place of existence? Of course, you would. Well, it is absolutely no different from the point of view of the woman. If you're initially a confident, ambitious, resourceful, hardworking, brave, mentally, strong, emotionally stable, fashionable, adventurous, humorous and competent leader of a man that she fell in love with the first time, but then as the relationship progressed over the years and your boss got emptied every day of the week, you get to complacent with where you are and you become fat, lazy, indecisive, insecure, unreliable, emotionally infantile, clingy, cowardly, desperate, and boring loser who remains stagnant in his life and refuses to grow further as an individual. Then let me ask you, gentlemen, if you turned out to be that kind of man, is it normal for your woman to eventually go dry in the bedroom and then be tempted to leave you and look for another man that can make her life a better place to live in? I'll definitely say so because you're no longer the man she thought you once were. You're no longer the man she's looking for and want to be with. You're no longer the man she looked up to and adored. Now of course, some of you gentlemen might think, well, it isn't fair. Isn't she supposed to be with us through thick and thin? Isn't she supposed to never leave us forever? Isn't that how loves supposed to work? Well, here's the thing, the world doesn't care because you are already expected to fulfill that role as the man in the relationship. In fact, she probably already gave you many chances to redeem yourself, but you got to complacent thinking that her disappointment in you will eventually subside and will forgive you in being a loser in a Disney movie. That may happen, but not a chance that's going to happen in real life, mate, here is the thing, gentlemen. Let's not look at intersexual relationship through a moralistic, spiritual or unethical lens. The truth is relationship is all about intersexual dynamics and it operates through a biological and evolutionary hardwiring ever since the hunter gatherer age, as much as we like to put so much emphasis or priority on personality and things in common when it comes to how a relationship will or will not work out, the truth is we, human beings will always be creatures of survival and we will always prioritize our survival and state of welfare first and foremost before anything, and it is no different to intersexual relationships. If from a man's perspective, a woman who is infertile to bear children is incapable of carrying the survival of our genetic legacy to the next generations because she's physically overweight, infectious, and incapable to nurture them towards good health, we would innately remove her from our selection of women that we want to bear our children with, and also our investment in paternity because she basically compromises the state of our survival. Similarly, from a woman's perspective, if a man who is physically inferior, unintelligent, unresourceful, incompetent and cowardly to protect and provide for both her and her offspring, she will instinctually remove him from the selection of men whom she wants to breed with, because those men threaten the survival of both her and her offspring.

Plus, women are the more vulnerable sex, and they have a finite timeframe to have children, so they are naturally way more selective and intuitive in choosing a mate than us men, so they can be literally more ruthless when it comes to leaving out the incompetent men that are not selected to breed with them. That is why there are way more men than women that are sexless today than it has ever before. No matter what spiritual barriers and ethics tries to oppose the way of our nature as human beings, most of the time, there will be utterly and ruthlessly abided by our survival instincts. She wouldn't care. If you are an actual romantic sweet pie at heart or if you're a quirky son of a bitch, when you absolutely got no pot to piss inmate, she will leave you for debt. Now, I completely understand that some of you may feel the anger after taking in all of this, and that is very much normal because you are basically in dissonance with your initial beliefs and conditioning. The worst thing you can do is deprecate yourself into the victim mindset and eventually hate on women for living within the loss of their own nature. Men and women are and will always be better together than we are on our own. Our specific and respective gender roles within the relationship complement each other's strengths and weaknesses, beautifully king and queen in perfect harmony, but in order to be better for the sake of each other, we must individually become better for our own sake. First, it is just a shame that in modern times, these respective gender roles are reversed and eventually wreaking havoc on the dynamic within the relationship and or marriage as a whole. Both men and women are suffering greatly because of this. Women unconsciously becoming the man that they look up to and want to be with all on their own while growing old and childless men becoming the women that they are looking for while being deprived of their masculinity and ridiculed for being weak, all because of society's ignorance, conditioning of female empowerment and oppression of masculinity that reverse the traditional roles that men and women are biologically hardwired to partake.

CHAPTER SIXTY-FOUR
BECOME THE BEST

Discipline and focus are extremely important to be adopted in order to further cultivate our sense of familiarity, adaptability, and eventually proficiency. With regards to a certain set of knowledge and skills within an endeavor or a craft, they are abilities necessary for our dedication to eventually become competent and seasoned. But for a lot of us, discipline and focus are either absent, forced, or they are divided among many different circumstances that eventually obstruct and impede our progression towards absolute mastery within our main commitment. This is what separates the good and the great from the best, or those who are on their way to becoming the best, the best lives and breeds their craft. Their levels of discipline and focus are already within the vicinity of obsession. So immersive and captivated are their minds that the other endeavors that are done within their daily routines are all purposely planned, adopted, and revolved around complimenting or supplementing their main commitment. So uncompromising are their attitudes that they are utterly prepared and willing to make great sacrifices that most people, like us gentlemen, would deem to be greatly impossible or unnecessary, like social lives and relationships, all in the pursuit of supreme mastery.

The slightly mistaken thing about focus that most of us believe is that it is all about the number of hours that you spent on a craft that will eventually get you to become skilled or proficient at something. Well, in actuality, to be more specific, it is the number of hours of intense immersion that actually counts towards your level of proficiency, the number of hours that you spent being thoroughly encapsulated within your work, where you will develop a deep and unprecedented level of rhythm and connection with them to the point where you will eventually lose all sense of time and space because your mental bandwidth is entirely occupied to the brink by the vast scope of your work. One could spend 12 hours daily on a craft, but if his mentality is timid, shallow, and easily preoccupied with other thoughts, but the work itself, the hours that he puts in would not realistically count towards his level of proficiency towards that craft. Practice makes perfect only if they are deliberate. That is why if any of you gentlemen are asking how to have an unprecedented level of focus while doing a task, the simple answer is make sure the tasks that you are doing are down out of your own profound level of sheer curiosity, enthusiasm, confidence and will because as much as many people told you to get rid of distractions or engineer your workspace in some way so that you have nothing else to focus on but your work, your state of emotions will still play a strong role in your level of commitment. If we are excited, passionate, and undyingly curious about something, our mind activates and innately redirect our entire attention towards it. But if we are uninterested, bored, and uninspired, our mind shuts down and eventually becomes passive. And as much as you want to stay away from distractions, you will eventually seek distractions out of your own innate impulse to occupy your mental bandwidth. Of course, there are always exceptions as there are multiple paths to the top of the mountain. Some people can force themselves to focus within an endeavor that they have absolutely no interest or passion in, but usually it is achieved out of a pure sense of extreme trusty urgency and necessity regarding survival and welfare. Achieving supreme mastery within an art or a craft or an endeavor is the moment where every action or response that you take surrounding the scope of that profession are all done in a swift, seamless, and instinctual manner. You don't have to bring yourself to think hard. It is all done through an innate habituated disposition achieved through thousands of hours of intense deliberate practice and this form of practice. It's not like your normal run of the mill type where your goal is only to understand the fundamentals and then go easy on your efforts. Absolutely not. This form of practice is demanding in every sense. You will discover your limitations and counter plateaus and experience tons of failures, setbacks, errors and frustrations. This form of practice requires you to never be satisfied or content with your progression no matter how far. Because the practice towards mastery is all about reaching and doing things that most people won't have the thought of doing or would never even dare to attempt in doing. The best people in their field have always created and enter a realm of their own. They have discovered, developed and extended the scope of knowledge, circumstances, and understanding within their field. A nice example is Muhammad Ali's Rope ado tactic, which involves leaning against the elastic ropes of the boxing ring to dissipate the energy of your opponent's punches while making them vulnerable to Countess and over expenditure of energy.

Ali experimented with this technique during his sparring sessions where he was trying to figure out how to better take punches in the abdomen. This type of practice and mindset is why the best people in their field are considered as exceptional or in the class of their own because they are always willing to go above and beyond their responsibilities. That is why, like I said before, if you have a timid, shallow, and limited mindset, you will never achieve exceptionality within your field to become the best or one of the best in what you do. You must treat your craft not as a job, but as a way of life. Of course, it doesn't mean that you have to spend every living moment in intense focus. No, we are all still humans. We need to rest and recover to come back more prepared and more adapted towards our work. When we spend too much time on the edge within focus, our mind becomes tight and eventually becomes inefficient and ineffective to process information. This is the reason why you often feel stuck during your work and could not progress effectively. Everything will start to go into a path of diminishing returns. That is why we need regular periods to unwind and recover so that our mind can expand once again and return to their primitive state just like muscles, but the difference between what the best does during their break or rest periods. And what normal people do is, like I've said before, they revolve their other endeavors as supplements or compliments to their main commitment. They do not engage in endeavors that will in any shape or form, compromise their performance and progress. For example, Miyamoto Mui does not engage in sexual activities and alcoholic beverages in his quest to become the greatest swordsman. Instead, he meditates, immerse himself in nature and visualizes his next opponent so that he never completely loses focus from the way of the sword. Often for Us, us, we tend to engage in activities and endeavors that completely takes our mind away or off of our main commitment, and we usually and unconsciously overextend the time that we spend doing those endeavors, ultimately sabotaging our performance and progress. This is like a mixed martial artist who indulge extensively in the drunkenness of their instant gratifications, that they lose focus to improve their performance. Where they're left off the best, always maintains their focus even when they rest. Being the best is a life not for everyone.

The pressure, the expectations and the sacrifices are incredibly immense, and you will always experience pessimism, doubt, and condemnation from people around you. Calling you terms such as you are crazy, you're a lunatic, you're just too much, and everything you are doing is completely unnecessary. Only few people, or even none will believe and invest in your work such as the master that you are learning from. People hate what they don't understand. That is why they are trying to prevent you from disturbing the scope, tranquility, and stillness of their judgments. This is where you will often experience times of distress, loneliness, uncertainty, and hesitancy in what you are doing. Because as social creatures, it is instinctual for us to compare and contrast with the opinions and judgments from other people to further strengthen the confidence of our own opinions and judgments, the temptations to stop and return to normality will haunt you time and time again. This is where you must become extremely self-reliant and self-sufficient and adopt a strong belief system to keep you in check, to never stray too far from your commitment. As much as I wanted to become a master myself, I have to admit I still do slip away from my work often and eventually lose focus on the progression that I've made and as admirable as the journey to become the best in what you do.

CHAPTER SIXTY-FIVE
MEN DIFFER FROM WOMEN

We're going to break this down to the bone, literally because men and women are not equal and will never be equal, they are designed to be complimentary to each other's strengths and weaknesses. This is an analytical and comparison chapter, so please understand the context. Now, what I'm going to be stating here are a collection of scientific and sociological facts of the difference between men and women. Some are common ones that you might be familiar with. Others are not so common that you might never even heard of them before. But I'm not going to waste your time rambling about them. Using all the scientific and nerdy terms is I'm only going to be stating what's necessary for you to know and understand. If you want to know all the details, the links are in the description down below. So firstly, we both have different anatomy and different hormonal profiles. Let's be honest here. We all know this one. But anyways, men have higher bone density and mineral content than women. That is why women are four times more likely to develop bone diseases like so osteoporosis and scoliosis. Men have larger skulls than women with wider and higher shoulders, which translates to greater upper body strength. Women have wider pelvis, which translates to wider hips in order to accommodate pregnancy. Men have more lean muscle mass than women, which are necessary due to larger bones and joints, which translates to men having more raw strength and explosive power than women, whereas women have more fat mass than men, which first of all is crucially required in order to regulate their menstrual cycle. Women who don't have a lot of fat mass can suffer from irregular periods, but this also translates to women being more resistance to fatigue than men, meaning women are better at cardio and endurance training than men because they produce more aerobic energy since they have a much higher fat mass than men, at least 10% more on average. And when it comes to aerobic and endurance training, the primary source of energy or fuel is fat, which again, women have a lot more than men when it comes to the difference of our hormonal balance. Reproductive, as we all know, men produces way more testosterone than women about 20 times more, and women produces more estrogen and progesterone than men. And these are all in order to facilitate each gender specific reproductive needs.

And they also help translate to each gender specific body composition, which I've mentioned earlier. Now, when it comes to neurotransmitters or the feelgood hormones in terms of dopamine, serotonin, and endorphins, or in other words, the main hormones that regulates and affects the mood, men produce more of them than women. That is why women experience this a lot more moot swings than men, whereas women produce more oxytocin than men, which firstly, again, assist in their reproductive needs, but also helps in social bonding and also sexual and intimate activities. That is why when women fall in love, they get more emotionally attached, significantly more than Men, men because they feel it a lot more due to having more oxytocin. Number two, our brains work differently. Yes, a lot of you might probably be unaware of this difference, and there is quite a lot of them. Now, again, I'm not going to bother mentioning the scientific terms and explaining to you guys each and every part of the difference in each gender's brain because it's going to take me an entire decade to do that properly. But essentially, it's all to do with the different sizes, activities, and tissues in various parts of the brain. Now, on average, women's brains were highly connected across the left and right hemispheres, in contrast to men's brains where the connections were typically stronger between the front and back regions. Women's brains also have more white matter tissue in contrast to men's dominance of gray matter tissue. Now, I know all of those sounds like gibberish to some of you, however, they need to be mentioned for what's to come, but essentially, men's brains are more suited to information processing or compartmentalizing structural work perception and motor control, which makes us better at cognitive abilities, analytical thinking, and endeavors that require physical adaptations.

Whereas women's brains are more suited to information integration, information assimilation, intuitive work, and emotional empathy, meaning their brains are more dynamic than men, which makes them better at multitasking, socializing, and remembering or recalling memories. Men's brains are also designed to cognitively process emotions in order to find solutions to emotional problems, which translates to them being more resistant to emotional pain and have more emotional control than women. Women's brains on the other hand, are designed to capture social cues better than men, as they have better capability to understand other people's thoughts and feelings due to their empathetic tendencies, making them more capable in detecting lies than men. Number two, our brains work differently. Yes, a lot of you might probably be unaware of this difference, and there is quite a lot of them. Now, again, I'm not going to bother mentioning the scientific terms and explaining to you guys each and every part of the difference in each gender's brain because it's going to take me an entire decade to do that properly. But essentially, it's all to do with the different sizes, activities, and tissues in various parts of the brain. Now, on average, women's brains were highly connected across the left and right hemispheres, in contrast to men's brains where the connections were typically stronger between the front and back regions. Women's brains also have more white matter tissue in contrast to men's dominance of gray matter tissue.

Now, I know all of those sounds like gibberish to some of you, however, they need to be mentioned for what's to come, but essentially, men's brains are more suited to information processing or com compartmentalizing structural work perception and motor control, which makes us better at spa, cognitive abilities, analytical thinking, and endeavors that require physical adaptations. Whereas women's brains are more suited to information integration, information assimilation, intuitive work, and emotional empathy, meaning their brains are more dynamic than men, which makes them better at multitasking, socializing, and remembering or recalling memories. Men's brains are also designed to cognitively process emotions in order to find solutions to emotional problems, which translates to them being more resistant to emotional pain and have more emotional control than women. Women's brains on the other hand, are designed to capture social cues better than men, as they have better capability to understand other people's thoughts and feelings due to their empathetic tendencies, making them more capable in detecting lies than men. And for women who are reading this chapter, please do not lie to yourselves. There is a reason why you put so much effort and thought into your physical appearance.

You are innately aware that men prioritize your looks more than anything else, no matter how much you want to deny it. That is why you take hours to get ready. That is why you go to the gym, to enlarge your glutes and legs, to make your hips look wider and make you appear more sexually healthy and fertile. That is why you wear makeups.

That is why you shave and zap your armpits.

CHAPTER SIXTY-SIX
SEMEN RETENTION REVISITED

Alright, we all know that going on retention transforms you into someone who is just adamant to take on your demons. And we all know the physical and psychological benefits that comes through undergoing retention, and we all know that it is works because there is research backed proof of its effects and even famous people doing it with eventual and evidential positive results. So, in this chapter, we're not going to be discussing the benefits like so many other people have been endlessly recycling. We are going to be discussing, in my opinion, the best method to prevent you from continuously relapsing time after time again. And this method is actually fairly simple but very rarely mentioned or even discussed in the self-improvement world. Now we all know it is important and necessary during retention to transmute your ever-growing ember of horniness towards constructive endeavors in order to take your metal captivation away from humping your own palm like lifting weights, building a business, and trying out fresh endeavors. However, there is one simple but crucial elements surrounding all of these that you may or may not realize that even though you've done all of these constructive things during retention, you are still extremely susceptible or vulnerable to relapsing. And that thing is the time you spent lying down on your bed when taking a short break, chilling and momentarily procrastinating. Now, let's not pretend to be entirely holy and righteous being shall we gentlemen admit it. A lot of us do get a bit lazy and tired at certain times of the day, either before work, during work or after work. And we just needed a bit of leeway to catch our breath before we do continue. But it's within these times that you are most likely to relapse and get tempted to start touching yourself, like going home after a hard day at the office, sitting in traffic, and finally reaching home where the tedious and the mundaneness gets the better of you. And you need a little bit of relaxation to refresh and reset your mind. So, you take off your dirty clothes, get naked and lie down in your bed, cradling your pillows and got nice and comfy. And as you lie there in peaceful serenity, slowly your thoughts drift off into an idealistic and imaginative world because you want to enhance your pleasant and pleasurable experience. And being a man with a dick, that idealistic world is having sex with a beautiful and sexy woman. Maybe it's your neighbor and before you knew it, you start to hump your own pillow getting hard and in desperate need for some dick stroking. That is when you impulsively open your phone browsing through social media, and eventually relapse. Now, why does this happen? Why do we become tempted towards sexual endeavors when we're in a deep state of relaxation?

Essentially, it's all to do with your parasympathetic nervous system. Now, in contrast to the sympathetic nervous system, which raises your awareness, sharpen your sensors, and basically puts your body in either fight or flight mode during work, exercise, or any other constructive activities, the parasympathetic nervous system is responsible for relaxing and loosening up your sensors, which will lighten and slacken the tension of your muscles and assisting you in going to sleep. Basically, it's the rest and digest mode of the body eventually putting your body in a sort of semi-comatose state. Now, what you need to know and understand about the parasympathetic nervous system is that it has a direct excitatory pathway towards erection because when or as you are incentivized into thinking about your sexual fantasies in your head, or even seeing your sexual fantasies through porn sites, or even just stroking your own dig for that matter, it emits an excitatory signal from the brain which relaxes the smooth muscles of your dick and fills it with blood, which inevitably leads to an erection. That is why it is only when you are feeling relaxed, calm, and comfortable that you can get your dick up, not when you're stressed out, obsessively focused and severely anxious. That is why all those massage parlors who provide extra services on their menu offers to initially give you a deep tissue massage to get you to relax so that when the lady starts stroking your dig, it's much easier to get it rock hard. Now, at this point, some of you might be thinking, alright, Mr. Forged, stop being a goddamn nerd. Just tell us the method. Well, in short, the method is to avoid putting your body and mind in an elevated or heightened sense of relaxation for the majority of your daily schedule. Or in other words, stay away as far as possible from your bed throughout the day in order to prevent getting tempted to relax. Do so only when sleeping is your soul and or final objective for the day.

That is why like I and many others have said before, filling up your day-to-day schedule significantly with constructive endeavors is extremely important. If you are working from home, separate your workspace from your bedroom as far as possible. Never work next to your bed or even on your bed, and for those who work outside, if possible, stay outside until it's time for bed. If you don't want to remain in the living room of your house until it's bedtime, because let's be honest, where do people rank the most? The bedroom, 87% of women and 73% of men do rank off in the bedroom. And as for those of you who ejaculate in the shower, stop showering with warm water and start showering with cold water to prevent your body from initiating the state of relaxation. If you want to relax or unwind for a bit, instead of lying down on your bed, just sit and lean back a bit on your desk chair or stand up and walk around. Just don't lie down. Another thing to mention is that you must have a healthy obsession or fixation over something to captivate your mind enough from drifting off into sexual fantasies when you are eventually in bed, whatever they are. Fitness history, cars, the lot because as tired as you can possibly be at the end of the day when it comes to sex, especially during long periods of retention and during nighttime, you best bet you'll be tempted to want to ejaculate even when your body's aching. But ultimately though it is your own tenacity of your will that will determine whether you'll eventually relapse or not. You must have a personally deep-rooted, strong, and clear enough reason of why you want to do it.

CHAPTER SIXTY-SEVEN
LESSONS FROM PAIN

Life is suffering. Gentlemen, we only have to know what those are that's worth suffering for? Poor, rich, short, tall, we always suffer either way in different forms. Everyone seems to dream and perceive that one day through dragging yourself through all the dark and painful trenches you'll fall into. The suffering will eventually end. Though when you reach the top of the mountain, there will eventually be eternal peace, but then you forgot to realize that there will always be more and higher mountains to climb afterwards and you can also slip and fall from the mountain you've climbed. When you are poor, the struggle is to get wealthy and clean your place inside the competitions. When you are wealthy, the struggle is to grow your wealth and stay ahead of your competitions. Life will always give you new and different problems to solve no matter the circumstances you are in. So don't ever get mentally surprised and discouraged when the pain never ends. When you have a clear direction of where you want to go or what you want to do, you must never identify pain as a pointless or meaningless interference. In fact, you know what? Even when you don't have a clear direction in your life, the pain is there to teach you something or point you towards that direction You are after your attitude towards pain and suffering must veer or diverge towards some form of devout zealousness in order to keep that focus and fire of enthusiasm towards your life burning bright. Otherwise, you'll eventually yield to the barrage of all the shit circumstances life will throw at you and succumb to the need for immediate pleasure and distraction. Like a child, we all learn much better and much more thoroughly through negative experiences and discomforts, small or big in terms of the magnitude of their impact on our physical, cognitive, and emotional state.

They compel us to adapt and adjust ourselves accordingly in order for us to eventually acquire the necessary wisdom, understanding, and consciousness to overcome them. Whether it is a heartbreak through a failed relationship, an unsuccessful attempt in a business endeavor, or even trying something new and conceding the first-time pain is the best teacher as they say it, and they're absolutely right. Pain is your most valuable ally, and you must treat it as such because they provide the much needed incentives for you to seek for selves. The answers to all your problems and questions, the only message and lesson that pain kept inducing you is to become better, and doesn't it excite you in some form of way? Hearing that? Don't you love the idea of becoming a better individual? Don't you love it when something drives or forces you to grow and become someone more than what you initially believed about yourself, a much stronger, smarter, wealthier, and more confident to you? Of course, you do. Don't lie to yourself. That's what failing a personal best attempt in the gym is telling you. That's what falling out of a romantic relationship with the toxic woman is telling you. That's what losing a large amount of money over a business venture is telling you. That's what the uncomfortable feeling of a morning cold shower is telling you become better. It's exactly like what Kratos told his son when he fails his hunt.

This is how I stay enthusiastic even during hard times. Call me a masochist. I don't, don't care, Sumi mate, because it works for me. I love pain because I love to become a better individual. You must transform your narrative towards pain from a shallow, hopeless, and deprecate antics into an appetite ambitious and persistent eagerness transform your narrative towards pain from, fuck this, it's too much. I can't do it to, okay, you got me there. I'm going back to the drawing board, then I'm coming back for you, and I'll beat you next time because here is the thing you need to understand. Gentlemen, we as men we're naturally stubborn problem solvers. It's just how we work and how our brains work, so whatever problems we face, however big they are and however emotionally damaged we become due to experiencing them, we are secretly and subconsciously driven to want to fix them even if we physically want to avoid them for however long we do so until we eventually find a way to overcome them. So don't try to escape our problem-solving tendencies, gentlemen, it's already hard wide within us. It's our opportunity to utilize them to the best of their abilities. It's only a matter of shifting your attitude towards better serving your innate problem-solving tendencies. Now, I know I've said that pain only teaches you one lesson, but I lied because there is another thing worth mentioning when it comes to the deeper lesson that pain can teach you, and that is it teaches you the value of gratitude and nourishment like no other circumstances could ever do. It brings into full, visceral, and intimate consciousness of what appreciation means when you constantly put yourself extensively in uncomfortable situations. When you have to profoundly exert yourself to the excruciating limits in your efforts, even the slightest form of gratifications can satiate you significantly. It's like fasting, I'm sure my Muslim audience can relate to this. When you withheld yourself from feasting on food, delaying your gratifications and resisting your natural impulses to want to satiate your hunger, the moment when you break your fast and take that first taste of indulgent even water tastes really good and I'm not messing about here. I've tried fasting for 48 hours to try and reduce the inflammation on my joints, and the moment I take that first sip of water, I kid you not even water has a taste. That's how bewildered I was because it makes me feel fulfilled given how relatively insignificant drinking water is in terms of gratifications, it's the same thing with regards to retention. When you abstain from sex for a long time and arduously resisting your natural impulses to procreate and ejaculate, the moment you have sex and eventually ejaculate, it's extremely satiating to a level you possibly never knew or experienced before. That's just how pain works. It resets your threshold of satisfaction towards pleasure the same way how pleasure works. It resets your threshold of tolerance towards pain. Today's world is just impeccably stimulated by too much destructive pleasures. That is why they cannot get satiated by mere simple forms of gratifications. That is why most people nowadays are finding it very hard to display gratitude and appreciation. I mean, you can notice them yourself. People who are spoiled rotten with constant stimulations don't even know the meaning of gratitude because they rarely or never put themselves in painful circumstances to earn and cherish those gratifications as all of those have been ignorantly given to them without any exertions of efforts, and in the end, when trouble eventually hits the door, they have absolutely no answers. Same way with people who watch us too much porn, they cannot bring themselves to appreciate and find pleasure in normal real-life sex because their threshold for pleasure is so elevated that they need a peculiarly significant type and amount to experience any form of satiation. So, appreciate the pains in your lives, gentlemen, because not only will they teach you about appreciation like no other being could, but they will also eventually bring and before you circumstances that you will appreciate for a long time coming. They may be annoying and unbearable at first touch, but that's their way to put a stop to your ignorance and stupidity and bring you into full awareness and forces you to understand and adapt to the circumstances around you. Pain pushes you to overcome them and prevail, and how could you not love them.

CHAPTER SIXTY-EIGHT
RITES OF PASSAGE

The governed civilization of the modern world has unquestionably numbed down our primal instincts. We have become so tamed from our phal origins to the point where we can be identified as domesticated as much as how our minds have evolved dramatically to be able to process and make more complex, reasonable judgments and establishing morality. We still innately possess those basic animalistic instincts to ruthlessly go after our desires. However, they have been utterly subdued, suppressed, and discouraged over time through the creation of modern civilization, as we've now been utterly conditioned to rely on the shepherds of the high society's commands to shut up, sit down, and listen. We've become so separated from our natural desire for independence and freedom. We no longer have to hunt when we're hungry because we are fed through the ease and convenience of Uber Eats. We're no longer encouraged to fight and defend for ourselves because we're told that the government will do that for us. We're much less capable, eager, and motivated to go after what we want because we're implied of the dire consequences that will face if we decide to do so. So tamed and domesticated, we have become that even when the cages doors are open, we've become afraid and reluctant to run free. This is how we remain psychologically enslaved and infantile. For so long. The transition towards adulthood and independence are so eagerly or agitated, expected, and anticipated in today's age, but at the same time are so underwhelming or insufficiently taught and encouraged. It's like expecting a flower to bloom without watering it and exposing it to sunlight. Back in the tribal days, the transformation towards adulthood were planned, cultivated, and celebrated. Today, they are barely implied and informed, or at the most, they are just hoped to occur in time as the high society wants to keep us remain enslaved through their convenient, degenerative, technologically induced conditionings, even leading to a lot of our parents' eventual neglection and discouragement of it. So, most of us modern men have no choice but to individually realize and initiate this process or transformation towards adulthood unassisted, leading to us having to face most of life's initially incomprehensible circumstances, the hard way, and seeking mentors on our own to help us find answers and clarify our destiny and independence. This journey is called the Rights of Passage. Rites of passage is basically a collection of circumstances that directly promote an individual state towards undisputed autonomy and sovereignty. Basically, anything that contributes towards achieving the position of self-initiative, self-reliance, and self-sufficiency. Trials that promote strengths and passions, endeavors that promote competency and dexterity and experiences that promotes wisdom and understanding. Back then there were set and predestined honorable rituals. Now, there can literally be anything that breaks you out that serene but deteriorating comfort zone that you are most likely sitting or lying down in right now, such as moving out and living on your own in a different environment of your choice in order to find out whether you are able to take care of your personal space and provide for yourself learning how to fight and defend yourself in order to increase your chances of survival, should your personal spaces invaded and threatened and quitting your current profession that obstructs your growth towards the mastery of your field and starting your own individual creative pursuits and establishments. If these circumstances are quite major and significant in magnitude, for some of you gentlemen, don't worry. You can all baby steps your way towards them. Like I've mentioned before, modern rites of passage can be anything that gets you to constantly break out of your comfort zone. It can be as simple as quitting a bad habit, like spending less time, or even deleting social media and porn. From there, you were sent towards building and forming good habits like developing physical and mental strength through going to the gym and cultivating knowledge through reading authentically good books. From there, you were sent even higher through trying out experiences and endeavors. They were too afraid to try before but had the burning desire to eventually want to like code approaching a woman and initiating a conversation with her, or joining a social activity and meeting with people of common interests like a hiking club or a fishing tour, or even competing in a sport. Sit down and just ask yourself honestly what other things that you have a burning desire to do, try and achieve, but are currently too fearful, anxious, and reluctant to do anything and everything that strikes a jolt of anxiety in you, but also a wave of excitement and enthusiasm at the same time. And that is the word I want you gentlemen, to pay attention to excitement. Because one of the hardest things to overcome in any rites of passage or self-improvement is bringing yourself to do them in the first place. And in my own experience, no matter how initially fearful and reluctant you are of anything, if the amount of excitement outweighs that fear and hesitancy, you will eventually and inevitably commit yourself to it. Regardless, nothing will stop you from eventually standing tall and proud. Remember that I mentioned about the innate, primal and feal instincts that we possess similarly to animals. This is the same thing. What do you think a dog is feeling when it's waggling its terror, while being involuntarily hesitant to enter a swimming pool? The trick here is to find out how to unlock and maintain that excitement, and every individual is different.

CHAPTER SIXTY-NINE
THE MAN-CHILD

The formation of psychologically or mentally infantile men stems not from our own inability to pursue and strive for independence. All of us always have the capacity for that. Instead, it is caused by our less fortunate and less optimal upbringings that significantly disparage and constraints their potentiality. We all know that our parents play an important role in the formation of our psyche during our adolescent years all the way into adulthood and how they assist us to properly function or live as a fully grown individual. Through examples and demonstrations, the father serves as a figure or beacon of guidance for us, mentors and paternal authority that instills the necessary disciplines on how to achieve eventual independence and fulfillment of potential in life. The mother serves as the caring and nurturing soul that over time providers with the perfect example in looking for, in developing healthy, long-lasting future relationships with other women. However, when the human dynamic relationship between our parents is crippled, insufficient, and decadent from the start, they will result in us having poor or any energetic relationships with them. And in fact, our mindset dramatically throughout our transition towards adulthood, hindering them down, obstructing their progress, and even counteracting them completely. Because as children, we are still vulnerable, curious, and excited beings. So, when we are conditioned and programmed in a certain way in terms of our thoughts and behavior patterns by our parents, we will inevitably adopt or instill that conditioning quite persistently even as time passes physically and emotionally. Absent fathers overprotective and demanding mothers and living in an extremely conservative environment for long periods of time are the main factors of why a lot of men today are still lost. Boys living in a grown men's bodies, fathers who are rarely or never been physically and psychologically involved in the development of his sons during the adolescent years, will absolutely disorganize and clutter their perspectives towards many necessary things in life that are important for them to know and understand, such as the need to cultivate physical strength, the necessity to have perseverance in the state of adversities, the value and courage in taking risks away from their comfort zones and the importance to find a purposeful direction or path in life. These are some of the many critical things that fathers need to induce into their son's mind from an early age in order to prepare and encourage them to form an attitude that is way more appropriate and adapted towards the ruthless and predicament circumstances of life when they eventually reach their adult years. Fathers that are really home from work to be physically available. Fathers that never put an effort to understand and connect with their sons by doing common endeavors to develop their relationship and fathers that compromise or relinquish their leadership position in the family by making the mother where the pan and the marriage, all of these circumstances will dramatically affect mean ability and confidence to verge towards self-sufficiency because he's simply unprepared unencouraged and unconditioned to become one. Mothers who are overprotective and demanding towards their sons will also profoundly hinder the development towards emotional maturity. Overprotective and demanding mothers are usually developed through physical and emotional unavailability from their husbands towards them, that they eventually starts to unconsciously shift their reliance heavily on their sons to provide those sensations of presence for them to the point where they will showcase and demonstrate an overly exaggerated and unreasonable amount of care and nurture, but also devouring commandments in order to keep their sons close, perhaps too close, discouraging their sons from taking big risks and wanting to be overly involved in their son's lives will inevitably encourage them to develop a mother complex, or in other words, an overly attached and dependent relationship with their mothers, even when it comes to making important life decisions that they have to contemplate independently, making them unwilling or reluctant to venture towards complete independence. Fathers who do not have a masculine and strong frame of mind or presence of authority, fathers who like mentioned before, voluntarily relinquish their position as leaders in the household in order to desperately please their wives will also result in these women doubting their husband's capability to protect, provide, and lead the family, eventually incentivizing themselves to take matters into their own hands and assume the mantle of leadership because they could not bring themselves to trust their husband's capability to take care of things. This will effectively put an indefinite stop to any intentions of encouragement and support from the fathers to their sons towards breaking free from the dependency of their family as now the mothers are in charge. So, both their husbands and their sons are operating from the frame of mind of their wives and mothers. And as we all know, a woman's mind does not naturally adhere to a man's mind because we are different. Like Brad Pitt said in Fight Club, were generations of men raised by women. Cultures, lifestyles, social lives and activities that do not adhere towards self-sufficiency can also significantly influence a man's decision to live in independence like the absence or lack of any rites of passage, whether they are individually initiated or collectively initiated by the people around him, friends and colleagues who discourage and condemns him in taking risks or trying out new endeavors together, and activities that have no direct contribution and impact for him to undergo a gradual process of self-improvement. For example, things such as refusing to move out and live alone in a different city or country, spending too much time indoors while playing too much videogames and watching too much porn, living a sedentary or a personally non cultivating lifestyle and being reluctant to participate or engage in any social activities. These accommodating factors can keep himself remain in the comfortable confinement of his previously induced infantile conditionings that will keep him at bay or even stray him away further from the process of individuation. That is why the more you get too invested and immersed in this modern world that is full of physically and mentally comforting, but degenerative, instant gratifications provided at the tip of your fingers through your mobile phones, the more you will shield yourself away from taking the necessary steps to eventually become an independent man. That is why you become a soft, feeble, cowardly, and feminine man that women do not want to be with because they could not trust you to lead, protect, and provide for her since you do not possess the attitude and capabilities of a properly mature man. Now, it is very important that you do not put every ounce of your hateful resentments and blame towards your parents because they have their own set of problems too, regardless, and it's just unfortunate that we got caught or involved in the middle of them. And as much as they've contributed quite significantly to our own set of misfortunes during our adult lives, most of them have no genuine and fully conscious intentions of doing so because as we know, oftentimes our parents only want the best for us regardless of the methods they've implemented to raise us that are formed over the years through their own, own good or bad experiences. As children in the care of our grandparents back in the day, misfortunes are inevitable sooner or later. And I understand that a lot of our anger comes from the fact that we have wasted so much of our youth being convinced that living in our comfort zones is the best way to live and have missed out quite a lot and actually living life through taking risks. So, most do we have to face unfamiliar circumstances the hard way, and the worst part is in technical and historical terms at least we are not entirely responsible for it. However, we have no choice but to do so in order to eventually break free, to make our future circumstances better than how they were. Because taking full responsibility over our own lives, regardless of circumstances, is the only way to eventually move forward in life and leave the past behind. Because again, no one is coming to save you. And as much as you want to despicably blame your parents and expecting a sort of obligatory, redeeming arc for them to enlighten your current and future circumstances, they are getting too old and wary for that no matter how much they desperately want to. So, forgive them because as much as they are put you through so much in life without them, there will be no you.

CHAPTER SEVENTY
BOLDNESS

Ever wonder how Andrew Tate k McGregor and Jake Paul are able to catapult themselves into superstardom in such a swift and rapid manner? One moment you don't know or barely aware of who they are, and the next day they're everywhere on the news through word of mouth and trending in every social media platform that me and you couldn't help but take a glance at. The simple answer is because all of them possess and able to display an unprecedented level of audacity, they speak induced stuff that most people wouldn't even dare to partake or get involved in, and sometimes speak induced stuff that most people wouldn't even thought was plausible or plausible. They are highly extreme and polarizing individuals that are not only capable to draw massive amounts of attention to themselves in such a short amount of time, but also captivate and retain them for long periods of time, even long after we stop seeing them or hear about them, they will still linger ever so comfortably within our minds. So why does hearing and seeing bold individuals speak and perform generate so much interest within us that we can't help or want to notice and be involved with them? Let me explain. We as human beings are so easily drawn by anything that generates some form of emotional arousal within us as they heightened our sensitivity to focus and recall intricate or selective central details of the circumstances that is happening in front of us rather than the circumstances surrounding us. Remember when I said that when you are excited and enthusiastic in doing something or speaking to someone for that matter, you become so immersed with it, her or him, that you tend to forget what time of the day it is. This is exactly the same dynamic occurrence. Ever wonder how Andrew Tate k McGregor and Jake Paul are able to catapult themselves into superstardom in such a swift and rapid manner? One moment you don't know or barely aware of who they are, and the next day they're everywhere on the news through word of mouth and trending in every social media platform that me and you couldn't help but take a glance at. The simple answer is because all of them possess and able to display an unprecedented level of audacity, they speak induced stuff that most people wouldn't even dare to partake or get involved in, and sometimes speak induced stuff that most people wouldn't even thought was plausible or plausible. They are highly extreme and polarizing individuals that are not only capable to draw massive amounts of attention to themselves in such a short amount of time, but also captivate and retain them for long periods of time, even long after we stop seeing them or hear about them, they will still linger ever so comfortably within our minds. So why does hearing and seeing bold individuals speak and perform generate so much interest within us that we can't help or want to notice and be involved with them? Let me explain. We as human beings are so easily drawn by anything that generates some form of emotional arousal within us as they heightened our sensitivity to focus and recall intricate or selective central details of the circumstances that is happening in front of us rather than the circumstances surrounding us. Remember when I said that when you are excited and enthusiastic in doing something or speaking to someone for that matter, you become so immersed with it, her or him, that you tend to forgot what time of the day it is. This is exactly the same dynamic occurrence. But regardless of followers or haters as extreme individuals, you must leverage every opportunity you can through all these awareness and recognition to build your own personal brands, establishments, entities, enterprises, and social status. Truly extreme individuals are simply unwanted in involving or exposing or marketing themselves as much as possible in as many places as possible because one of their main goals is whether you love them or hate these individuals, you will without a doubt notice or acknowledge their very existence. And that is pretty much what you need to do in order to have a good chance to swiftly catapult yourself into the upper echelon of society. Of course, don't expose or market yourself just for the sake of it or just to say hello and bounce off hopping that people would want to eventually support you long term for heaven's sake. Please don't do that because you will only make an utter fool of yourself and make yourself look like an absolute limp wrist at halfwit. Drawing people's attention in order to captivate them enough to make them become your loyal supporters is not exactly an easy feat, especially in today's age, where literally everyone is desperate for attention. There is an overload of commonality in the market. So, you must find a way to stand out on your own. You need to have a strong foundation before you actually expose yourself. There must be actual distinct substance integrity, entertainment, and uniqueness in both your polarizing words and actions, or at the very least possessing and demonstrating two of them because without substance and integrity, you will be nothing but a slight insignificant unmemorable, momentary gust in the wind. Just like what happened to Dylan Danis. And without entertainment and uniqueness, it's only a matter of time before people divert into other more appealing options. Now, another very important thing to mention is that the life of an extreme, bold and polarizing individual is not what most people ought to want them to be. As most people only fantasize of the circumstances that they want to before them, like money or fame and not the circumstances that they do not want to before them. But as with every decision or choice, there will be rewards and there will also be consequences. You see, gentlemen, life at the top is not free of problems. It only gets rid of, or at least significantly relief the problems you are facing back when you are still in the rut or still climbing the ladder. Like previously, you may struggle to pay rent and now you're able to finally afford a nice house. However, with new life circumstances comes a set of new life problems in this case of life at the top, the ever. So, increasing amount of expectations from you to deliver your promises to your supporters, the endless provocations and pressures coming from your enemies towards you fall or die. And the necessity to constantly protect your image and reputation to appear perfect, they all can inevitably become too hard to accept and too much for want to handle, especially for those who are both physically and mentally fragile or unprepared to do so. And it is more common to those individuals who've risen to the top too quickly for their own good.

That is why often you hear young celebrities or public figures getting addicted to drugs, engaging in questionable misconducts and developing severe insecurities or mental health issues because they just could not handle the sudden dramatic changes in their lives and eventually wishing to go back or at least contemplating to go back and live a normal life. One may wish for greatness, but one also may fear greatness to a much greater extent that can result in them falling from grace. You have to eventually learn to not give a fuck about pesky little things. And to achieve that, oftentimes you have to be utterly selfish for your own wellbeing, even if it means putting a little bit of stain and strain in your reputation. And to be honest, you need to be most of the times because firstly, you will not be able to please everyone. And secondly, life at the top is ruthless. The standards are even higher, and competitions are even fiercer. You can't afford to lose yourself in the moment for too long. You must demand more from yourself to keep yourself relevant in the game. That is why only few could handle and sustain such intensities in their lives. Now is being extreme, bold and polarizing the only way to achieve success? Of course not. There are endless ways to the top of the mountain, gentlemen, but this is by far and so far, the quickest way to get there. Just look at Kobe Covington. He was deemed as unappealing and no one knew who he was because he was so neutral in his approach and didn't want to hurt anybody's feelings, which caused him to get nearly cut from the UFC because he wasn't drawing enough eyes, ears, and butts for the business. But one flip of a switch through an extremely controversial, offensive, and provocative interview changed the entire cause of his career and life forever. The only question that remains is, do you gentlemen fear greatness? Obviously, most of us would casually say, of course, not living a life, being unwilling or unable to unlock, explore and maximize once for potential is a way worse form of existence than death itself.

However, as much as every single one of us desire to be great, a lot of us greatly underestimate the challenges that will be imposed onto us, such as the immense sense of responsibility that one must possess to become one and remain one, and the profound changes in one's life that may isolate him entirely from normality. If you wish to become such an individual, this is something you need to take seriously because as quickly as you can rise, it is even quicker when you fall.

CHAPTER SEVENTY-ONE
DEFEAT

You know, there are some points within our lives where we will inevitably receive our very own asset tests. Essentially, these are the trials that we experienced when we are at a very vulnerable and compromising state, both during our highest highs and our lowest lows. The tests to measure our vigilance and ignorance despite the luxuries we experienced when we are well up the ladder in life and the tests to measure our resilience and perseverance despite the bleakness of our circumstances. When we are still in the rut of life or when we do fall from grace, this is what we will all encounter during our individual self-improvement journeys. Our extent to resist indulging in the onslaught of temptations and gratifications after an extensive period of time of personal growth and abstinence and our extent to wanting to redeem ourselves when we do slip away while at the same time getting overwhelmed with disappointments and regretful actions. The latter of which is exactly what falling off from your self-improvement journey feels like. You know the last full urges to undergo a nuclear ejaculation after months of not wanking your dick off and then having to dwell in your own failure after voluntarily giving into your impulses towards the thing that you initially sought to destroy forever and the cravings to quench our desire for all the pallets of taste within processed foods after months of undergoing body recompositing through lifting weights and eating clean with bland organic foods and then having to withstand our never-ending compulsion to consume more of the devil's fruits once we've tasted them after a long while. The reason we fall off from self-improvement journey is simple. We unconsciously become too comfortable for our own good. We put ourselves in delightfully comfortable positions for way more and longer than necessary, and we forgot to keep ourselves mindful of the circumstances surrounding us, like for example, mindlessly and cautiously scrolling through Instagram and encountering pictures and reels of hot women getting invested for too much and too long into that shit, and then finding yourselves rock hard and eventually touching yourself because your testosterone level is through the roof after long periods of retention. Now it is normal to want to reward ourselves after all the time and work that we've put in to cultivate ourselves into a position or state where we initially never thought was possible. However, we're humans, we always will gravitate more towards pleasure rather than pain, and it's no different when it comes to self-improvement. Our elevated sense of self-worth that is cultivated through self-improvement can turn on us should we decide to underestimate the extent to which it can blind us from the seductive dark forces of temptations until eventually we are too late to realize that we've regressed far back to where we started or because of the snowball effect of one ignorant decision or choice. And the worst part is the psychosis and superstitious extent of our disappointments and remorse on ourselves for our own misconduct and failure will tempt us even further to bask ourselves deeper in all the gratifications that we initially want to avoid, especially when it comes to the endeavors that we spend a lot of time and effort working on, like retention and diet. The moment where your mind says, fuck, what have I done? Can't believe I just did that I'm such a failure man or any other sorts, is the moment where your fall from grace begins because it's instinctual for us to seek any form of means, usually pleasure to get rid of the painful feeling that we are suffering from. The greater the pain and agony, the more we will be tempted to want to eliminate it as soon as possible by any means necessary. That is why you find yourself engaging in a train of masturbation after relapsing on your year-long retention streak that caused you to experience a cataclysmic level of self-accusation and self-condemnation like you've never experienced before. That is why you find yourself stuffing your mouth with candies, donuts, and ice creams after you realize that you've consumed more cheat meals and junk foods than you actually should or initially planned on consuming that eventually caused you to spiral into an emotional whirlwind in despising your own abilities and self-imposed ethics. It's that extreme feeling of revulsion and repentance towards ourselves that got us to experience our steep and deep fall from grace that eventually leave us in the pool of our own tears and the ridicule of those gratifications that we ended up consuming more of. Rewards and gratifications are infinitely and endlessly seductive. They're pretty much like a hot woman in a lingerie persuading you to come to bed and bang all day long and the moment you want to get up and go to work, it poses you back into bed, gives a nice stroke on your dick, and you ended up emptying your tank before the day even started and eventually doing nothing and going nowhere for the entire day, week, month, or year. This is especially important to take note of specifically when you are well up the ladder in your self-improvement journey and where all the temptations are pretty much at your disposal for you to relish in. You must maintain a relatively high level of self-awareness when it comes to reaping your rewards because one oversteps slip can get you caught up in a seemingly comfortable but consequential downward spiral, and this can happen in professional circumstances as well where you got too comfortable and arrogant in your own way that the quality or outputs of your work eventually sees or drop. One way to develop self-awareness is to become utterly self-critical, constantly identifying or pointing out your strengths and weaknesses, your tendencies and vulnerabilities without your fragile ego getting in the way of you being brutally honest with yourselves.

The moment you feel like you are slacking or hesitating to put yourself even in a slightly uncomfortable position is the moment you must put yourself in an uncomfortable position or at least a position where you aren't unwinding or loosening up in order to activate your sympathetic nervous system. For example, if one afternoon you look at the time and you make a mental note to yourself to go to the gym in two hours, but then suddenly out of nowhere you start to feel somewhat doubtful, uncertain, or reluctant to go like, should I go to the gym? Should I just skip this one session? It won't make much of a difference, would it? I'm already chill right now, and I don't think I want to get away from this. That is the moment you must affect it immediately Go to the gym or at least take a walk or do an endeavor that engages your alertness and vigilance. Same thing with regards to retention.

The moment your dick tells you, "man, I'm so fucking horny." If you're really sweet of Tunisia and Tatiana, were here and then you find yourself start humping your own pillow is the moment you should immediately do 200 pushups or submerge yourself in an ice bath or do anything that gets you to become alert and not feeling relaxed or complacent. I personally did the same thing in terms of diet as well. At night. Often, I get cravings for sugar and what I did to signal the hormone to stop telling me that I am hungry is I chuck two full beer mugs of water just to make me feel full and quite a bit nauseous. I'll have to admit, bad habits are a lot easier to develop than good habits. That is why they're a lot harder to unlearn or withheld because a lot of bad habits are natural animalistic impulses for us human beings as for those of us who do slip off the ladder and then ended up completely at rock bottom or at least significantly far off from where we've fallen from. This is where at least personally; the real acid tests are going to be imposed onto our will possibly more than ever before because the realization that we've basically tripped onto a landslide and regressed far back into the position where we first started is certainly not an easy feat to its stand. It's agonizing, heartbreaking, and morally damaging all at the same time, and this is the part where I've mentioned that you engaging in a seemingly unbreakable sequence of indulgence in pleasures and gratifications in order to desperately numb or get rid of the agony will occur because imagine experiencing the disappointments of your own failure, coupled with realizing that you have to do all the hard things all over again from the start and experience all the pain all over again. Like if you are on a yearlong quest to abstain from ejaculation and then completely relapsing on the last day of the year, wouldn't you be disappointed in yourself initially or the willpower you have to muster up to resist your natural impulses and all the work you've done to get you to that point in your goal only to have all of them slip away at the last moment. It's pretty soul crushing initially, if I'm going to be honest. However, good news for you, realistically, it's only your mythical spiritual and superstitious attachment to them that got you to think and feel that way. Like if you didn't go to the gym for two weeks, simply pick up where you left off. It's that simple because you haven't fallen that far off, and if you didn't go to the gym for three or four months and then having to start all over again, all of your precious work will not be in vain. Sure, it will be as painful as when you first started, but your progress towards the stage or level that you left off will be much, much faster and easier than when you first started because of muscle memory. And this not only applied to your body, but your brain as well. Like if you've learned and polished a skill and then having to forego that skill for a long while, yeah, you will be initially be a little trippy, rusty and clumsy, but you've done this many times beforehand, so it won't take that long to get yourself back into the rhythm of where you left off because your brain has already been periodically predisposed of that particular circumstance and stimulus. All you need to make sure is that you must not enter that morally self-deprecating state where you engage in those stupid, unnecessary and mentally damaging negative conversations about yourselves that does nothing but gets you to underappreciate your efforts and denounce your own potential. The road to redemption always begins with a reignited and deadly, a form of determination, not with a darkened and lackluster form of disapproval over one's own capabilities that has already been proven significantly. And if you need to find the motivation to do them all over again, remind yourself of all the reasons why you started doing them all. It may sound cliche but take a moment to bring those reasons back into clarity and impose them back into the forefront of your mind. And if you find yourself thinking, oh, what's the point I've failed when I tried my hardest? Why should I bother trying again? Well, this time when you do try, treat those temptations as your nemesis, compile bad narratives about them and make them utterly noticeable to you on a daily basis, like posting notes about them on a war's side or in front of your workplace because when you acknowledge that you have mortal enemies, they could push you beyond the norm of sanity. You will be sharper and more focused than ever before. As losing or conceding to your enemies means that your dignity is as frail and worthless as your enemies mocked it to be. Uh, no man in this world wants to have his dignity being utterly shamed in front of his beloved peers, especially to those who believed in him. What we need to constantly remind ourselves is this gentleman self-improvement in and of itself thoroughly is not exactly a delightful term where we usually associate it with feeling good about ourselves through experiencing growth that happens after self-improvement. Self-improvement is a process, a process of basically going through vast array of discomfort in order to unlock and cultivate the necessary attributes that we want to eventually possess and utilize to our advantage. The word improvement or development does not come or is not achieved from moments and circumstances of solace. It comes from moments and circumstances of struggle and resistance. Improvement or development does not happen and will not happen within comfort and luxury because there are no circumstances to comprehend, adapt, and overcome only circumstances. To relish, benefit and appreciate. Self-improvement is all about constantly putting ourselves in uncomfortable positions. It's a lifelong quest. It's not a momentary phenomenon to eventually season doing and then reaping all the seemingly infinite rewards without considering the consequences that comes after it.

CHAPTER SEVENTY-TWO
WHAT YOU NEED TO KNOW
ABOUT MONEY EARLY ON

Now, before I start though, I would like to say that this is not a financial advice. I'm far from a financial expert because I'm not a walking multi-millionaire or billionaire, and although I have a banking and finance background in my previous employment and also back in university, I only took the job because I was pretty good at mental math and I only took the course because I wanted to party with hot girls because as we all know, business, school, business degrees in university are all just cool excuses to tell our parents for us to secretly party hard and get drunk. This chapter is my personal take on developing financial literacy and responsibility in your twenties based on my own set of past experiences and current perspectives. When it comes to money or wealth in your twenties, all the focus should be put on maximizing your cash flow and building sustainable and scalable business entities that will both enhance or amplify your credibility and reputation as time passes. Now, I know some of you may be impatient to know about my take on investments, real estate and cryptos, but bear with me here because this first thing here is without question the most important when it comes to building a strong financial foundation and accumulating wealth in your twenties. That is why you have to know and understand this first, maximizing your income or cash flow from your primary entity should be your utmost priority. Build a personal brand or business that showcases your credibility and proficiency to deliver highly valuable products or services in any field of your choice, as this will significantly assist you to establish that strong initial foundation and exposure that you desperately need in the beginning and today, it has never been easy with the power of social media and online shops. This is where having a sales background would really boost you tremendously. Your main goal here is to get as much exposure and deliver so much value and care to your customers to the point where they would not hesitate or think twice to part themselves with their hard-earned money in exchange for the value you're giving them and also make them become significantly enamored by your products or services to the point where they will come for repeat purchases and spread their positive reviews through word of mouth and social platforms, which will inevitably increases your exposure customer base and eventually market share. This is also where focusing on developing a single good quality product or service, not a barrage of average products or services, is absolutely critical in establishing your reputation in the market. If your product or service is that good, almost any form of publicity is good for business. Don't worry about money if your product or service is shit because it will never come. Remember, the higher the value you can deliver, the more effortless the price become to pay for it. In terms of working nine to five, personally I would rather die than go back to living a corporate lifestyle because no matter how high you go up the corporate ladder and how much you earn, let's say 30 grand a month, you are still contractually an obligatory bound to the corporation. You won't have a lot of time to enjoy the fruits of your labor or do all the things you want to try out. And as we all know, time is our biggest asset and our most valuable commodity. Like if you want to go on a long holiday with your family and friends, one call from the boss to get your ass back to the office and you have no choice but to oblige otherwise, you'll risk diminishing your reputation or even losing your job. Plus the fact that corporate politics play a huge role in most nine to fives, if you're not a proficient ass licker and cocksucker, your employment status pretty much hangs in the balance of the boss's own personal appreciation of your efforts and their internal conflicts generated by their own or the collective disapproval of you. But of course, I'm biased here because my experiences in corporations have always been significantly negative, more than positive. But in all honesty though, not all corporations are like this. If you are currently struggling to make ends meet at nine to five is your only option to pay the bills for the time being, then by all means is the right thing to do. And what I would also do if I was in that situation, but of course do that while also slowly building your brand on the side outside of work. But if you do love your corporate job and they treat you well while also make your career very scalable, then fair play you made. I am never an advocate of saving money, as I'm sure most of you gentlemen also are because for many years I've tried that and it doesn't get me anyway. It only devalues my money as inflation kept on rising through the years by not putting them to work for me, putting them in banks and deposits only protect them from inflation and are combating against inflation. And it only looks nice on your bank account when you check the balance on your phone, but after that it's not much. That is why in your twenties you should absolutely prioritize and not be afraid to invest significantly into yourself in terms of skills, knowledge, and experience. And for those who are wondering endlessly about how to start building value for yourself within your chosen field of craft, this is it. If you are confused about how to start a strong foundational brand or business, you have to first build value through cultivating your proficiency in your craft. And today, as we all know, information is everywhere. You can literally find mentors online and learn from them. Go on an apprenticeship period with those mentors and learn as much as you can from them vividly absorb their knowledge, experience, and practice like a kid mimicking his parents before. You want to put your own creative and objective twist in your brand. So don't be afraid to spend a significant amount of money investing in yourself because they cannot be taken away from you. As those skills and knowledge, you accumulate over time will be deeply embedded within your mentality, instincts, and muscle memories. The only way those investments will go to waste is if you invest in the wrong mentor or you put yourself out practice for long periods of time. Honestly, from my point of view, investing in yourself is much cheaper and way more worth it than taking out a massive student loan to go to college or university because college and university teach you what they think they want you to know without considering your individual specific needs and precious time. Now, in terms of investments and passive income, when it comes to most of us in our twenties, we're like desperate and hungry lines, but at the same time, lazy, in irresponsible bastards. We want gargantuan amount of money fast to snatch and flex because we're just too lazy to put in any work that here's why we jump onto the bandwagon of stocks and cryptos. Now, my own experience on stocks have been overall positive, but I wouldn't say the same on crypto because of their extreme volatility. I mean, I lost 20 grand on crypto due to its crash back in May, and it's all because of my childish GRE to achieve a double on my initial capital. I was like little bit more, little bit further maybe, and before I knew it I already lost seven grand in a matter of hours. All in all, though, I will not recommend you gentlemen investing a large portion of your net worth into stocks and cryptos if you want to invest in them, just make sure it's a portion of your money that are sitting ducks and most importantly, that you are prepared to lose in case of a major crash happening. But of course, if you profoundly understand how they work, unlike me, and you can capitalize on the opportunity for massive gains fast without succumbing to your own greed, then fair enough, take more risks if you want to. If you want the safest bet on your money, index funds are your best option in my case. Now in terms of real estate, young men get overly excited about this, but as we all know, house prizes are rocketing at the moment and forming a massive real estate bubble. So, if you invest in real estate now, assuming you have the money, probably in two to three years' time, the bubble will explode and house prices will come crashing down. So all your hopes of appreciation and value on your initial investment will be down in the water in a short period of time. Everyone fantasizes about the passive income real estates can generate and yes, it's very appealing. However, when you are young or if you're not born in a family of generational wealth at the disposal, most likely you won't have a lot of dough or $500,000 comfortably just sitting in the bank. And if you want to invest in real estate, most likely you're going to be investing about 80 to 90% of your wealth in one real estate property and not 10, because you're not a millionaire yet obviously, the biggest problem about passive income of real estate is the abysmally long amount of time and it will take to eventually break even. Even if you do decide to rent it out like an average two-bedroom house cost around $400,000 and assuming you rented around $3,000 a month, it will take you more than 10 years to eventually break even may. And if your cash flow is appalling, chances are you'll most likely be forced to sell the property rather early to cover up your lack in cash. Real estate only works if your overall cash flows are already in check and when you can purchase multiples of them without worrying about breaking even as the matter of breaking even will be taken care of by your main income sources. That is why, again, like I said before, the best investments to make in your twenties is building a strong foundational brand or business to solidify and stabilize your income. Like if you earn 20 grand a month after tax from your business, plus a three grand rent on the property you bought, breaking even will be done in less than two years, mate, depending on your personal expenses, it might take two years at most. So, when you are young and still not having much dough coming in every month, forget about real estate investments. Just rent out a place that can keep you warm and sheltered for the time being. Because as men, we don't need a lot of small and unnecessary things around us to satiate us. We can comfortably rent a small studio apartment and be completely fine whilst we build the foundation of our income sources. So that's pretty much my personal take on finance, gentlemen, not as in depth as you probably would've wanted, but as I said, I'm no expert.

CHAPTER SEVENTY-THREE
THE DARK SIDE OF MAN

Do we live our daily lives struggling to cover up and protect the seemingly sinister properties of our dark secrets? I'd say so human beings wear a lot of masks daily because they possess qualities that may be considered as both socially unacceptable and morally unethical qualities that the social norms and the laws of civilization will claim to be unfit and dangerous to the serenity of societal living qualities that these powerful people also possess but refuse to admit, to make them appear pure and righteous to not jeopardize their own reputation, but behind closed doors and the comforting wars of their own home. They release those dark qualities without hesitancy as nobody is watching them speak about or perform their most wicked and disturbing conducts. We are always told to embrace and showcase the virtuous and upright qualities of our psyche, like the ability to love and empathize and to reject and repress our malicious and ill nature qualities from ever servicing and wreaking havoc towards the circumstances around us because the world told us that they should not exist and yet what we resist will always persist no matter the masks that we wear in public. There will always be times where we both subtly and inadvertently reveal our dark side qualities because they are and will always be a part of us. Violence, greed, lust, deception, vengeance, narcissism. These dark and sinister qualities are one with us and they have both close and selfish relations to one another. We all possess the capability and capacity to perform these selfish, hostile deeds and you know what will trigger and cause these dark qualities of ours to go unleash and uncontrollable. It's their lack of expression and demonstration and or being overly and unambiguously expressed or demonstrated. For most of us in our dark qualities, it's usually the former all strong or significant thoughts and emotions are meant to be expressed in some form of way to instinctually satiate the nature to convey failure to do so will result in the slow but sure buildup of neurotic and eventually psychotic attributes. As those thoughts and emotions will start to violently revolt against one another and disorganize the structure of our psychological order. That is why you always experience a profound amount of stress, anxiety, and agitation whenever you can't or unable to express what needs to be expressed, like the need for you to convey your brittle frustration of waiting in a public line for too long. For example, we've discussed aggression before in this book and it's profoundly close association with anger or rage when it remains unexpressed or withheld for too long and we'd be right because violence is what happens when the rage accumulates past breaking point and becomes unable to satiate itself through the right form of expressions. Utter destruction of properties, physical harm, and even semi intentionally taking lives will be the penultimate result of a long unexpressed aggression. Aggression is our need to convey strength, dominance, and control over our circumstances and to achieve that, oftentimes it comes with us needing to impose our physical and mental will to assert our sense of supremacy and authority in order to satiate our need for self-esteem and self-actualization. That is why you must convey them through endeavors that allows you to impose your physical and mental will. Like lifting heavy weights in the gym, learning martial arts, playing sports, hiking a mountain, or even getting proficient in a difficult, complicated, and strenuous skills like cooking or tailoring. Aggression is our natural need to conquer and bring difficult circumstances into our command and understanding to achieve a state of self-reliance or self-sufficiency, that is why you must convey them in such a way that is worthy and worthwhile for our physical and mental demands.

The state of obsessive, extreme yearning and impatience happens when greed gets both repressed and overly exercised, and we all know why. The narrative always portrays greed as a despicable quality that leads to nowhere but humiliation and regret. We all want more and most of us want them fast and through wanting them fast, we often rush into unanalyzed and uncalculated conclusions which will more often than not result in tremendous consequences. However, without greed, there will be no curiosities, no excitements, and no inspirations. The state of discontentment is what makes us human beings strive for more in life, bringing in unprecedented levels of progression and evolution within civilization. Discontentment is a natural gift. It's what tempt us and eventually incentivizes us to take risks to achieve and acquire more, and that is the word I want you gentlemen to pay attention to risks. Because extreme and uncontrollable greed can stem from our lack of exhilarating anticipations through taking risks in life. The exhaustingly prolonged state of profound mundaneness, tedious and complacency generates an absence of physically and mentally stimulating sensations to satiate our discontentment, which will inevitably and instinctually bring us to seek those sensations in hastily and thirstily manner. Often out of sheer hopelessness like a dehydrated man in a desert, desperately seeking for water to drink. That is why the world of gambling is designed to provoke our state of discontentment because they seemingly offer the satiation that we crave. But as we all know in gambling, the house always wins in the end. On the other hand, greed can also stem from getting too deeply caught up in the momentous occasions of positive experiences or opportunities leading to the similar rush of impatience for more as the desperation due to a lack of positive sensation, greed is our natural need to continuously explore, experience and acquire.

That is why you must convey them in ways that continuously involves adequate risks and rewards to neutralize the restlessness that comes from extreme or prolonged monotonously, like the adoption of a new and interesting endeavor in your routine and pursuing an extension or expansion of your current routine like going or turning professional on a constructive hobby that you like. However, when you are riding a momentous occasion of positive streaks like winning, you have to learn not to bite off more than you can chew, or in other words, you have to know when to stop and readjust because your overwhelmingly escalated level of confidence or metaphysical reliance on luck wave can put you at a much less of an edge to remain objective and concentrated, making you more vulnerable to making mistakes due to carelessness and underestimation caused by over excitement. That is why you must learn to set predetermined limits on your wave of momentum before it comes crashing and dragging you down along with it Rave sexual violation and assault, basically our rapist's tendencies are a result of a sexually unsatiated and unfulfilled life back in the tribal age. Rape is the grim result from men who are not sexually selected by women to protect and provide for them, and their lack of sex translates into a forceful and nonconsensual action of sexual violations on women from another village that successfully rated to satiate their sexual cravings and today it is not much different. Men who lack sexual experience in their daily lives for such a long time will accumulate an intense and dangerous level of sexual cravings and it is only momentarily negated or neutralized by the presence and access of pornography and or prostitution. For those men who lack sex on a regular basis due to our prolonged sexual frustration, we often look at women objectively to an extreme level as there are no intentions for meaningful interaction to develop deep personal connections, only the intention to unleash our raw, visceral, and fear lust onto and into their bodies, to explosively spread our seats and release our sexual cravings.

For modern men, the extreme fear and anxiety to get rejected and taking rejections too personally are the main cause for the massive buildup in the raven of your frustrated eroticism. Sex or procreation is an essential need to be fulfilled for human beings because it is one of our main natural and instinctual purpose to exist Besides eating, sleeping, and excreting our fecal matters. In order to express lust properly and carefully, you must firstly not be embarrassed or feel disgusted with your intentions and desires. We are all humans, and we have our own unique set of sexual preferences and fetishists. Secondly, you must not hesitate or abort for too much and too long to express lust through your natural flirtatious tendencies in the presence of the opposite sex of your interest in order to proceed ever so closer to fulfilling your desires in which your lust is instinctually pursuing. Regardless of whether you eventually consume it or not, it's all up to you, but the most important thing is to convey those growing sexual tension through gradual seductive invitations during the interaction. Let's not pretend that we've never done this to someone else, shall we? We've all been there and done that when it comes to deceiving others, even when it comes to something small like an opinion or a needless matter because believe it or not, deception is actually one of the most important strong traits to have as a leader because it's about being able to manipulate, seduce, and convince people as thoroughly as possible the world of politics and social hierarchies, or revolve around deceiving others and winning them over to your side. The extreme case of this dark quality going out of control usually does not come from a lack of expression because deception is often utilized in normal social situations like preaching an opinion from a perspective and even humorous, sarcastic and nonsensical or comical interactions, but rather its rebellious nature stems from too much utilization, exploitation and getting away with too much of it without ever facing any form of repercussions, criticisms and consequences to the point where it becomes a normal part of your behavior or personality or character just like speeding on the highway and never getting a speeding ticket for doing it continuously for long periods of time. That is why highly deceptive people are usually extremely insistent when refused and extremely defiant when accused and would always want to justify their claims regardless of what is true or what is not. Your lack of exercise or expressions in your deceptive capabilities on the other hand won't eventually result you in becoming highly deceptive, but rather the opposite. It gets you to become more ignorant and vulnerable to the selfish intentions of deceptive people in order to utilize deception properly and less exploitative meaning for it to be beneficial to your own intentions as well as appealing or being harmless and even beneficial to others. You must learn to appeal to others' best interests first. Then slowly align them towards your own best interests, making the interaction or negotiation a win-win situation. This is why learning how to sell is the best medium to exercise your deceptive capabilities. Always remember this gentleman, the best way to ask for help and making an offer to other people is the first figure out and understand what their best interests are and make sure that you can significantly fulfill them within your compensation and offer. If you gentlemen want an example of a cleverly deceptive and cunning leader who is exceptional in his ability to manipulate and negotiate, look no further than our very own captain Jack Sparrow, as he was always able to find a way even in harmful and life-threatening situations to negotiate his survival while appealing to his enemy's best interest. Even though in the end he basically lied to them all Throughout the history of mankind, revenge or vengeance have been deeply ingrained in our social calibration as it is our default instinctual response towards a wound caused by another individual, both physical and emotional. It is a defense mechanism against the anxieties towards survival, stimulated by the reactivation of memories involving major injuries and losses experienced earlier in the lifetime of a person and driven by the desire to repair through neutralizing or eliminating the threats that caused a previous wounds vengeance comes from all individuals own apparent degree of paradigm towards moral rationality and justice.

This is why if one's code of moral ethics hasn't been properly developed and solidified through the acquisition of further conscientious knowledge and teachings like religion, he would always submit to his natural instinct to relentlessly seek and achieve retribution instead of forgiveness. Vengeance is vividly similar and related to aggression as they involve the accumulation of rage the longer you bottle it up, but the violence that resulted from accumulated vengeance is more saturated, directed and passionately intended than the violence that resulted from accumulated aggression, often leading to vicious uncontrollable moments of sadism to express or channel vengeance constructively and harmlessly, you have to shift from a mindset of personal retribution towards a mindset of general competition instead of physically harming the individual that hurt you through an act of savage and consequential retribution, revitalize your vengeance towards an act of superior reconstruction, such as building a stronger physique, becoming more capable and knowledgeable, acquiring more resources and material possessions, meeting with more physically appealing and fertile women and getting more established and recognized in various territories, rejuvenating your competitive spirit and tendencies through participating or engaging in mutually antagonistic endeavors such as playing single-minded driven competitive sports like boxing is the best way to transmute your vengeful tendencies as it still involves you. Trading blows with another individual whose aim is also to harm and injure you. Narcissism involves around us having a dramatically elevated borderline delusional sense of self-importance while almost completely abandoning our natural born gift to empathize and sympathize with other people. Again, we've all done this at various point in our lives, oftentimes unconsciously until we either get called out or everyone started distancing themselves from us. Our obsession and ruthlessness to bring circumstances to the way we want them to be in our thirst for attention, validation, and appraisal from other people to fulfill our never-ending vessel of self-esteem oftentimes result in our complete neglect of other people's wellbeing. The most common example is spending our time immerse within our own priorities too much while ignoring or insulting the needs of other people close to us, compelling someone to do our dirty work for us while simultaneously questioning or attacking their moral decisions if they refused and taking all the credit for someone else's hard work, using our superior position and exposure in the social hierarchy just for the sake of fulfilling our thirst for cloud, captivation and circumstantial obedience or convenience. We all love social attention and recognition as human beings and narcissism can stem from a life that is absent or lacking in constructive attention and appraisal to assist in the formation of one sense of self-esteem leading to an individual's desperation and yearning to seek for them. But for the most part in today's world, it comes from an overwhelmingly ridiculous amount of complimentary or gratuitous attention and appraisal that causes an individual to develop a new paradigm regarding their own seemingly superior and special existence in this world, which leads to that individual's eventual and utter fragile dependence for those attention and appraisal to have any form of self-esteem oftentimes going to great lengths, even demonstrating morally or ethically questionable conducts. To obtain any form of attention and validation to help neutralize or maintain narcissism from overcoming your rational and objective perspectives, you have to always maintain a high level of consciousness regarding your own worth for commendable, whether you are lacking them or getting showered by them, you have to realistically know when, where, and why you are deserving for attention and praise. Thus, keeping yourself reasonably in check before you think of humiliating your own reputation and be remembered as a completely deranged individual. If you want to be self-absorbed or egocentric, earn it. Prove that you are somewhat credible, respectable, and reputable so that your self-centeredness will be overshadowed by the overall positive impact of your deeds. But then again, human beings are selfish creatures and for the most part, it is only the severity of the consequences that can force them to become aware of their own missteps, to reconsider their decisions. There is no escaping these dark qualities of ours, gentlemen. No matter how much you want to reject their existence, they will always eventually break free and demonstrate themselves either in front of you or even in front of other people, both consciously and unconsciously. As I've always said before, human beings are capable of demonstrating sinister conducts and the high societies telling you to get rid of them because they want to easily control you as submissive puppets due to your lack or absence of selfish attributes that comes from your dark side. Do not think of these dark qualities as quote unquote evil or bad as all they want is an adequate amount of expression. Just like any other forms of thoughts and emotions, they only turn evil when you try your hardest to disregard their existence and when you let them run free without a leash. Controlling them is only a matter of acknowledging their existence inside of you and finding proper ways or mediums for them to fittingly and appropriately express themselves to satiate their nature. Our dark side hides our true potential because they contain the origin of our deepest desires, thoughts, emotions, perspectives, capabilities, and imposition of will that we often conceal due to the narratively induced fear of being socially rejected and punished if we do express them. You must not be afraid to become aware of their existence as your other half and utilize their nature to serve you in opportunistic and challenging circumstances.

CHAPTER SEVENTY-FOUR
ONCE UPON A NOBODY

Let's go to the chase. Life as a man feels absolutely terrible when you're out of shape, broke, unemployed, lonely, incompetent sexless, and entirely dependent on another person to live the pressure to succeed. And your collection of insecurities just consumes your thoughts day and night. And people sense that from you and they just decide that they don't want to associate with you or have anything to do with you. Women couldn't care less about you alive or dead, nor do they want to bother themselves acknowledging your insignificant presence. Everything. And everyone will go completely south on you and leave you to care for your crippled self on your own, a fucking nobody. That feeling of utter uselessness, worthlessness, and ineptness slowly start to spread their tentacles of darkness, embracing themselves to claim their authority and identity within you. You start to feel that your mere existence is nothing more than a rusty vessel for the world to shit on and ridicule upon the feeling of despair, overwhelms your judgments and puts you in a position of constant self-deprecation. You're not born in a supo family with generational wealth to play with. You're not genetically blessed for aesthetics and athletics, and you're not exceptionally gifted with a gargantuan hippocampus that you bring. It's all unfair. The world is cruel, and people are evil. What's the point to keep on living when my existence is only nothing but a wasted effort? Why was I even born? Only to live as both a laughingstock and a hindrance to our evolution? Is there absolutely no way I could turn this darkness around? Should I just end this pointless existence of mine because I just feel like I'm more useful, beneficial when I'm dead? Should I just end it right here? Your set of misfortunes all can be undone and all it takes to start is a simple shift in your attitude and mentality. You'll often underestimate the impeccable impact attitude can give into your life. Attitude is everything. It is literally the single most important difference between those who fail and those who prevail. This one very crucial mental shift is what ultimately saved me and most likely many others from taking our own lives. Took me a while to decode it, but this is what I've been wanting you gentlemen to know. Never let a single significantly bleak and dire moment in your life define the value and worth of your entire existence. As every man's merit is never definitively established within a single specific moment, they are cumulatively established from all the conquests in his own unique lives. Voyage, let me repeat that once more. Never let a single significantly bleak and dire moment in your life define the value and worth of your entire existence. As every man's merit is never definitively established within a single specific moment. They are cumulatively established from all the conquests in his own unique life's voyage. So never let your current circumstance of being out shape broke and lonely, permanently determined the entire scope of your identity within your lifetime. Because they only exist in a particular moment within your life unless you let them become forever. You are not utterly worthless. You are just temporarily redundant. You are not completely useless. You are only briefly dormant. These are not mere hopeful and metaphysical incantations to motivate you or make you feel good about yourself because we don't do that shit here. These are realistic and objective driven relics of what is both plausibly and practically possible. You are never utterly worthless or entirely useless, no manners. You are only worthless and useless if you decide to remain so or be so because every man in this world has the power to transform himself over time. Every man in this world has potential and it is your duty to discover that potential and impose them into building the life that you want. The world you are living in is not an idealistic and fantastical wonderland where you can live and enjoy every single ounce of your make beliefs. This world has its own natural mechanics of operation, and if you do not bend to its will and align them with your own, you will never make the necessary changes to see things for what they are. And you will be forever occupied and bitter about how the world could never be to you. Only the men who willingly submit conceit and affirm their fate to their misfortunes, who will eventually be forgotten by everyone as both utter and complete failures in this life. Because there is only one thing that is worse, much worse than being a loser or a nobody. And that is being a sheer coward to fight against your misfortunes. At least you will have absolutely no regrets and people will respect you enough if you die trying to be a winner rather than accepting your miserable fate to die a complete loser without fighting back the 300 Spartans, were fighting a losing battle against the Persians. But at his day, whose sheer courage and determination to stand and fight until the end makes their deed worthy to be echoes of eternity, they never retreat, they never surrender. As long as you are alive, you will always have the chance to be able to make something out of yourself. Let me repeat that one more time. As long as you are alive, you will always have the chance to be able to make something out of yourself. And all it takes is the voracious will of a single man. What is exactly the point to keep on living when life itself has been nothing but constant suffering for you? Well, if you ask me personally, gentlemen, I'd say it's to prove that I am so much more than just a waste of time and effort because I know that I am not. And similarly, I know that you are not.

CHAPTER SEVENTY-FIVE
CRISIS

Facing a crisis is probably one of the most, or even the most hair pulling, gut-wrenching and ball breaking experience we could never felt in our entire lives. Crisis in simple words is basically the dramatic meteoric and abrupt end to a fortunate circumstance or a serious or unfortunate circumstances. Whether it is about losing our jobs, breaking up from a long-term relationship, suffering from a convoluted or vacant sense of identity and confidence, or a hellish combination of all of them and more, they all just make us feel this enormous, seemingly never-ending, momentous wave of dread and agitation. Panic is probably the best word to definitively describe it. All of us will definitively encounter these sensations one way or another in our lifetime. Crisis is just a part of life. All good things sooner or later will eventually come to an end. What goes up must come down in the end. What is a life will eventually cease to exist. Again, that is just how the world works. Very hard to swallow. For some of your idealistic absolutists, but love me or hate me, you'll absolutely thank me later. But anyways, those things are a much later, so let's not become pathetic defeatist here, shall we? How can we better handle the crisis we are facing or will be facing in the future? More specifically, how can we diffuse the psychological turmoil that we experience during a crisis or when a crisis is looming in the far distance? I think some of you gentlemen already expected this and for good reason because this is actually the most important thing to instill into your mental firmware. Most people find it very hard to simply acknowledge and admit that misfortunes have befallen them, and they spent precious amount of time and energy pointlessly debating and wishing that the clock would magically rewind itself before the crisis and circumstances could and should be different. And when I mean different, I mean things have to go exactly the way they idealistically want them to be. When a crisis happens, people usually tend to overthink and overreact and try their best to find ways to restore or fix their circumstances as quickly as possible. Like if your long-term relationship abruptly ends, you will tend to desperately try to fix things and work things out to get back together. Same thing when you lost your job. You tend to desperately try to renegotiate your case to be reinstated or hastily. Send your application everywhere to restore that employment status. And it is understandable because it is instinctual for us to respond that way as we humans are creatures of habits and routines, and when that long developed structure collapses, we lost that sense of command, control, and order. That is why we panic and become headless chickens, hopelessly trying to rebuild or reconstruct that torn structure like after your relationship suddenly ends the following day, you're going to be physically and mentally fixated on your missing daily dose of cuddles, blowjobs, and intercourse. The same thing with losing your job the following day. You're going to be physically and mentally fixated on your missing daily dose of meetings. White shirts, tie spreadsheets and paychecks going into your bank account, and the same thing happened to us when covid hit and changed nearly everything with regards to the structure of our lives. The speed in which you can move on from the occurrence of the crisis and the extent to which you can remain mentally sound during the crisis will almost entirely depend on your ability to simply and sincerely acknowledge or admit that the crisis has happened or will be happening and that they are out of your control. Because most crisis are literally out of your control, there is nothing you could do to reverse what has happened. Time only moves forward. Don't panic when you are panicking, your blend of negative emotions will cloud your judgments and you will inevitably become impatient and start to say stupid things and make irrational decisions, which will more often than not cause you to involuntarily amplify your sense of misfortunes. Relax for a bit. Your tendencies to want to fix the damage done will always be there to haunt you but understand that you will get the chance to do that eventually time only moves forward, but it doesn't move at light speed. Okay? So, there is no need to jump into ill prepared and uncalculated conclusions or actions. The same thing applies to facing future incoming crisis. You must intelligently concede that it will happen regardless of what you do. You must educate yourself about it and adapt accordingly during the crisis. Which brings me to the next important point. This might make you feel at ease at first, but I must insist that if you don't get the first point right or be able to achieve a state of admittance in a crisis, there is no need for you to move on to the second point because you may actually end up in an internal crisis manufactured and escalated by your own immature and incompetent mentality. But anyways, during a crisis, it is all about continuous adaptation like the economic cycle, no matter at what stage it is at, it's about constantly adjusting and restructuring yourself so that you can fit your current circumstances better and adjust yourself. You will just like the three crises of the human life, the quarter life crisis where it's about finding your place in this world and trying your best in getting your shit together, which most of us are in right now in our twenties. Then after conquering that as you go older, you'll face the midlife crisis where it's about acknowledging your own mortality and finding out you're declining physical and mental capabilities. Then after conquering that, you'll face the late life crisis where it's about dealing with the losses of all your loved ones, friends, family, and contemplating the regrets you may have in your life. It's all a continuous cycle or encircling process from crisis to recovery to conquer until your demise. Single, divorced or widowed will eventually turn to taken, engaged, or married and vice versa. Unemployed or retired will eventually turn to employed or self-employed and vice versa, and being shy, awkward, or anxious will turn to being confident, charismatic, or savvy, and vice versa, so on and so forth. The cycle continues until it eventually ends with either your timely or untimely demise or your own self-sabotage and other extreme uncontrollable circumstances affecting you. The main point here is for most of us providing that we are able to accept and move on from the occurrence of the crisis and make the necessary adjustments needed to eventually recover from it. The cycle will return to our desired state once again, thus completing the loop. Once again. Speaking of adjusting, this is probably one that you gentlemen are very familiar with. They say that one man's trash is another man's treasure. I'd say that one man's trash paves the way towards many treasures for the same man. Remember what Tyler Durden said in Fight Club. It's only after we've lost everything that we are free to do anything. This is the burn knuckle genesis or origins of the abundance mindset, and it's completely true. When your life's order is completely destroyed, that is when you will become utterly free to establish a new order from scratch based on how you like your life to be moving forward into the future. When you lose your job, you have all the time in the world to pursue other valuable endeavors of your interests. When your long-term relationship failed, you have all the options in the world to find and build a new and better one. When your reputation is tarnished, you have the freedom to either reclaim that back or the much better option, go into a new territory and establish a new one, so on and so forth. Like when Covid happened, a lot of us are in financial crisis, and we have to find other opportunistic means to help us survive through the crisis. Businesses have to adapt and go digital and utilize that opportunity to expose themselves further in the market in order to survive, and I bet most of us went into learning both investments and cryptos and took advantage of its blast off and wiring to the moon during the pandemic itself. Even many small temporary businesses were created to circumstantially adapt during the pandemic itself, like developing unique military or terrorist mass designs For God's sake, the next financial crisis is coming pretty soon, so educate yourself as much as possible so you are more prepared and can adapt way faster according to your own circumstances when the crisis eventually happens. This is what I meant by being an opportunist, learning, adjusting and adapting to your circumstances so that it will turn into your favor no matter how bleak it is. Like if you are absolutely broke with no skills at all to earn a living, pursue physical labor, and slowly rebuilt from there. A lot of organizations could use some muscles, bluntly speaking, adapt, don't stay where you are or desperately hoping to restore past glories that have already gone. It's such a simple analogy. Why force yourself to continue doing or pursuing the things that don't want to or can't serve you anymore? Let them go pick up what's left of you and construct a new structure of order in your life with new endeavors and people. I believe that being mentally calm during a crisis is more than just being able to remain psychologically functional, progressive, and objective, but also being able to significantly understand what you are dealing with and what you are getting yourselves into. Because eventually and ultimately, those are what makes you reliable during a crisis and gets you to have the confidence to take control and not ally beat around the bush for too much and too long.

CHAPTER SEVENTY-SIX
NONE OF YOUR BUSINESS

I think it's currently safe and appropriate to say that we've all been guilty of this particular mess in this social media age. We are always going to be exposed to the grandeur and mischiefs of other people around the world. We've never felt so connected before, yet we've also never felt so out of touch with the physical manifestation of our own individual lives. Just because we're spending more of our times daily, immersing ourselves and worrying about what other people are doing, what they're eating, where they're going, who they're hanging out with, what activities they're doing, what countries they've been to, what they're wearing, how they're looking, who they're dating, et cetera. Literally endless classifications and categorizations that you can name. And I guess at some point when we are eventually overwhelmed by all the insecurities and indignations that we've created and accumulated for ourselves through being captivated by other people's collection of merit, we will inevitably question ourselves, why are we still doing it? Why the hell are we still spending eight to 10 hours a day scrolling through social media and making ourselves feel even more miserable for the day before we went to bed, even when we know that it is bad for us to do so? World gentlemen, the simple answer is because you've been utterly plugged in into the world of self-esteem porn, and just like regular porn, nearly everything is escalated and manipulated. This urge to extensively consume these idealistic portrayals comes from a place of significant level of lack due to the sense of fear, laziness, incapability, impatience, dissatisfaction, and unavailability or inaccessibility to manifest our desires into physical demonstrations, we just want to feel somehow hastily stimulated, ass satiate our own desperate and convoluted emotions. We watch porn because we are either fearful, lazy, incapable, impatient, unsatisfied, and or in shortage of real-life physical intimacy. Similarly, we pay too much attention to other people's lives online because we are either too fearful, lazy, incapable, impatient, unsatisfied, and or seemingly insufficient to become the main star or the main protagonist in our own lives. Pursuing and experiencing both physically and mentally cultivating endeavors. That is why, again, just like porn, you ended up making the deliberate choice to stimulate yourselves, impulsively and precipitously through experiencing them from other people's point of view because you are lacking and or unable to experience them yourselves. Now, having said all of that, the main question and also the most crucial question you should be asking yourselves is not why am I doing it or why can't I stop doing it? Instead, it should be, how is it going to be beneficial for me and my circumstances if I keep doing it? You must shift your attitude from a bemoaning and dubious perspective into an acquisitive and uncharitable perspective. In other words, be selfish and let's not pretend to be good little boys here, shall we? Doing self-improvement in general is all about how each specific endeavors that we are doing can benefit or cultivate both our present and future circumstances for our own sake. Self-improvement is a selfish path, and your point of view must originate from your own objective judgments that fulfills your best interests. So objectively speaking, you can now ask yourselves, how is paying attention to other people's lives going to be beneficial for me and my circumstances if I actually just keep doing it?

If you are struggling to answer that question, then let me answer it for you, because if you ask me a site from trying to establish new legitimate business connections or network, which are quite rare, and being able to partially help in revitalizing or clarifying your competitive drive, should you be able to properly utilize the emotions that you get from your insecurities, I literally don't see anything more useful or beneficial or purposeful you can get from doing it. There is absolutely minimal ROI for most of the time, and worst of all, you are exhausting the most precious commodity and resource that you have your time, and we all know time does not add. Once you lose it, you lose it forever. So just try to calculate the amount of time that you spend sitting or lying down, going through literal portfolios of people's documented moments that you could instead use to make your life just that little bit better every day. Which one would you prefer in your quote unquote self-improvement journey? So again, objectively speaking, it shouldn't be your business because it is none of your business apart from your own family members. One person's life is their own concerns to account and their own blessings to enjoy, and so is yours. So, keep it that way. Too much paying attention to or immersing selves diligently in other people's lives put you in a very disadvantaged position where you will eventually start to live your life subconsciously and involuntarily in accordance with other people's terms and metrics. It's a natural response due to our instinct to conform as social beings where you start to do things because other people are doing them, wear clothes because other people are wearing them. Go to places because people went there before, so on and so forth, and it does not apply only to your friends or random people you've met, but it also applies to the people you are currently aspiring from. Celebrities, athletes, and other people of both great credibility and publicity.

If you ped or idolize them too much, you start to morph yourselves to live in their shadows again, doing what they do, saying what they say, wearing what they wear, and acting how they act. You are literally becoming the cheap knockoff or rip off version of that individual, trying desperately to become exactly like them, which you never will and emulate their way of life, which you may not entirely prefer. It's not a bad thing at all to take aspirations from people. In fact, you need it to make circumstances clearer for you to assess and judge, but don't try to entirely replicate them. Cherry. Pick those traits, the ones that you like the most, and the ones that you can relate and associate with the most. Put your own twist on them and apply them to your own life so that they can help you manifest your own specific desires relative to your own individual circumstances. Don't be a total mimic. Don't live predominantly or entirely in other people's shadows. Create your own character and lifestyle from which you can make it simpler and clearer to envision and pursue by aspiring from other people, but not obsessing or fixating on trying to become exactly like them. It's like one man said during his prime winners. Focus on winning losers. Focus on winners.

CHAPTER SEVENTY-SEVEN
MENTAL AUTHORITY

Emotions are no question the most complicated part of the human race, trying to completely understand them. It's like trying to know exactly how many stars are in the Milky Way. You could spend an entire lifetime trying to uncover their entire layers. And when you think you've done it, there is always another undiscovered layer taunting you with its incomprehensible properties. But regardless, our efforts to keep them from entirely influencing our decisions and actions will always be appreciated, not only by ourselves, but also from the people around us. Now, before we begin, I'd like to point out that this is not a universally acclaimed method. This mental conditioning is basically what I've learned and utilized personally to manage my impossibly irresponsible anger that I've suffered from for more than a decade. A method that according to me at least, could effectively become a substitute or a supplement alongside your meditation work. This method is not to extinguish your emotions or to completely remove them from existence because you can't ever do that. As emotions cannot be destroyed. It's only to momentarily neutralize them and keep them at bay until you found a way to express them properly and constructively or compensate for them. Because as much as you like to wish that you could suppress your emotions as much as possible and as long as possible, to the point where they will go away forever, they will eventually resurface sooner or later whether you like it or not. The first and foremost thing that you must do is to find your trigger points or what incentivizes those emotional reactions. And as simple as it sounds, it's actually very hard to do initially if you've never done a thorough objective introspection regarding yourselves before, especially those trigger points that can make you consider hurting someone because it literally involves you calling yourselves out for your own ignorance and weaknesses that you often don't want, don't care, and too sensitive to admit and comprehensively work on. You must fully understand that negative emotions are the defensive or coping reactions that are generated by both internal and external provocations and conflicts surrounding your un insecurities, uncontrollable irritations, and unrealized expectations, but also oftentimes it can be just your own hormonal imbalance affecting your mood. Now, your trigger points can be identified in the ranges or scope of those three categories.

What they are is down to your own responsibility to introspect and identify to make your introspection process easier. And I've always said this many times is to make them more plausible and tangible to your five sensors. I e write them down so that you can perceive them a lot clearer and more definitively than just relying on your mental notes. If you can't find your trigger points and fully acknowledge them, i e, you are able to know the visceral conditions of why they are able to generate negative emotions from you, then half of your problems are already solved. Because again, the main problem with identifying your trigger points is simply your fear of a diminished sense of self-worth afterwards because it literally involves and revolves around you pointing out your own shortcomings and vulnerabilities. And if you kept rejecting or ignoring or avoiding those trigger points, you are basically running away from the problems you're trying to solve. Your rejection or ignorance towards your weaknesses and deficiencies are what's causing the constant outburst of retaliation because you are trying to avoidantly contradict yourself evidential reality. On the contrary, your acceptance and acknowledgement of your trigger points will generate the subconscious and intuitive understanding or sense of control and anticipation that you need to realize about yourselves to reduce or neutralize the internal conflict between your ego and conscience when you get provoked. Of course, this is a lot easier to do when it only involves minor provocations or circumstances that you can easily tolerate without much mental effort or exertion like getting your windscreen shot on by birds or someone pulling a small prank on you, for example, as you can simply acknowledge and dismiss them because they barely scratch your ego. But when it comes to major provocations, i e, those that makes you tick and become fully aware, those that really gets underneath your skin and deep into your nerves or those that triggers you a lot and puts a huge dent on your ego, like someone blatantly insulting your physical limitations and status or losing a crucially substantial amount of money, for example, then you need more than just acknowledging those trigger points to effectively neutralize those fast and momentous buildups of negative emotions. This is where the other half of our problem lies in this case. You also need to counter those momentous negative emotions quickly or swiftly with convicted future conception or narration and or eventual execution of positive circumstances, ideally as soon as possible in order to generate a wave of positive emotions so that they can help neutralize your wave of negative emotions, acknowledge and counter for irritations and most unrealized expectations. It can be literally anything from eating your favorite dish to treating yourself with something personally gratifying. Like for example, personally, if I get massively irritated to the point where I want to punch someone, I simply shift my thoughts into getting my favorite ice cream afterwards to redirect my focus away from the provoking negative circumstances towards the rewarding positive circumstances.

Now, when it comes to your insecurities being significantly provoked, which is possibly the hardest thing for all of us to emotionally handle, it's quite a bit more specific. You must redirect your thoughts towards positive circumstances that not only generate positive emotions, but also can help compensate the dent or cut in your ego. Like for example, if someone blatantly insults your height, which you are very insecure about, you need to neutralize those negative emotions that have been generated through that provocation by shifting your thoughts into positive carbon sensory circumstances that you are going to manifest ideally later in the day or afterwards, like lifting weights and getting a PR or a PB or working extra hours through the night on your own personal project. Whether you want to respond or not to the individual who provoked you is entirely up to you. But the most important thing is to calm yourself down before saying any word or expressing anything essentially. It's relatively similar, like trying to calm a baby down from crying, by making funny faces, singing him or her song, or giving him or her nice treats. Now, maybe some of you would say, wait a minute, isn't that relatively similar to toxic positivity? No, it isn't because toxic positivity is when you firstly Diluted and ignorantly refused to acknowledge your weaknesses to eventually work on them and compensate for them. And secondly, toxic positivity is all about positive thinking and not positive performing. Notice the difference. Now, would this method have a thoroughly immediate effect on you? No, it wouldn't because just like muscles, you need to mentally condition your mind consistently through time to experience the full workings of this method or any method to be honest, because again, this is not the soul and absolute method for emotional control. In order to eventually achieve emotional strength, you have to practice or train emotional control long enough to the point where it becomes a predisposed instinctual response for your mind to simply flow through. A lot of people still think that controlling your emotions or being emotionally strong means that you are entirely neglecting your emotions. That is absolutely not the case. You have to understand them first and foremost before you built an attitude around them so that you can have total authority, although your natural impulses. And one of the main important essences of masculinity itself is being able to control your emotions no matter the circumstances, so that you can remain consistently objective. And that I'm very much sure is what you gentlemen want to eventually achieve.

CHAPTER SEVENTY-EIGHT
WINTER WORKHORSE

Winter translation, the season to engage in comfort, good food and warmth. A blissful moment for all of us to just sit in our homes beside the fire and reflect the long year that have passed. A lot of us buy gifts for ourselves and our loved ones, while feeling the touch of the friendly and familiar hands that we've grown so accustomed to for many years. And some of us went on holidays to escape the blistering coal from jeopardizing the remaining droplets of enthusiasm that we have from the warmer days. It's a season cultured for celebration, appreciation, and reminiscence of the good times that we've had the whole year alongside the people that we love, respect, and enjoy being around with all the while enthusiastically awaiting the dawn of a hopeful new and better continuation of this beautiful life that we are eager to enjoy further. Lovely, isn't it? And if any of you gentlemen already have plans to relish in this winter, please have an absolute ball with them all. Enjoy them to the absolute fullest. As for some of you gentlemen who don't have any plans for this winter, who don't have anyone to enjoy or celebrate winter with, or who are just relatively wary, tired, and uninterested with what winter brings translation, it's the season of minimal distractions or the time in the world and relentless progress. You see the main reason why I think winter is the better season for making progress. It's not because summer or spring can't get you similar progress that you want. No, they certainly can. Instead, it's simply the matter of absolute periods of free time during winter are relatively way more available than in warmer seasons. And again, as I've said before, and I think I'm starting to sound like a broken record at this point, I'm always, always against wasting time. In summer generally, you have loads of activities, loads of moments to socialize and network loads of options to try something new. The sun is out, the sky is clear, and both your mood and demeanor are energized because of it. You basically have more to enjoy or benefit in and out of your regular routine. During warmer weathers, holidays and distractions are made for warmer weathers and are certainly more amusing and delightful during warmer weathers. Whereas during winter, similar to extremely cloudy and rainy days, outdoor activities are pretty much dormant unless you're into winter sports, which let's be honest is a lot less appealing to participate in. Majority of people are staying inside to get warm and killing time by watching Netflix or doing other mundane endeavors, or they fly to a warm tropical country to relax until the winter had passed. A lot of people are going shopping, and because we're men, we don't need 20 different types of shirts and 50 different types of pants.

So how much time are you going to spend during the year end sale if you do decide to shop? Probably half a day maximum. Other major events are only Christmas and the new year, and let's be honest here, how many Christmas dinners are you going to have with your family and friends and the new year? Realistically, it's just another day, mate. Just a subtle reminder that you are getting older and have done nothing major nor gone anywhere significant in your life. That is why I personally think winter is the better, more opportunistic and suitable season for you to just put your head down, isolate yourself, and just make leaps of progress in whatever it is you are working on. You have three whole months to yourself. Imagine three whole months locked down in a prison cell or three whole months living within a minimalist style fight camp with nothing but a voracious mind and a burning heart. You will inevitably compel yourselves to work your agitation, boredom, and restlessness due to the lack of physical and mental stimulation, will eventually force you to cope by engaging in the most convenient endeavors available at your disposal. That's unnerving and unsettling sensation to impose your desires and will into something worthwhile, productive, and meaningful. Just consumes your every thought. You just can't sit still for much longer. You have to do something to advance towards a certain form of development. That's why prisoners do hundreds of pushups, pull-ups, read and write a lot during their time being locked up. Winter is also the perfect season to test and reveal your current mentality as the lack of sunlight naturally will make you feel more lethargic and warier. And this is the supplemental battle you would want to voluntarily undergo to cultivate your capacity and capability for dedication because as we know, it's already, it's not easy fighting your natural instincts and tendencies, especially when it comes to dealing with your declining moods and eventually turning them into constructive habits. And before you think "damn winter, sure does sucks. It brings anything but good news." Well, first of all, I can't fully disagree on that because statistics do have shown that winter is the least preferred weather for most of the population. However, secondly, there is actually one good news for you gentlemen who are looking to lose weight. As in winter, our blood pressure rises to regulate our core body temperature to produce heat and keep us warm, thus, naturally allows us to burn more calories than during warmer weathers. So, if any of you gentlemen are looking to accelerate your weight loss journey, then winter is the perfect season for you to work on it. I'm fully aware that this is a highly personal opinion, but I'd just like to make the most out of my available time despite the seemingly unfavorable and uncooperative circumstances. And I think so should you gentlemen because there is just this sense of great reward and supremacy that you feel afterwards just through the conscious acknowledgement that you are able to bring yourselves to carry out challenging, constructive activities despite some annoying and inconvenient hindrance or resistance from your environment. While most people have conceded to their basic instincts, because at the end of the day what matters most is you are the one who is progressing.

CHAPTER SEVENTY-NINE
LIARS

Lies. Lies, lies. Yep. We've all been on the receiving end and also done them countless of times in our lives. So, let's stop pretending to be the self-proclaimed most pure and righteous men on this planet, shall we? Because I know that a lot of you will still ignorantly claim yourself that you never lied once in your entire life, and that you don't have the capacity or capability to lie whatsoever. Well, you're lying already, so that simply proves my point. But anyways, why do we lie or why do we decide to become dishonest? Now, I know for most of us, the word lying or lies have been culturally and morally ingrained within our psyches and egos as very antagonistic or hostile terms. And yes, of course, so have I. But for the sake of this chapter, I'd like you gentlemen to firstly try and loosen up that firm ego investments or biasness of yours regarding the human being's natural gift and capability for dishonesty, so that you can further understand the role and scope of its relevancy and appropriateness or inappropriateness with regards to different context and circumstances within the human life. Because I know when it comes to lies and dishonesty, there is always an everlasting lingering spiteful taste in your mouth that simply signifies it as bad for everything known to man. Now, as humans, we communicate with each other via various verbal and non-verbal signals, such as spoken language, facial expressions, tone of voice and body gestures. But her ability to communicate is further enhanced by our understanding of what is going on inside someone else's mind through our capacity to empathize with each other. This natural gift or ability of ours to empathize is a product of being able to sense or recognize other people's minds as separates from our own. And lying or dishonesty is a fundamental part of this empathy, a byproduct of sorts that comes from our ever-growing and extensive understanding of other people's thoughts and feelings that we've developed through the years of social interactions and communications within different social circumstances. Basically, we've acquired an almost instinctual response of interpretations regarding someone else's frame of mind, just through a brief observation of all those communication signals, again, both verbal and non-verbal, that they've demonstrated either previously or concurrently. Now, making the choice to be dishonest or to lie always comes after those specific interpretations. I mean, if you want to purposefully deceive someone, you first have to be able to understand what that person might be thinking or feeling to objectively assess whether this person can be deceived, at least roughly to some degree. But behind all of our acts or conducts of dishonesty and deception, all of that revolves around these three crucial metrics. One, protection of self-interests, two, avoidance of conflicts, and three, manipulation of perception. These three metrics are very closely linked to one another, and very rarely one occurs without the others or at least one of the others. Now, as we know it from previous chapters, human beings are naturally selfish. Despite our capability to empathize with other people's thoughts and feelings, not all of us could relate or would want to relate and eventually reciprocate with support physically, emotionally, or even financially. That is just the brutal reality of this world, like the current war that is going on. Some of us actually cared and provide support, and others just continue to go about their own lives without any care in the world. Mostly, they just pretend like they care when they are asked about it in order to protect their image. But in essence, all of us have our own priorities and desires, and majority of our thoughts, decisions, emotions, and actions are allocated towards fulfilling them. And if we encounter any form of obstacle, hindrance, or resistance, we wouldn't naturally want to either get rid of them from existence or outsmart them in a way that minimize losses or damages from our side. This dynamic is evidential everywhere in politics, infidelity negotiations, and even in subtle daily social interactions, escalation of credibility, protection of wrongdoings, management of reputation, alleviation of announcement, concealment of truth, you name them all. It's built within our survival instincts. Now, at this point, as I'd expect, I'd say a lot of you would find this utterly preposterous and unnecessary. Why can't people just don't lie? Be honest and tell the truth? Well, the answer is not because people don't want the truth. It's because they cannot handle the truth. People love ideals and they love being promised a better good while ignoring all the dark days there may lay ahead of them and telling the truth or revealing the truth, utterly destroy those ideals and will often send them into uncontrollable emotional reaction due to the massive cognitive dissonance they're experiencing, and often would get confrontational to defend their ideals against opposing contradictions. Human beings say they want the truth, but often they cannot comprehend and handle complete disclosure. That is why being objective amps and understanding this, oftentimes we become tempted to engage in dishonesty and deception in order to take advantage of or opportunistically exploit this tendency for vulnerability and ignorance in order to manufacture ideals to keep people positively occupied while we fulfill our own desires and priorities. An example can be one person's plainly obvious, desperate attempts to attain respect and acknowledgement can effectively be exploited by us to incentivize him or her to carry out our dirty works and keeping him or her around with a false promise for eventual friendship and affection. Now, I know all of that sounds really twisted, but what if I tell you gentlemen that dishonesty is not all dark and dreadful, that it could also be intended for non-exploitative intentions and sometimes even pro-social intentions because in truth, dishonesty can also effectively bail us out of awkward situations, spare the feelings of others, preserve or strengthen alliances, keep us out of trouble and even save our lives. Remember, when you try to maneuver a blunt statement that you've made to avoid a colossal misunderstanding with one of your mates, I did remember when you hold out your frustration to call out your boss for being an absolute wanker in front of the whole office in order to protect your reputation and employment status. I did remember when you called your girlfriend's sister, who is massively overweight, beautiful. When she asks you how she looked at that particular day, I did remember when you pretended to be sick when asked by your mom in order to avoid going to school. I did. Okay. The last one might be a bad example, but hey, no harm was done at the end of the day, so we're all good. So, you see gentlemen, dishonesty is not all utterly degrading and demeaning, contextually and circumstantially. They can also be crucially necessary to implicitly benefit all parties. It's not a malicious move, rather more of a smart one. Now, some of you may still be extremists in your perception regarding dishonesty and think that everyone should still say the truth out loud and adhere to the truth no matter what, and ideally speaking, so do I, gentlemen. So, do I. But unfortunately, objectively speaking, it is not always plausible all of the time since in order for you to be completely honest, you must have utterly nothing to hide, nothing to protect, and nothing to lose. And in the real world, in real life situations, most people always to some extents have something to hide, something to protect, and something to lose. So, you really can't entirely blame them for trying to best serve their priorities, even if it means minutely exploiting an opportunity to do so, because let's be honest, we all will do the same.

CHAPTER EIGHTY
CHANGE IS HARD

It's no longer a secret that we as human beings love to revisit old, bad, or unfavorable habits, either consciously or unconsciously, even though we deliberately made ourselves countless. A promise to refuse or never to concede when temptations strike. Occasionally we just can't help ourselves but to voluntarily or involuntarily loosen up and let our basic instincts take over our rational and objective decision-making process, or rather overwhelms them to let our minds relax for a bit and not be so uptight and strict on ourselves. Because for most of us, it does eventually get quite monumentally tiring and taxing to always be mentally on guard and uncompromising. Now, realistically speaking, for most of us, unless we're extremely obsessed, immersed, and focused on attaining a live goal, it is not an utterly preposterous or unacceptable circumstances at all for us to occasionally or momentarily decompress, unwind, and relax for a short period of time just to enjoy a selection of some of the justifiable temptations around us in order to refresh and restart our minds so that they can become more cognitively effective and efficient. When we do get back on track, eating a bit of junk foods, watching a little bit of Netflix, drinking a little bit at a social event, sleeping a little bit in the afternoon, playing a little bit of videogames, it will be far from the end of the world. And as far as I'm concerned, most of us are actually pretty capable of not sleeping completely out control. When we do enjoy ourselves alongside our selection of reasonable bad habits, we often simply just dust ourselves off the temporary obstructions, pick up where we left off and we're back where we want to be. There is absolutely no critically endangering problem with this particular circumstance. It's literally your cheat day if you want to call it that way. It is only those who are unable, incapable, or desperately can't help to remind themselves that they are being too overzealous in rewarding or basking themselves to the point that they are literally losing themselves within the whole paraphernalia of distractions that they eventually regress, too far downhill to pick up where they left off and lost nearly all of the progress they've made or most of the progress they've made. Basically, they're in too deep and too fast to make the easy U-turn back to the surface, and now they've become negatively buoyant, which makes it much harder for them to swim back to the surface. You are literally getting too comfortable and unaware for your own good regardless. You falling repeatedly too far back into the comfortable but dangerous realm of your old habits and having to work your way back up much harder to the point where you previously left off could stem from either one and or a combination of these four factors or reasons. The first one is pattern recognition. Now we human beings are creatures of structures and habits. We need some form of constitutional order in our lives in order to feel safe and secure and removing or changing that order will instinctually cause us to become convoluted and yearning for an establishment of disposition or regulation that we can live by.

Oftentimes, it always results in us trying to desperately save our old order way of living that we've been accustomed to and conditioned in for so long. It's just a survival and safeguard mechanism. That is why trying to steer away from old habits to build new ones is a bit like trying to get used to living in a completely different house around a completely different environment after staying in only one house for your entire life. I mean, what can you say? Old habits do die hard. Making crucial changes is hard. That is why we often always get tempted to revert back to our old ways of thinking and behaving because they feel safe and comforting, especially when we talk about our bad habits. They're much easier to form due to the absence or lack of any resistance. It takes quite a significant amount of time to become fully established in a new order or structure of life. Imagine playing videogames daily for 10 years straight and wanting to completely get rid of it in the first week. Not that you couldn't, but chances are you won't be able to unless you experience. The next reason I'm about to explain, which is lack of drastic and severe consequences. This is probably the most important point out of the mall. Nothing induces immense dread and the desperate need for immediate changes as experiencing a traumatic or devastating life circumstance that results from our own misconducts. When we experience a traumatic event, especially the one that is caused by our own action or inaction, we tend to reflect on them deeply and extensively to try and figure out what went wrong and distinguish whether there are any patterns to our mistakes. Such a toll of physical and or emotional damage will almost always incentivize us to conscientiously avoid making that same mistake again and or try to find a way to thoroughly fix that mistake in case it happens again in the future. Now, most traumatic events outside of our control happens abruptly like an anvil being dropped onto your head, making it more effective objectively for us to form a new structure or order to live by. However, the consequences of most traumatic events resulting from our own bad habits and mistakes are often slowly accumulated over time through minuscule and seemingly unnoticeable, yet actually noticeable cracks and deformations that we often mindlessly ignore or ignorantly dismiss because they lack the momentous magnitude or rather being too understated to bring you into full attention for your own mistakes until it eventually accumulates into that giant anvil that drops onto you one day.

Smoking and lung cancer, for example, sugar and diabetes, porn addiction and erectile dysfunction, alcohol poisoning, extensive procrastination, lack of emotional control. Now, some of these consequences are temporary and can be fixed over time, but others can become lifetime critical, and trust me, you don't want to be on that end of the scale. It is arguably necessary to indulge in temptations once in a while, but it is absolutely necessary to remain mindful of your own limits. That is why I think it is important to induce a sense of sensitively profound dread plausibly and tangibly into yourselves regarding the narrative towards your own bad habits and old mistakes to compel you to think twice or even more before making any decisions. Next is the natural response to emotional distress. This one is very obvious, and I'm sure most of you gentlemen have experienced this as well. When we are clouded or overwhelmed by negative emotions, our first instinct is to immediately vent out and react and or try and find a way to numb those feelings, utter distress, and torment. Again, an innate defensive response from our survival instincts and the fastest and easiest method is to either emotionally react to release those profound emotional tension and or seek some form of comfort or salvation through instant pleasures and gratifications lashing out, sobbing your eyes, chugging an entire bottle of liquor munching off one full bucket of ice cream, snot some powder jerk off sleep the whole day and doing nothing for the whole week. It's not an uncommon scene to become caught in this web of spiral after a massive breakup, getting fired, losing a loved one, life-changing injuries, destruction of reputation, lack of results, and extensive loneliness. No matter how far you veered away from your past mistakes and old bad habits through completely developing a new frame and structure for your life, all it takes is one very bad day for you to become seductively tempted to revert back to your old destructive and degenerative way of living. Even in the early stages after experiencing trauma could lead you to this circumstance once again, unless you have options of methods and constructive endeavors that you could effectively utilize to distract yourself from or controllably, convey or express those negative emotions building up inside of you in order to put a halt into die proceedings, there is a high chance you will inevitably succumb to your innate temptations and finally, unsupportive environments. Our environments contribute significantly to shaping our identity, whether complimentarily or derogatorily. Mostly it comes from the external influence of friends, family, and culture. A lot of us who are still young, lack a profound sense, are having an underdeveloped sense of individuality and mostly are also lacking the ability to make decisions purely for the productive sake of one's own existence. Even if we do have a strong sense of individuality, we still occasionally become societally seduced and peer pressured into conformity due to the fear of loss of community and or reputation. And human beings innately hate feeling isolated. Now, it is utterly beneficial and wonderful for us. If our environments entirely support and escalates the better structure of life we are trying to construct for ourselves, it just takes away the unnecessary resistance and makes life easier for us. But if the opposite occurs, it gets unbearably arduous to try and endlessly resist the constant nagging ridicule and threats from our environments to come back to how we used to live like that fits their degenerative ideals or narratives. Here you really have no control over their decisions or perceptions since they are still deeply rooted within the comfort of their old order way of living. The best thing you could do is either move to a brand new and mutually constructive environment, or at least try your best to re-engineer your environment to better suit your new way of life. And yes, I'd also say having the right friends and or companions is crucial. Remember, treat your past mistakes and alt bad habits as critical options for you to always consider when you feel like you are slipping away. Because most of the time we always underestimate their effects until we eventually taste the bit of flavor of regrets. And because at the end of the day, it is your own decision, your own responsibility, and your own consequence to face. That is why in my own experience, the best method to prevent yourself from slipping too far away in repeating the same mistakes again, is to constantly condition yourself by inducing a profound sense of immense dread when thinking about or performing your past mistakes, especially the ones that have the most personal impact so that it could obstruct the momentum of the slip. Fear compels us to question and reflect more than any other negative emotions because it puts us into a state of having something major or significant or meaningful to lose, and that is why it is arguably the best effective tool for influence.

CHAPTER EIGHTY-ONE
IT IS POSSIBLE

I genuinely think that being able to distinctly know and discover the one thing that we are exceptionally good at is one of the most critical and desperately sought after moments for every single one of us young men in our twenties and thirties. Although realistically, it is not always necessary to discover it for us to become proficient or successful at something, nor is it always opportunistically available or accessible for everyone to discover it. It is without a doubt one of those significantly lingering questions that often presents itself in the forefront of our minds, especially for us who find it hard to endure dispassionate efforts that eventually gets us to have a deep, often frustrating introspection with ourselves of trying to desperately decide what endeavor we should entirely commit to. What am I really good at? I don't know what I really like doing. I have no clue what really excites me and all those amplified skeptical narratives that we generate for ourselves. Finding our potential is a very tempting feat as most men never get to conscientiously explore them, yet alone admittingly, discover and acknowledge them in their lifetimes. Now, the old me would've said, well, just try everything as much as you can and find out eventually what clicks the most for you. And although that is quite a masculine driven advice, now when I think of it, it is not exactly the cleverest nor the most efficient strategy to try and discover your potential as when it comes to potential. It's quite rather a semi-abstract existence as you can never really exactly or plausibly fathom how much of them you actually possess within a specific endeavor until you practically demonstrate them to a high extent. That is why mindlessly and randomly exploring its extent without any sense of focus or specificity, it will more often than not deviate you from accessing its magnitude. And also, there are so many factors influencing its magnitude, such as inherited inclinations, natural predispositions, cultural adoptions, specific upbringings, life-changing events, and many more. So, you can never really exactly decipher the scope of its reach until you've actually reached it. You need several specific methods of approach when it comes to discovering your strengths that can also properly serve and relate to your current unique circumstances. This is an approach that literally everyone can utilize and should try to utilize. In my opinion, especially for those of you gentlemen who are currently completely lost and utterly perplexed on endeavor, you should start committing to or at least highly consider in committing. The primal roots approach is about recollecting important pieces of your times during childhood, of which there are many of course, but this is about those moments where you became totally enamored by a subject or an object where you inadvertently and wondrously immersed yourself deeply into its core. It's those things that occupied your entire scope of attention intensely whenever you looked at it, touched it, heard about it, and performed it, and it's often those things and endeavors that you spent unrecognizable amounts of time with and got lost within it on your own. During your free time outside of school, videogames and movies, things that profoundly spark a deep level of connection, sense of heightened awareness and irresistible attraction from within you. Things that initiate a sense of deep wonder fascination and vast constructs of imagination within your mind, beyond what's initially plausible of that particular subject or object whenever you spend time on them. Like Albert Einstein's eventual fixation and obsession towards understanding the hidden invisible forces within this universe like gravity and energy all started when his father gave him a compass when he was five years old, where he became utterly fascinated by the needle, which points at a different direction wherever he goes and turns. This was what touched him to the core of his undying fascination in the beginning. When we are children, our minds are fluid, dynamic, passionate and curious. We purely do things for our own sake to fulfill those endless thirsts in understanding the circumstances around us. As we grow up, our minds become more structured, conventional, systematic, but at the same time rigid and cautious. This caused us to play by the rules that are set for us extensively. Our matured and judgmental minds allow us to make better decisions for ourselves, but at the same time, utilizing too much of them for too often will bury or shove that childhood creativity, curiosity, and playfulness into the back of our heads. You must unlock this sense of dynamics back by becoming single mindedly adventurous for your own sake, regardless of outside influence and judgments. The evolution approach is for those of you who are already relatively proficient in a certain field yet struggles to find that massive leap to strongly identify your own unique place within that and never. The evolution approach is literally about specialization where you identify a particularly small yet crucial or critical subject within a scope of a skillset set and redirect a great majority of your focus towards that respective subject through delving way deeper into the much smaller worm holes that most people operating within your craft rarely explore or yet to discover. Narrowing further down your niche will allow you to create or develop your own distinct space of operation, which will separate you from the rest as your skillset becomes way more saturated and tailored for specific needs, which will ultimately make you more sought after as you become extensively proficient within that particular scope of skillset. An example of this is Leonard Lonsdale, a tailored based in New York who pretty much make relatively similar, luxurious, bespoke tailored suits for men just like other tailors in Salva Row in England. But what makes him unique or distinguishes him from other tailors is that he had extensive knowledge and experience within the style of suits produced during the era of the 1960s and 1970s with white lapels, flake trousers, flashy colors, and big pockets. This is the main reason why he was one of the only sought after tailors to be selected to make suits destined for many big and major Hollywood motion pictures. Over 30 of them, in fact, ranging from the Wolf of Wall Street, American gangster and Bridge of Spies. The fusion approach on the other hand, is similarly for those of you who are already relatively proficient in a certain field yet finding it extremely difficult or obstructed in pursuing a higher degree of expertise within that field, maybe due to financial or political or personal reasons. In this case, the fusion approach is about discovering another interest outside of your field, of which when you eventually become proficient with, it could be effectively utilized to complement or become a driving force to alleviate your other field into new heights or dimensions of demonstration and even expertise. This is actually a lot of what people utilize nowadays, combining the skills and experience they've accumulated over the years through corporation employment and utilizing another skill to further promote their expertise into a new dimension of demonstration, allowing them to discover and penetrate new markets or opportunities like for example, cooking and editing, finance and writing, language and literature or engineering and journalism just like our favorite car presenter, Jeremy Clarkson. It is extremely important that these fields are flexible enough for you to utilize codependency, so to speak, in order for this strategy to work. Nothing is more potentially sabotaging than being proficient in two fields that exist on completely opposite ends of the skill spectrum such as medicine and mechanical engineering.

For example. We learn more from negative experiences than we do from positive experiences because negative experiences race way more questions needed answering, and because we human beings innately respond defensively towards threats, the more dire the experience is, the more we either tend to avoid it completely or the more we want to try and create solutions towards it due to the strong emotional callings, this particular approach involves capitalizing on our own protective response towards our traumatic or distressing experience in order to develop potential sources of resolution and redemption towards that experience, those sources then become tools and outlets for us to both mitigate and or prevent previous damages from repeating themselves and in turn can help in serving or assisting other people who faced similar experiences or damages. The late Chester Bennington was sexually abused by his own father at a very young age of seven, summoning various forms of insecurities, spite, and frustration, and caused them to experience further malice in his personal life, such as bullying, writing, poetry and music became his outlet to mitigate the psychological damages that scarred him for life. Music was his tool or outlet to passionately express his thoughts and feelings, which later served as the outlet for millions of other people around the world experiencing relatively the same physical and psychological damages as heated. This allows those who listen to his music feel a sense of comfort and relatability, which help them break out from the feelings of isolation and loneliness, solving your own major problems and utilizing those solutions to try and help others. Facing relatively similar circumstances, compels you to develop a profound sense of righteous duty to try and make the world you're living in a much better place than when you found it, allowing you to go to great lengths and extend to assist others as much as possible.

It's a very powerful driving force. One only you can understand as it is deeply rooted to your emotional core, which allows you to extensively understand and empathize with others going through similar circumstances. Most of us tend to stay away as far as possible from negative or traumatic experiences as they trigger a dreadful response through profound and blunt emotional rush. But to understand that running away from those experiences will only further amplify your sense of dread towards it as what you resist will always persist. This is probably the hardest one for me personally to accept as I've always believed it. In order for anyone to excel at a particular craft or a trade, you always need to have some form of devoted obsession and fascination in order for you to sustain in developing the necessary skills and knowledge to eventually become successfully proficient. But again, I was wrong and this was practically proven by my own uncle. He was born in a family of medical trade, a line of acupuncturist to be exact. He was taught about the trade from an early age by my grandparents and went to America to pursue his further education on the trade. He's currently a very successful acupuncturist, way more successful than my grandparents ever were, and also a lecturer at a medical university. And when I asked him personally whether he genuinely have a deep level of passion and curiosity in his craft, he said these words to be frankly honest, I don't, not one bit. It's heart and arduous and sometimes borderline enslavement as you don't get to sleep very much and you're always busy day in and day out. Now, of course, hearing those words got me extremely perplexed and I asked him next, so what made you spend over four decades mastering this craft? There has to be some sort of reason for your motivation from your end. And his answer is What caught me off guard? He said, honestly, I have no idea. I think it's just the sense of responsibility that I had ever since I was introduced to this trade by your grandparents to just get good at this shit, even though I'm not talented, to provide a better life for them. And of course, myself. It was never about passion or obsession. I didn't know anything else but this. This was my only ticket. I mean, getting the respect, acknowledgement, and gratitude from those people I cured is a nice little boost to get me up in the morning. And of course, the money is very substantial, but in all sense and purposes, it's all just about being a responsible man and being responsible for your duties and circumstances. Really nothing spiritual or metaphysical is influencing me. It took me a while to digest all of these, but in essence, it's all about getting things done with minimal emotional attachment. Oftentimes, when we want to commit to something, we wonder extensively about the reasons of why we are doing it, whether we'll be successful at it in the end, or whether we are making the right choice, which are basically all the things that I've mentioned in the beginning of this chapter. Of course, it is crucial to weigh in your options in order to make the most optimal decision. However, sometimes you don't have all the options when your entire back is against the wall and your only choice is to push through it regardless of how you feel, either because you are in need to keep your head above water in life, or because time is against you.

You just have to do what is necessary and avoid all incoming doubts and questions creeping up your mind. Don't feel, just do what is needed to be done and do it well like your life depends on it. Men need a sense of purpose in life, passionate or not truth be told, it all depends on our own perspective towards it. Our own realization of our true potential can only be practically acknowledged by us when we put tremendous amount of time and effort into whatever we choose to commit.

You won't ever know what you are really capable of by just sitting ducks and trying to get that aha moment through introspection alone. You have to know the extent and limitations of your circumstances and apply the most appropriate strategy to optimally explore your potential with regards to the amount of effort and time. It won't always be as ecstatic of a sensation as you tend to imagine it will be, but again, it is entirely your choice to commit.

CHAPTER EIGHTY-TWO
REASON VS. EMOTIONS

I've always emphasized how important it is for us to be able to have a significant level of control over our emotions and impulses as its unhinged. Nature could leave us vulnerable to making poor decisions and eventually drown us in the wallows of regret. However, looking back at it, I've realized that what I've told and explained to you gentlemen are merely simple tools on how to manage it or neutralize it, which is fun on their own, but they won't necessarily allow you to have a sense of confident authority over your emotions and impulses. In this chapter though, I'm going to explain pretty much the only weapon potent enough for you to eventually achieve that sense of authority and control, which is cultivating your ability for rationality. Now, in a hindsight, you might think, well, we're already capable of rationality, mate. Isn't that what makes our brain different from that of animals? And the answer is, yes, we do. However, our brains do still possess the yield primarily impulsive, reptilian, and mammalian attributes to sense, feel, and process emotions even before the evolution of the neo cortex that allows us to perform cognitive functions. Emotions will always be the innate priority for our brains to process. That is why most of us often unconsciously make decisions and judgments based solely on how we personally feel about the circumstance. Our ability to rationalize things will need to be trained and practiced over time. If we do want to eventually develop that mental capability to interfere and restrain our emotions. To develop our rationality, the first thing we need to do is to become fully and acceptably aware of our own impulsive and emotional nature. Emotions originates as chemical reactions and sensations that is biologically designed to capture our attention and take sharp notice of our environments onto which we are intrigued enough to want to understand where they come from and interpret them into language. However, because they are processed in different parts of the brain from our cognitive functions, most of us don't get to know where they come from or the reason why we react as such to them making our interpretation of our own emotions oftentimes inaccurate and vivid. That is why oftentimes we do not know the exact reason why we feel angry, sad, or depressed. Now, I got a lot of bashes from people who think that controlling our emotions means that we should completely shut down our reception to our own emotions like a robot. No, absolutely not. You cannot completely separate yourself from your emotions. It is utterly impossible. You cannot fully separate your feelings from being involved in making decisions. Even the most rational people of the mall is unable to do so. However, what makes rational people different from most of us and more effective and successful in decision making the nurse, is that they have a deep sense of introspection to deduct emotions substantially from their thinking and contract. Their effect, their sense of awareness is what make them able to vigilantly control their impulses. Irrational people on the other hand, have no such awareness. They always rush into conclusions and make decisions based on whatever accommodates the needs of their emotional biasness that also suit their egos. You can actually distinguish someone who is rational or irrational or at the very, very least notice which one they're more inclined to or dominant by simply through the nature of the decision making, rational people do what needs to be done. Irrational people do what they feel like doing, which today often comes in the form of defensive excuses to avoid responsibilities, the existing nature of our impulsive irrationality below our own level of consciousness. That is why it is difficult for us to become innately aware of them operating. However, although we may not be conscious of its nature, we can be conscious of its activity, scratching the surface through our physical responses and reactions. This is how you develop that awareness. Pay attention. I've talked about emotional trigger points before, but never in a way that is descriptive enough to help you become more mindful of their existence. Try to catch yourself off guard by noticing behavior from yourself that is suddenly off character and moments where you can feel a sense of emotional pressure, brittleness and leakage. Usually it is in the physical sensation of a sudden buildup of tears, a difficulty to swallow, a heavy feeling on your chest, a sudden hesitancy to speak or monitoring up words and your immediate mental withdrawal from a situation i e un inadvertently went into a brief and sudden self-reflection mode and or you shift your focus away from the circumstance by slightly looking down overside you essentially circumstances that trigger a subtle accumulating sense of sensitivity, vulnerability, anxiety, agitation, irritation, and stress that momentarily disconnects you from your sense. You also tend to freeze, shutter, stop whatever it is that you are doing or even got sloppy, careless, and unaware of what you are doing during this moments. These slow grade emotions will slowly compel you to react, and a further provoked or remain unchecked can turn into high grade emotions where you will completely enter into tunnel vision and culminate into unsupervised rash actions. Like when we experience strings of losses or defeats, we often start to feel that we are somehow eternally cursed for misfortunes. This can get us to become extremely fearful, hesitant, and nervous, and become more prone to making even more mistakes and experience more failures. When you finally become aware and conscious of your trigger points that create all those subtle tendencies, this is where you must bring yourself to withdraw physically and completely from the situation, especially in the beginning. Or if you are a beginner, find yourself a place where you can be alone like the bathroom or your own room, and focus on trying to dig deep into those trigger points to see where they originate from. It is much better to displace some situational awkwardness through physical withdrawal, especially when there are people around you than to utterly embarrass yourself through a sudden outburst of emotions. This is something you need to constantly practice as the more you are able to imminently step back and assess yourself, the easier it will be to eventually tame your emotions without having to physically remove yourself. Now, this is where the challenge can be quite substantial for most of us, especially if you've never done a deep, raw and brutal introspection into the roots of your own weaknesses. Our rationality is able to innately recognize and acknowledge our discrepancies, but our ego and irrationality prevents it from ever being brought into full consciousness again, pain versus pleasure. The reason why you experience all those understated sensations is because you have a vivid notification of your own weaknesses, but your ego decides against them ever being taken out of their shelves, thus creating the mental friction within your mind, resulting in your failure to effectively interpret those weaknesses and master your response towards them being provoked. Your biggest enemy and challenge here is bringing your ego to come to terms with the reality of your circumstances instead of allowing you to maintain favorable and soothing illusions about yourself, your weaknesses, the root of your major high-end emotions, especially in today's age, they all originates from a collection of underlying unresolved insecurities. Provocations of our insecurities gets us to go into a protective or defensive state as they are innately perceived as existential threats to our need for self-esteem, either from the social and or our own perception of ourselves. Acknowledging and accepting your deep-rooted insecurities in being able to dissect and pinpoint their origins will be the key to you eventually recognizing with clarity their components and pattern to the surface objectively and achieve the state of rationality. Being able to fully know and understand something give us the sense of control and confidence that we so desperately need towards the chaos and unpredictability of our circumstances and a high degree of our rationality allow us to achieve that state. We all have our own insecurities. That is what makes us human. No matter how godly or untouchable someone appears to be, they have their weaknesses. They are just way more viscerally aware and understanding of them to the point where they have become proficiently capable to stop. Its surfacing for other people to notice and take advantage of rationality and irrationality, reason and emotion. They are like riders and horses. The horse is our emotional side with the power, the energy, and the passion. The rider is our rational side with the restraint, the control and the direction. Without the rider, the horse is wild, aimless and destructive. Without the horse, the rider is lifeless, inactive, and stagnant. When they work together, they can become extremely productive and capable of amazing feats. The effective and objective rationality is an ability developed through constant practice and maturity. They do not come naturally. Assess every circumstance with your rationality first and foremost in order to come to an objective, conclusion and or decision. Once you know what to do with the situation, with utmost clarity and confidence, your perspective and attitude towards that situation simultaneously changes, and yes, so does your emotional reaction or response. Your initial whiff of negative emotions will transform into a wave of positive emotions filled with enthusiasm. As you now have a clear direction of where to go, and also as your your ego has come to terms or see eye to eye with the reality of your circumstances, this is exactly how you effectively tame, transform, and utilize emotions to your advantage. As useful momentum, emotions provide the components to develop effective reasoning. Reasoning provides the means to utilize productive emotions.

CHAPTER EIGHTY-THREE
HOW LIFTING WEIGHTS SAVES LIVES

One of the most mentioned components about self-improvement is the profoundly momentous and infectious effect that introducing and adopting fitness into your life can contribute not just for your own physical and mental benefits, but also how those particular effects can carry over both tremendously and extensively towards other important aspects of your life, like your career and other creative pursuits. However, one of the most seldomly elaborated parts about fitness to a significant degree in this self-improvement space particularly, is how exactly does a mere basic form of physical exertion could ever had such a positively, significant and crucial effect in drawing the fine line between one man's decision involving life and death. How does plainly moving your body against forms of resistances and opposing forces could ever summon such a compelling and metamorphic form of resolution towards keeping our existence in this world? Well, there are two reasons. The first one is because physical exercise is the simplest and most viscerally tangible form of conquest, all men need a sense of worthwhile and worthy purpose in life, or at least a sense of sincerely, confident, appreciable and honorable series of efforts that is propelling himself in the right direction within his life towards a desirable and gold. Basically, the conscious acknowledgement of the light at the end of a long and dark tunnel and physical exercise specifically is the most unambiguous, accessible, and purest form amongst all of those worthy and worthwhile conquests that provides the highest degree of conceivable clarity towards that particular end goal. As every man in this world secretly wishes to become strong and capable, completing a worthwhile conquest or achieving a state of progression within it will always give you an immense sense of satisfaction and fulfillment, not just narratively, but also biologically as well.

When it comes to hormonal release, which is always inherently essential for both our sense of self-esteem and self-actualization and fitness or physical exercise provides you with this particular sensation more effectively and efficiently than any other forms of conquests, simply because of its lack of complications and also due to its very preferably palpable effect for us human beings, as we all innately prefer things that can be perceived more viscerally by our five senses, physical or tangible conquests will always be more preferred and effectively perceived by us than mental or intangible conquests. However, as we all know it, cultivating physical strength is the most effective way to cultivate mental strength as its tangible nature provide us with the material blueprint to carry over into the intangible and complex world of our thoughts and feelings. A strong mind could lead to a strong body, but a strong body always lead to a strong mind, which brings us to the second Reason.

Physical exercise allows us to tap further and deeper into our survival instincts, particularly involving our own sense of self-preservation. The self-preservation instinct is primarily focused on the body itself and its wellbeing. This includes health, strength, diet, fitness, and endurance. It's like a management system for your body. It seeks to find a root cause for problems in the body and it can seek to test the body's endurance to harm or stress. Pain and fear are the integral parts of this mechanism as they act as forms of resistance into which we will inevitably respond to as we all know it by now, our bodies naturally gravitate to pursue pleasure and seek to avoid resistance. However, the imminent presence of resistance innately compels and motivate us to improvise, adapt, endure, and overcome when we have no other choice or options are when our back is against the wall, which will call for the effect of increased strength, mental sharpness, and heightened from us. Physical exercise, especially lifting heavy weights, though not as profoundly potent in producing the significant or extensive degree of pain and fear than let's say suffering and nursing and injury or being stranded on a deserted island full of predators still could relatively an analogically emulates those sensation that compels us to exert ourselves tremendously to eventually allow us to overcome them like the worrisome sense of fairness due to the risk of failure and injury when trying to attempt a PR or a PB and the pain stemming from the immense exertion in order to lift that heavy weight complete. The exercise compels us to push ourselves harder than ever before and summoning new feet's of yet to be explored, capabilities of which will inevitably be established as we slowly adapt. You don't necessarily have to enjoy it, but you have to do it regardless in order to eventually overwhelm that sensation of pain and fear yourself. This is how the analogy of physical exercise mentally help us prepare to face adversity and how it carries over to other life endeavors. When it comes to facing and encountering resistance or obstructions, it unlocks or rather expand and extend our capacity and capability to endure and eventually adjust ourselves to suit our circumstances. It doesn't have to always involve lifting heavy weights. It can also involve running, swimming, or climbing just as long as you are willing to constantly push yourself beyond your initial limitations, no matter how minuscule as this is extremely critical because if you're not willing to push yourself further beyond your comfort or safety zones, just like anything, it won't allow you to cultivate the necessary attributes to help you overcome the degree of adversities or limitations you are facing. Never underestimate or disregard the evoking effect that physical exercise could bless you with. It is inadvertently transmuting as it certainly was able to solely and effectively prevent myself from jumping off a balcony and stabbing myself to Death, death with a kitchen knife many years ago, and I'm very confident that a lot of you, gentlemen and women for that matter, have relatively experienced such a circumstance as well and get to witness your own metamorphosis or rebirth into a much more compelling and polarizing individual. I owe pretty much everything to physical exercise or lifting weights in general. So much so that although I'm not religious by any means, I do pledge my eternal loyalty and commitment to it till the day I no longer exist.

So if any of you reading still skeptically wonder how physical exercise can cure the absolute majority of your personal issues, I highly suggest you try it out and take it seriously, because trust me, you won't ever regret it.

CHAPTER EIGHTY-FOUR
HEROES

People love to be promised to better future and existence. I mean, why wouldn't we? In this cold, chaotic, and unpredictable world, we all struggle to make sense out of everything. That is why all of us need the acknowledgement and assurance of the right direction to go and the right place to eventually reach so that we have a calming and confident inducing feeling that no matter what form of adversity the life throw is at us. If we just keep pushing our limits, if we just keep on adapting and adjusting ourselves towards our circumstances, we always have a subtle lingering sense of hope to hold onto, regardless of if they are true or false, for us to eventually arrive at that satisfying and fulfilling future that we dream of. That is why most of us commit to a religious belief. That is why most of us love self-improvement, and also that is why most of us are easily manipulated by charismatic and powerful politicians, but more of that in another chapter. Human beings have the desperate need to believe in something, a higher power or entity to act as a safe space or place to conform to and a beacon of guidance towards a specific promising future. That is why we easily get so inspired by people of high authority like celebrities, athletes, businessmen, famous authors, basically, people who have achieved a lot of merit throughout their lives, display desirable and honorable character traits wherever they go, and worked their way up the ladder to live a life that most people can only ever dream of. In this current time where masculinity is simply being constantly diminished, ridiculed, and condemned, we no longer have that abundant source of inspiration where our fathers were supposed to be our first and main source of inspiration. Most of them have been utterly repressed by the centric social order. By the time we enter kindergarten, as little boys we're not encouraged to be strong, to take risks and to dream high. Instead, we're punished. If we ever showcased our sense of adventure, we were ridiculed and laughed at. If we ever reveal our dreams, regardless of if they sound ridiculous or unrealistic, and we're isolated from any other masculine influence through inducing denigration about them, we're told to just sit down, shut up, and listen. We're told to not be like those toxic masculine men We're insisted to just stay inside, be safe, and be comfortable not to go outside and discover what we want because it's dangerous. There has never been a more crucial time in our lives before when us men desperately need to seek legitimate sources of inspiration and guidance to help us navigate through the brutal reality of life and to unlearn the narrative that caused us to be incompetent, undeserving sensitive, lazy, delusional, and empathetically irresponsible for our own lives. We need mentors that could help us develop a strong sense of conviction within us, educate us with practical information, and incentivize us to start taking actions, and that last part is a lot harder than it actually sounds because we've been conditioned for decades to just wait for the right moment until a light bulb magically turns on inside our heads hats one Sunday morning. Now the main questions are how do we choose the right mentors for us? How do we narrow down our judgments on them and what metrics should we base our judgments from to establish the legitimacy in our perception of them? Your mentors should first and foremost be significantly relatable to you. They ideally have undergone and overcome relatively similar circumstances in the past as you have and or they share and have achieved relatively the same objectives that you personally want to achieve. This is important, otherwise, you can't build or will lack the identifiable and empathetic connection with them because as men, common grounds, values, and functions are the healthy building blocks or foundation of our bond with other men, whether they are close or distant, especially in this fatherless age. For men, we tend to seek other father figures and or elderly brother figures externally through the internet, which means our mentors are almost always going to be distant. Second is that they have a realistic appraisal of themselves and the weaknesses. Everyone loves and desires to be perfect, but no one actually is. Sooner or later, people will dig and find out the cracks to your inconsistencies and utilize them against you. Perfection is ideal, but in the real world, it is impossible. Your mentors should never self-proclaim themselves as eternal absolutes, as colorful as their merits are. The worst thing that they can do is letting their ego completely cloud their judgements and belittle others in an attempt to keep themselves relevant and stay longer in the limelight. Their grounded acceptance of their own major insecurities or weaknesses and their desire to improve on them is a great example of their own sense of humility and being able to still put themselves in our shoes despite their achievements. Third, they have a loyal devotion to truth and reality. No one likes a liar, and no one likes to be manipulated into believing or following a lie. No one wants to waste a lot of their time and have to live facing the dire consequences later on. Your mentor must have an obligation towards objective truth, no matter how painful it might be for you to take in. It is their responsibility to make you realize the raw and brutal mechanics of how the world works. In order for you to disconnect from your previous conditionings, the truth hurts, but they are necessary for you to have the much-needed tangible clarity on that hope you are holding onto. Instead of clinging onto the enigmatic and vague estimation of sugar-coated lies, your mentors must be factual absolutists rather than fictitious obsessions, they have enemies and have their own history of controversies as many truth preachers do. Fourth, they have a tolerant attitude towards people once in their lives they were in the same place to those who currently looked up to them, people do what they do and become someone who they are now good or bad because of a collection of underlying and understated reasons or problems that they've attempted to solve. Your mentor should have a profound acknowledgement and understanding of these mechanics in people. Oftentimes, mentors look specifically for those who are good listeners and literally informational sponges easy to manage and taught. If we were still innocent children, then sure, but as young men, we've developed our own critical thinking skills that allow us to make our own independent judgements. However, because of this extensive narrowed down perception of ours, we tend to unconsciously develop an escalated sense of conviction and superiority biasness towards our own judgments, which basically caused us to become stubborn and sensitive dickheads who are disagreeable and easily triggered When challenged with a new perception, your mentors must understand this and possess their own methods in dealing with such an individual systematically and persistently. Otherwise, it'll showcase their lack of intent and their own reluctance to help, and finally, they are able to reach the goals that they have set for themselves. Tangible evidence and results are what matters the most. At the end of the day, whatever your mentor preaches you to do, they must also practice them with their utmost loyalty and pride and be able to display or showcase effective and desirable outcomes that emerge from those practices. Nothing is worse than someone who tells you what to do but does not do the particular endeavor himself. Everyone despises a fraud. Your mentors must not allow you to do whatever things that they themselves hasn't done or will not do in the future because they themselves have very little understanding and mastery of those endeavors. This is utterly crucial. You don't want to become someone's sacrificial lamb or experimental rat towards an endeavor. That one is too much of a coward to try and understand himself. The right mentors can incentivize us to finally spread our wings or grow them back where they were once clipped off. Just make sure that we do not eventually live under their shadows when we are finally able to fly on our own. Because although the most preferred, effective, and efficient method of learning during an apprenticeship is imitation, if we get carried away with the momentum, then we'll just be the discount, knockoff, and copycat of our mentors who only exist in the dark edges of the limelight. We won't have the opportunity to stand in the middle of the limelight with our own unique twist.

CHAPTER EIGHTY-FIVE
TOUGH LOVE

A lot of the times when we're trying hard to solve our own personal problems, we often beat around the bush rather too much. We try to associate them with anything but our own sense of accountability and responsibility. We often let ourselves float and glide around the emotional waves that our problems spawn from within us. And you know what? Like I've said many times, this is actually our default response towards distress. We still possess the innate animalistic qualities to process emotions and react accordingly to our surroundings. However, unlike animals who don't have that higher degree of cognitive abilities, we possess the evolved and systematic a ability to solve problems. Now, this can be either a gift or a curse depending on our level of awareness and competency to utilize them. Our tendency toward want to translate our emotions into plausible language. Nine times out of 10 will always result in an inaccurate interpretation due to the constant interference of our own unconscious egos causing us to lose our crucial sense of control and authority over ourselves. This lack of understanding in the inability to interpret the source of our emotions is what lead us to spiral further into self-deprecation and desperation. Again, we hate and are afraid of those that we cannot understand, and our most feel emotions react to them, and they're gone. We, on the other hand, dwell on them, intensifies them extensively to the point where we feel constant anxiety well beyond the moment of occurrence. This is our curse as human beings, if you want to call it that way, and because we lack that personal understanding and mastery over our emotions and their sources, our selfish nature kicks in and we then start to point fingers on external circumstances such as other people, unfortunate events and metaphysical entities like spirits and bad luck to try to desperately make quick sense out of everything, or we completely dismantle ourselves from our own sense of self-esteem by pointing and voicing out all of our problems while desperately hoping for sympathy to lick us in the yes instead of rationally finding effective ways to fix our problems. This is where the brutal tool of tough love is necessary. Reality does not care about your feelings, nor does it care about the mountainous number of fears and insecurities that you have created for yourselves or because you couldn't accept their unfavorable effects on you. Hate and cry all you want. It won't care even if you die begging for it to change. It will treat you in differently like you never exist. Reality only favors those who blend into its nature and find ways to leverage from it. Every problem has a source, just like every effect has a course, and it is your responsibility to find that source. This is why tough love is so effective for moments like these because it skips over all the touchy feely you wallowing bullshit hits you with the big slap in the face and brings you face to face directly in front of the source of your problems, which more often than not always involve your own derogatory and pitiful attitude towards facing adversities. A lot of people treat tough love as a harsh and insulting method to consult someone into self-improvement.

Even calling it bullying harassment or verbal assault. I mean, if it goes way too often and far from the problems at hand, then yes, but other than that, I completely disagree because it's just your sensitive, delusional and egotistical answers that are unable to take the visceral and unrelenting entirety of your circumstances, especially those mentally stifling ones that you create and maintain illusions for sympathy and empathy do not solve problems. They only negate their effects over you momentarily, while also debilitating your tolerance towards them. If you are a rational person or a person who is objectively driven, regardless if you were initially offended by the blunt and ruthless way, someone calls you out for your personal irresponsibility and incompetency, deep down you will actually feel a great sense of relief that someone actually points out the source of your problems because now you have unlocked or discovered that much needed sense of awareness, understanding, and authority over them, even if it is only a minute sense in magnitude, all it takes now at the practical actions you need to undertake to eventually solve them or at least mitigate their effects on you. Tough love brings you into full attention and renders you completely and necessarily powerless as they viscerally illustrate the natural consequences of your behavior, which is the perfect way to get you to submit or coe your hold on any ideals that are withholding you from making the necessary changes to save yourselves from repeating the same mistakes all over again. Do not hate those people who gave you a bit of tough love because although they might look and sound like they're bullying or insulting you, in actuality, they're actually care about you enough to want to must drop all that rational passion to give you the incentivization that you desperately need.

They may seem like assholes, but they are the necessary assholes. That is why I also highly encourage you gentlemen to find mentors that occasionally give you some tough love, because if they really don't care about you, they wouldn't say a damn thing and will just ignore you or let you dwell and wallow on your own problems for as long as you like. While secretly laughing at and capitalizing on your misery, pay more attention to the content of their words, not the context, so that you don't mistake applicable, constructive criticisms for personal attacks or irrational feedbacks.

CHAPTER EIGHTY-SIX
DUTY

A man's strong sense of duty and commitment towards a profession or an endeavor. In times where he does not even want to undertake the tasks that were assigned for his commitment, it is only bred when a man can finally learn to understand the clear and crucial essentiality or necessity of his livelihood, ambitions, and character that dependent ethically and morally on him undertaking and completing those necessary tasks. In times of today, most of us only express our desires to commit to an endeavor or a profession only through the face value of our enthusiastic words and spontaneous promises to try to convince ourselves and others that we are actually someone that is worthwhile to be around. However, when the time actually come for us to demonstrate our commitment, we then compromise ourselves to slack off the momentum by creating gradually cumulative, subtle, and silly excuses for our own fears, incompetence, laziness, and arrogance towards those tasks that we chose to undertake in the first place. Oh, I've got a bit of headache right now. I'll do them tomorrow. Oh, I'm a bit sleepy today. Maybe when I'm feeling fresh as a ripe apple, then I'll do it. I don't really know how to do it. Yeah, I'll figure it out later when I'm ready. I'm not really in the mood right now. I don't have the energy to do it, but I'll get it done as soon as I can later on. Today becomes tomorrow. Tomorrow becomes next week. Next week becomes next month. Next month becomes next year. Why does this happen to us? We say we want to achieve the things that we want to achieve here. We waste and sacrifice a lot of precious time doing nothing or other unimportant dopamine inducing and degenerative things instead of completing the tasks that are necessary to be completed in order for us to gradually get closer to achieving those goals that we've set for ourselves. We know the things that we need to do to get there, yet we simply didn't want to do them. Is it the fear of the mountain that you have to climb? Is it because you are reluctant to face any adversity, resistance, or discomfort in those tasks? Is it the anxious feeling that you're not good enough to complete the tasks with merit? Are you afraid that you might not make it in the end? Do you think it's a total waste of time doing them or that it would not make a big difference to your life even if you do them or not? Regardless of whatever irrational and subjective excuses you've created for your own failures or lack of progression, it all comes down to two things. Whatever you do, you acquire, accumulate and maintain. Whatever you don't do, you conceit, dissipate, and mistreat. Some tasks are much less appealing than others, but nonetheless, still essential. Whether it is doing the arduous and painful L session in the gym or the monotonous and boring administrative and bookkeeping work in your business, they all are necessary tasks to be completed. If you want to achieve your dream for Zeke, or if you want to know exactly how your business performed this year, month, or week compared to last year, month, or week, sure they may not always make a big difference to your progression, and they certainly won't always be the work you're jumping out of bed in the morning for, but they are certainly the work that you must do in order to contribute directly towards your livelihood, ambitions, and character, no matter how minute their effects are.

As a man who genuinely wishes or striving to become someone more than what you initially thought of an estimate yourself to be, it would disturb you with doubt, agitation, and disappointment at night, knowing that you have not completed any necessary tasks that you've set for the day because it disrupts the state of progression that you are after every single day. If you want to talk about morals, it is morally a dishonorable act to run away from your responsibilities and break your promise that you've made for yourself and for your own sake, or because you just don't feel like doing them. How you feel about not doing the work has absolutely no leverage or association on what's the work itself will contribute to what you've decided to commit your body, mind, resources, and time into must be sincerely and completely whole. There should be no compromise or at the very least, very minor amount of them. You need to be very harsh and critical about your attitude, morals, and ethics towards work. Put pressure on yourself to compel your body and mind to fight for survival. Otherwise, you revert back to your selfish nature of running away from pain and seeking pleasure, set demanding deadlines or manufacture them for your endeavors as a critical and objective measure of your competence or incompetence towards them. The pressure from the slender amount of time to reach your goals compels you to not have the luxury to procrastinate, be fearful, and contemplate about your current mood and feelings. The continual rise in intensity as you approach closer to the deadline becomes an intense everyday challenge and fight to maintain your momentum that you must push yourself for in order to survive narratively. This will viscerally teach you how to work under pressure and incentivize you to start working immediately. The feeling that we have endless amount of time to complete our work has an insidious and debilitating effect on our minds. Our attention and thoughts become diffused, and we become ignorantly dismissive as the lack of intensity, tension and pressure makes it hard for the brain to jolt into a higher gear, to solve problems and take initiatives.

This is what I meant in the beginning about that crucial sense of essentiality when it comes to your duty and responsibility. This particular attitude and behavior towards work is certainly not for everyone as most people always ask the question of when we get to rest or when are our breaks. People nowadays overly celebrate minor and meaningless achievements like their 18th birthday or their graduation out of university, while having absolutely no idea and plan of what is next for them or how they want to end up in life 10 to 20 years from now. They take long rests or holidays to prepare them for God knows what, and just let fate direct the course of their lives. You don't do that. You know what you want. You sit on the captain's chair, take the wheel, and regain control of where you want to go, to reach the destination that you want to end up in. You get things done and you only rest when they're done. Similarly, in real daily lives, you only rest when your daily tasks are completed so that you know that you've earned that rest. Instead of trying to hopelessly sleep away your disappointment and uncertainty in yourselves, do the work. Don't leave it hanging, finish it. Be honorable for your own sake, and if you want to for God, God loves those who go to great lengths to help themselves, so please him the best you can, even at times when you don't feel like it.

CHAPTER EIGHTY-SEVEN
DOMINANCE

We do not like to talk or point out explicitly about relative power positions, and we are generally uncomfortable when others talk about their superior rank and the hierarchy. That is why we often dismiss it, even though we can clearly notice the position one has within a social setting, whether it is within friendships, professional settings, or intimate relationships. And yes, speaking of hierarchy as the most complicated animal on the planet, we also develop socially perceived hierarchies on the people around us based on physical prowess, position, money, status, knowledge, experience, popularity, and made selection. Whether we like it or not, judgments will be made on us, and we will make judgments on other people in order to select our level of association with them. It is inevitable. I mean, we are social creatures working for our own survival and prosperity. Remember now to clear things up. The purpose of this chapter is not to teach you how to be dominant or alpha as the state of dominance in a man often comes through gradual character maturity and competence as they navigate a choir and experience further circumstances in life. This chapter is mainly to assist you in social settings, in terms of spotting or showcasing someone who is implicitly considered as the dominant individual in the group or the one who is in charge of the whole situation. As it can also turns out to be you if you observe this about yourself and around yourself. The idea is that when someone feels that they are in a superior social position and is actually the superior one, it will radiate upwards in the nonverbal communications towards others and or from others towards them. In other words, it can be clearly perceived through their body language, gestures and micro expressions towards one another.

Dominance is demonstrated not explicate. It is very important to know who you are dealing with in social situations. If you have the reassuring intuition that someone else is more dominant than you within a group, do not let your big ego in the insecurities embarrass yourself by trying to subtly or expressively out for the man. Know your environments thoroughly. If it is a social situation that you are significantly competent in, it will naturally give you the confidence to take charge. If it is not, then back off. Remember, your reputation is on the line, and you must protect it at all costs by being vigilant on everyone who is present. The best thing you could do when someone else is more dominant than you in a social situation is to simply observe him and learn from him. If you can spot his inconsistencies and weaknesses through time, it will be advantageous for you in the long run. But anyways, here are the 15 signs of social dominance based on my own extensive observation on someone who is a perceived leader of the group Whenever he goes, some of them are quite obvious and some of them are not so obvious.

NUMBER ONE

they have a strong but relaxed stature and demeanor. The state of dominance is that you have an impeccable feeling of control, confidence, and authority over your circumstances. And when you feel like these, you are naturally more relaxed and carefree. Your movement is slow, you sway more when you walk. Your eyelids are relaxed, or half closed, and you tend to lean back more. When you sit in contrast to someone who is overwhelmed, anxious, or nervous, their gestures are tense, their movements are sudden, and they cannot maintain a fixed position for a long time.
Their eyes are fully open, and they sit more upright or leaning slightly forward with a closed or defensive posture.

NUMBER TWO

They make eye contact and stare with anyone they please for as long as they please. Dominant people or people who feel superior to others rarely put their heads down or look down for extensive periods of time. Their chins are always up in the air and they're always looking around for things that interest them. Their feelings of superiority make them develop this sense of arrogant disposition whenever they interact with someone, and yes, that includes eye contact. Their reassuring acknowledgement of others inferiority towards them gives them the sense of entitlement to judge others at their own will and pace, which may make others feel uncomfortable, but they won't give a shit because chances are they fully know that people won't or don't dare to do shit about it either.

NUMBER THREE

they smirk more than they smile. Smirking could be a subtle sign of approval or dismissal depending on the context. Regardless, dominant individuals are hard to please and disturb. They usually are non-reactive and very rarely laugh out of control or expressively display too many emotions whether they are positive or negative.

NUMBER FOUR

They touch people a lot more. Remember what I said about dominant people feeling entitled? Well, this is another one. Dominant people will not hesitate to cross other people's physical boundaries, whether it is a pat on the back, a slap on the shoulder or a hold around the waist. Invasion of people's physical space is a subtle indication of an attempt to gain some form of direct control or influence on that person like a puppeteer. That is why oftentimes when you see a person wrapping his hand around someone and walking towards a certain direction, the person who is being held will inadvertently follows the direction of the person that is wrapping their hand around him.

Again, depending on the person, this can make some people feel uncomfortable, but again, chances are people won't or don't have the courage to do shit about it unless the individual also has a dominant personality.

NUMBER FIVE

They take up more space and leave more space between them and others. This is one that most of you would know of and notice, as I've said before, superior people love the sense of control and authority. It is almost like a constant necessity for them. This reflects in their need to oversee everyone from a clear vantage point. Thus, that is why they take lots of space when they stand or sit and leave lots of space between them and others by leaning back and pushing their chairs slightly away from the table or sitting at the far end or edge of the table. This is the reason why inside the office of most high positioned executives, their tables are large and wide to maintain space or distance from any individual sitting or standing in front of it, and this is also why they are always located at the far end or corner of the room as far away from the entrance door instead of in the middle of the room or right beside the door. This is so they can see everything that is within the room or coming in and out of the room from a secure vantage.

NUMBER SIX

When they speak other people's head turns rapidly towards them. Their eyes fixate on them, they become suddenly silent, and they listen attentively. Superior people are both respected and feared. Their high level of competence in many areas of life gets people to become naturally intimidated by them, so people often feel the need or pressure to give them complete attention, either to not get called out or to not display behaviors that will upset them.

NUMBER SEVEN

When they interrupt people, no one dares to argue, and they get away with it easily. This might offend some of you, but this occurs quite often. As said previously, when they speak, others went silent and give them full attention. Thus, when they interrupt a conversation, no matter how exciting it is or how annoyed one might be, they all still turn their heads and are prepared to listen to what they have to say.

NUMBER EIGHT

People walk behind them, and they rarely glance back to check if anyone is still following them or not. A lot of the time when we are in charge of a social situation, say leading a group to a restaurant within a mall, we often unconsciously take a brief glance behind us to know who is still following us or if anyone decides to break out of the group. This is actually a common primal sense of insecurity. You're not wanting to feel isolated or separated from the tribe, and it is also self-esteem and competence. Check to see if people value or trust your leadership. Dominant. People don't need to check because they know people have to and will follow them because they often already set the tone and took charge from the very beginning.

NUMBER NINE

They will not hesitate to state or display their displeasure with someone that is present. Their sense of entitlement and their confidence that people will not dare to question them leads them to feel comfortable and non-threatened in saying whatever they want. Even explicit criticisms and insults towards those that they dislike because they know most people around them would by default agree to their statements or be dynamically peer pressure to agree even if they actually don't. This is the power of influence one's own' authority can have when they are highly respected and feared.

NUMBER TEN

They talk with a deeper voice and never overexplain or justify anything. High pitched voice can signal either excitement and enthusiasm or insecurity and anxiety. Dominant people never need to strain themselves to be heard. As I've said previously. When they talk, people will listen. They only say what is necessary and never have the need to overly justify their statements because usually those who tries really hard and extensively to make a point are the ones that are dishonest and ort in their statements.

NUMBER ELEVEN

When uninterested in someone, they tend to subtly demonstrate them by half assign. When dominant people get bored or mildly annoyed at someone's presence, they usually don't give those people any attention or they direct their attention somewhere else more interesting to them and they demonstrate explicitly without any sense of remorse. A lot of us sympathize a lot even with people we're not interested in. We continuously try to entertain them or maintain our attention towards them even if we secretly are desperate in wanting to get out of there just to not hurt their feelings or discredit their efforts. Dominant people don't care. They show or imply that they're not interested regardless of how you might feel afterwards.

NUMBER TWELVE

People around them compete in a system and earn their approval. This is probably one that you often see in corporate settings. People often lick the boss's car, soaking wet to earn their approval and get closer to them in order to attain further status positions and benefits. The need to continuously appease dominant people becomes imminent when you realize that their approval means that you are given a certain probability of being invited within their social circle or get rewarded for your efforts by earning their trust in the form of their approval. It's opportunism for survival and prosperity. Whenever dominant people need some form of assistance, you can easily notice that the people around them subtly compete to raise their hands first and be the ones' chosen to do favors for them.

NUMBER THIRTEEN

People match and follow their demeanor. We all know this. Energy and demeanor radiate and becomes contagious. Conformity towards respected authority is inevitable.

NUMBER FOURTEEN

They rarely second guess their decisions and often subtly insistent, dominant people are masters of getting others to just concede their ideals or fears and follow them. Instead, they are able to make complicated and nerve-wracking things sound simple and relaxing. A lot of us are quite emotionally fickle when it comes to making decisions because either we want to get the most out of it or because we are afraid of misfortunes happening or interfering dominant. People don't care about all those things. They just want a decision that make the most sense and give them the highest yield, and they get us to concede by taking advantage of our fickleness through escalating the fears and downplaying the rewards that our decision presents.

NUMBER FIFTEEN

Their characters interests and outlooks make them always valuable. I save the best and most important for last. This is probably the one that most of you gentlemen do not realize and probably the most impactful out of all of them when it comes to dominant people, the real ones, how they are able to maintain their sense of confidence and superiority, despite other people's condemnation of them is quite simple to understand, yet hard to spot, but it's this, their authenticity and devil may care attitude in themselves and the things they do in their lives never completely disservice or disqualifies them of their livelihood and essential need regardless of other people's disapproval because regardless of people love them or hate them, people still need them for the competence or resourcefulness that they possess in high demand and highly sought after endeavors. I used to say in the past that we should not look for other people's approval, and yet deep down as social creatures secretly we still do no matter how subtle that sense is, and this is how dominant people of authority create that balance. They utterly know that people will come looking for them regardless of what they do or how they feel towards them because they possess something that a lot of people are looking for. In other words, you need to have skills, knowledge, and experience that you personally want to do and possess, yet at the same time highly valuable enough for people to come looking for you for compensatory assistance. For example, the individual who might base this chapter upon possesses a skill and competence that ensures that he is always needed by others. That particular skill Is his, his ability to develop and maintain connections with different people of different social backgrounds. He always said that he personally loves to get to know other people and their unique lifestyles, and little did he know that that passion of his could turn out to be the most valuable thing he could ever possess in his life. We all know the term, your net worth is your net worth, and that is evidential in this individual's life. His vast connections of people of different backgrounds and competence allows him to develop tons of business deals and get highly compensated for it, giving him access to even more connections and opportunities. People always need people, especially in business, they always want exposure, reach, consulting, service, marketing, finance, logistics, loyalty, and exclusivity. So, no matter how much people to dislike him for his attitude, opinions or outlook, the same people will come back looking for him for a much needed favor or assistance. So, it is important that the endeavors, at the very least one of them that you personally commit to or are passionate about, are highly valuable enough and sought after enough for people to want to constantly look for you because as I've said before, the market will determine how valuable you truly are, not your own isolated and often biased estimate of it.

CHAPTER EIGHTY-EIGHT
WHY MEN LOVE FIGHTING

The main reason why we as men are drawn to combat so much is the same physiological and psychological reason why we are generally attracted to be somewhat involved within conflicts in the first place. It's the arousal that comes from both the anxiety and excitement of being involved in something primarily subservient to our innate hierarchal and territorial nature. The assertion of dominance and the imposition of will determine someone's state of superiority or supremacy within a social setting or space have been evolutionary, inherited and acculturated both into our biology and society. As men, our greater muscle mass, stronger bones, foster reactions, thicker skin and greater tolerance towards pain are all purposefully God-given to better equip us for combat, conflict, and self-defense ever since the dawn of mankind. That is why men are the ones who goes out hunting. That is why men are the ones that go to war. That is why men are the ones who do construction work. That is why men are the ones who work in protection and distress response. Because we are naturally and hereditarily much better equipped for all those high-risk endeavors. Our primitive disposition towards combat and conflict makes us highly intrigued and captivated towards witnessing or even engaging in fights. That is why the 75 to 90% of mixed martial arts audience are all predominantly occupied by men. In today's time, obviously much has changed, civilization has evolved, and everything has become a lot more controlled, restrictive, and prohibited. Thus, we become a lot less inclined to want to engage in combat, let alone meticulously prepare ourselves for combat, or even purposefully expose ourselves towards combat unless and only if the circumstance caused for us to do so. That is why many of us today have absolutely no idea how to defend ourselves or crumble in the face of personal conflict with another party because we are no longer often exposed to its circumstances that compels us to learn or be taught how to defend ourselves. From a very young age, most of us were born in supremely comfortable, censored, and civilized world as opposed to our ancestors who were born during the times of bear, constant disputes and antagonism. Now, today, generally we learn how to fight at a much later age and for slightly different reasons and purposes, often much more intrinsically or metaphorically inclined and involved than before. Also, a lot more civilized than before, such as our high admiration towards fighting or fighters in general is because we secretly want to possess the physical capabilities, mental attributes, and character traits that fighters have or that are derived from the results of learning how to fight. And we'd be right because if you think lifting weights can develop or cultivate your physical capabilities and characters substantially, fighting takes that particular issue into a whole new dimension. Because you're no longer trying to overcome an inanimate object of a certain magnitude that does not pose a direct and conscious threat towards your safety in a fight, you're not trying to overcome an individual whose sole purpose or intention is to physically and mentally damage or incapacitate you completely. It's a completely different realm of facing adversity than merely enduring the arduous but salvageable pain of an endeavor. Here you are facing actual threats or the type of pain that can seriously or brutally damage your wellbeing and existence, narratively speaking. So, it is a lot more complicated task to quote unquote overcome or withstand than to just merely quote unquote complete through enduring aches, which you also have to go through in a fight. By the way, fighting is not just a test of character or willpower. It's a test of everything, including your skills or knowledge of the art, bad tendencies, intelligence, and even your attitude in a much more justifiable clarity.

There is only so much pain you can quote unquote just endure in a fight before someone takes them to a level that is too much for you to handle. And unlike lifting weights to stop, stop when you reach failure, more of your primal instincts will be reawakened during an actual fight or even in a normal hard spa against someone. A lot of fighters say that you'll know who you really are when you engage in combat against someone else who is willing to impose his will against you. And it's true. Everything that is perceptible, quantifiable, and noticeable about you will be evidently exposed before, during, and after a fight. Your physical and mental weaknesses, bad habits, level of patience, fear, persistence, endurance will power, confidence, and your attitude towards success, hardships and failure will all be exposed, especially if it is your first time engaging in a fight or a hard spar because you have no time to think and we're a social mask When you fight. It's all about survival in there and everything is done at a very fast pace. Thus, you will only do what your current predisposed or conditioned instincts tell you to do, whether it is to cover up, crumble, and eventually yield or to hold on and eventually muster up the courage to fight back fighting. Or in this case, learning how to fight is the most bare, pure, and visceral form of self-improvement and competition. I'd say even more than lifting weights or any form of physical exercise because it makes you become more self-conscious than ever before, especially when it comes to identifying your own practical weaknesses through constant, brutal, humbling process that occurs way more than lifting weights. Because you are now consciously competing and measuring yourselves against other individual's capabilities and traits which will make you become more viscerally aware and apprehensive of where you stand amongst all your peers.

You will often feel like you are nothing or don't know anything most of the times, but that is precisely why most men with a strong enough desire kept doing it because they constantly learn something new about themselves and about others through sharing combat time with one another, and eventually develop a much deeper bond with one another all while cultivating themselves and fixing their weaknesses through healthy competition. Plus, the confidence boosts of knowing you have the capability to defend yourself and defeat someone is quite a nice addition to your social presence. So once again, for you gentlemen reading that are into self-improvement or more importantly, are having a hard time in introspection and putting your ego to the side. Learn how to fight. Just sign up to a boxing gym or an MMA gym. Just try it out for three months and do a hard spa with someone who is also looking to hard spa. Most likely you lose badly and quickly, but don't take it personally.

Rather catch yourself in your thoughts and feelings afterwards and see practically for yourself whether it had helped you to become humble enough and conscious enough to spot the strengths and weaknesses in both your practical capabilities and character.

CHAPTER NINETY-EIGHT
THE ONE PERSON YOU MUST ALWAYS AVOID

Throughout our lives, we've encountered different types of negatively impactful individuals that only brings further unsolicited dire readiness and gloominess to our existence. There are the pessimists, the chronic complainers, the bewildered blame us, the exceptionally envious, the notorious procrastinators, the bad losers, the cowardly, carefree bums, the delusional incompetence. The lot life is already hard enough for the most of us. And the last thing that we want in our lives are a bunch of limped, pessimistic, and insufferable defeatists to roll us up into one massive snowball and push us down towards the valley of self-doubt and deprecation. I've said in the chapter once before that's having an unproductive and degenerative circle of people around you will only escalate your probability for self-sabotage. And after you do so, you'll become your own personal wrecking ball of utter, despicable, and disreputable existence. You'll hate yourself to the point where you become the worst person that you can never imagine yourself to be. Honestly, it's like wearing a ventilator where instead of being pumped oxygen, it pumps a decadent and decaying mixture of both piss and feces. You'd much rather ask someone to shoot you in the face than getting your face slowly decomposed with pure wretchedness. Now with that being said, amongst all of those wickedly, unbearable individuals, there is this one particular individual that you should pay way more careful attention to because this particular bastard of a pest, for a lot of us, it's like an unnoticeable parasite or leech. They don't tend to portray the noticeably obvious traits and behaviors. They will prompt us to confidently categorize them as someone with a massive red flag waving in the back of their heads. However, over time, you'll realize These men or women are what I call the nit pickers. Now, some of you have probably already heard the term before, but my guess is most of you have not. But in essence, nit pickers are those individuals who always managed to somehow conjure up a collection of subtly needless and gratuitous form of excuses. For every positive circumstance that occur or have occurred, basically, they will somehow make every positive event and situation big or small, collectively, or personally sound like a depreciative liability to us. For example, if a man said, Badman, good news, I've managed to make an extra 10 grand for the month, and his nitpicking girlfriend would say, yeah, but it's not 20 grand, isn't it? Babe, if you made 20 grand, we could go on a holiday to Miami, and you could still keep the 10 grand. Or another one, if a man said, "yo, bro, I finally got myself, my dream car, a new Beamer", and his nitpicking friend would say, "yeah, but it's the old version that just got replaced at the end of last year made. So, it's not exactly new, is it?"

Now, I don't know how you gentlemen would react to those answers, but for me personally, the first two things that pop inside me here are, was that really necessary? And where the hell did that come from? It's quite hard to put it into words, but essentially, these individuals will make every personally worthwhile effort that we've done sound like a completely futile and ineffective waste of time. They will turn the narrative of a heroic, wholesome, and meaningful event directly into a complaint letter without any suitable and applicable complaints in them whatsoever. No, the most dangerous thing about these individuals is that we don't get instinctively incentivized to call them out on their infectious deeds or because their offensives are so subtly executed that we don't get tremendously bothered by them at all initially. That is even for a person with a strong sense of awareness, only a small bitter of taste of spite, but nonetheless dismissible. But of course, as time goes by, like everything, small things add up and they accumulate into one mass effect. And similarly, with this, you'll eventually be instilled a narrative by these individuals that nothing you ever do will ever be enough or significantly satisfying for you to reap and relish. The worst part about this, it's not the moment when you realize that you've become a successful self-deprecate but is the profoundly valuable amount of time that you've wasted, forgiving, and tolerating these individuals slowly poisoning you over the weeks, months, or years that you'll wish to the heavens that you could get back. A couple of things that I could say that I think could possibly help you gentlemen in spotting these types of individuals early on, and these are not absolutes, is that they often have high expectations, and they rarely showcase a sincerely enlightened form of gratitude or appreciation, both towards other people doing them favors or giving them gifts, and towards circumstances working in their favor. Their form of gratitude and appreciation is usually quite noticeably more inclined towards necessary formality rather than genuine sincerity. This you can spot by noticing when they say thank you or I appreciate that to you, either by completely avoiding eye contact with you or their eyes. Do not smile along with their lips when they say those words, because when people genuinely smile, their eyes also smile or become much narrower and the smile on their lips with a much longer, with a delay instead of instantly disappearing back into their resting faces. Now, you could objectively argue that the individual may be just shy or extremely reserved, and you'd be right, but if that's the case, you may have to sacrifice some valuable time before you notice or spot their behaviors taking an effect on you and realize what they've done. Either way, when you do run, do not feel sorry or sympathetic for leaving them alone because remember, misery always loves company, and they will always fight to keep it usually by any means to summon your sympathetic traits to accommodate and eventually tolerate their actions further.

CHAPTER NINETY
CONCENTRATE

Right. Let's get straight to it, shall we? There is absolutely no fancy tips and tricks apart from re-engineering your environment that can be done to help you improve your level of focus and concentration. A high level of focus either comes naturally from an individual's immense sense of curiosity, interests, and fascination towards an object or subject and or actively from regular training and practice in order to improve its level of intensity and duration. As I've said many times, we all live in this age full of cheap and instant distractions leading to the endless Sikh for novelty, lowering our tolerance for dopamine dosage, and eventually turning us into people who always set to experience massive withdrawal or symptoms. Every time we ran out of stuff to look at or listen to on our phone, i.e., severe cases of ADHD or ADD, I bet most of you couldn't even stare at the ceiling for five minutes straight without frantically and agitated looking around you for any signs of novelty that you can utilize so your brain can inject that much-needed dopamine search. That is why most of you, when you put your phone down or back into your pocket or pouch, you'll find that it will only take you me a seconds before you inevitably reach for it and turn it back on again. Our lack of focus and our insatiable thirst for constant novelty is primarily the reason why we cannot withstand even a slight bit of boredom and mundaneness. That is why more and more people today tend to quit or delay on their tasks very early on in the beginning, even tasks that are necessary. That is why most of us are not able to become relatively proficient at something because we ourselves are unable to enter a high level of immersion without inadvertently diverting our thoughts and concentration to somewhere something and or someone else. That is why a lot of us now really display or feel any form of gratitude because our minds are always actively looking for the next hit of dosage. The best example being we now often always busy capturing moments on our phone to get as much positive validation online for our entire self-esteem to depend on instead of being actively present to both immerse and cherish the moments that we are experiencing at the time. Now, whether your lack of focus and ability to pay attention for long periods of time are doing you a disservice in life. It's all subjective. I can't have an absolution that everyone whose attention span is equal or lower to that of a goldfish would constantly suffer from unfavorable circumstances in their lives. But for those of you who are actually suffering at work or in your personal life because of it, you will have to realize that this particular trait is an ability that must be trained and practiced over time in order to cultivate and eventually instilled as a retroactive habit. It's not a trait that you can simply catch or develop out of thin air. You need to actively utilize it day in and day out, like trying to grow your muscles. And let me tell you, it's not that easy. Most of you listening to this wouldn't even bother to put in the extra work even after reading this chapter or because it's quote unquote boring or mundane. Yes, I do mean that because if you think developing focus and attention span at work is crucial, it's actually even more crucial to put effort into developing them outside of work when you are bored to death. Because during work, at least there is already something readily available for us, us to try and impose our focus on. But outside of work is where all the distractions will seduce you. And if you cannot develop a relatively strong tolerance against them, it will eventually affect or infect your level of focus at work for the worst, which is why being the generous man that I am, I present you with one simple exercise to help you improve your focus and attention span. And you can utilize this exercise in your free time as well, or even extend the duration by reading the chapter at half speed. Look at this candle. Try and focus all your thoughts on this candle for one full minute. Yes, it's not a measly 15 seconds or 30 seconds, we're going to go the full home run. Yeah. Now what I mean by focus, it's not just to stare at it or think and imagine something else completely different while staring at it. No. What I mean by focus is to immerse yourself in both the inner workings of the candle i e its properties, how it's ignited, how it stays ignited, and how it will eventually be put off on its own and its possible practical applications. I e what circumstances and occasions can the candle be utilized for? The purpose of this training is not only to improve the intensity and duration of your concentration, but also to improve your accessibility, to focus in moments where you don't want to focus your thoughts only on those things that involve or evolve around and having something to do with the candle itself for one whole minute, and no, I won't be putting a timer beside it, otherwise, you gentlemen will only focus on the clock and force yourself through the process

CHAPTER NINETY-ONE
STRESS

It's quite rather preposterously, hard to wholeheartedly accept, especially in today's time of ultimate sensitivity and emotionalism, that the credibility and relevancy of the male life is utterly dependent on his ability to perform with merit. The male burden of performance always correlates perfectly with our innate instinct to want to have a function or purpose or multiple functions or purposes. The masculine world is a world of action, adventure and conquests, a world of problem solving, constructionism, invention, and discovery. And with that comes both at tremendous collection of risks and expectations that are attached. Along with it, we've already talked about and discussed the often disregarded and overlooked risks that comes from taking on colossal and monumental conquests many times. Now it's time we discuss about the often overly idealistic and escalated expectations that comes from those conquests. We all know in today's world of constant stimulation on social media and everyone's unrealistic attempt to portray the perfect and flawless life has resulted in the creation and implementation of a new norm of perception in terms of life quality, where anything under the accepted standard of mass attention and compliments is considered redundant, irrelevant, or even utterly worthless. Thus, also creating a mass global pandemic of constant social insecurities and comparisons among everyone with a cell phone in their hand. And the worst part is we can't do anything about these expectations. If anything, they will get progressively more idealistic and unrealistic since human beings will never ever be satisfied. For us men, it naturally instills a tremendous amount of pressure on us as we are the ones that are more expected to perform with merit, to eventually need those standards or at least hover around the tolerable limit of those standards. And yes, I'm not only talking about how we look, but also our financial position, accolades or achievements, material possessions and popularity or social connection. Otherwise, we are slowly going to be sidelined and receive less opportunities for even more financial prosperity, resource accumulation, productive collaboration, and mate selection. Basically, the less we are able to perform and meet the new standards of living, the less we will have the opportunity to survive in this world and pass our genes to the next generation. Now, for a lot of you, this might sound utterly ridiculous or unacceptable, but I know that you also feel the same immense pressure and anxiety to perform, even though you may not actually viscerally acknowledge it, because secretly, you also desire roughly the same things in life as any other men, the six pack abs, the nice car, the big house, the beautiful women. You are only desperately attempting to cope against the realization of the mountains you need to climb through attempting to go completely your own way. We are expected to perform, and we must perform as it is our job to adapt to our environment so that circumstances can favor us, whether you like it or not, especially in this current hypercompetitive world, most of us men today may be surprised, or gob smacked about this issue.

Since the centric society has softened a soul into shallowly, irritable dependence, but actually the male life has always been like this since the dawn of time perform and be respected and rewarded or yield and be exiled and forgotten. I've always said it before, that your value as a man in the eyes of the world depends on what you have accumulated, possessed, and contribute through the works that you have committed to throughout your life. Whether it is a great physique, millions in the bank, being able to speak five languages, or even building a huge loyal community, this is the ruthless game that you are playing. Gentlemen, afraid, shocked, stressed, anxious, angry, bitter, hateful, desperate, clueless, helpless, no one cares. The high pressure and demand that the world bestows upon you will always be there. Whether you like it or not, I'd say by this point, some of you could be mentally rattled as most normally would. After hearing all those rough bells and whistles, some of you probably already start visualizing the worst that could happen endlessly and anxiously contemplating what the future would look like for you. Probably already measuring the time you've wasted fooling around in your twenties, and some of you may already one step away from breaking or giving up completely as you feel everything is already too late. I completely understand the high amount of stress and pressure you are feeling, the sleepless nights, the gloomy mornings, and the sore demeanor that you've experienced due to agitated worrying about the future on whether you would make it or not, and enviously seeing some of your friends doing really well in life. I understand that. I also went through all of them, that stress is your survival instinct kicking in and constantly attempting to find the solution to your problems. When our brain perceives threats in our social environment to our status or autonomy, it reacts in the same exact way it does to physical threats. However, despite everything I've just said, not everything is bleak news for us all. One of the good news is that, as gentlemen, we always mature far later in life than women. Performing and accumulating good values takes a much longer time and requires going through much longer and bumpier roads. The other thing you need to know is that you cannot completely control what will happen. Also, obsessing or worrying about the future in other people's lives does nothing for you, but drain you from the much-needed time and energy required to improve your own. Eventually, you'll fatigue yourself off of the worries and start to care less of the things you can't control. No matter how bleak or prosperous you want to visualize the future to be, both gifts and shits will be thrown at you as you go through life, and they can always either delight or interfere with your life further most of the time, and I mean 99% of the time, your high expectations will not be met exactly the way you thought or visualize them to be, so don't overly obsess over it because you'll be immensely disappointed. Be grounded and realistic with your own expectations. The only thing, and I mean the only thing that you can do is to do your absolute and complete best in the present moment, day in and day out. Fulfill your commitments, duties, and responsibilities. Capitalize on every opportunity presented before you decide wisely, and most importantly, act immediately. Whatever the results will be in the future, good or bad, remain ruthless and keep improving. Whether you choose to embrace the pressure and demand from life or completely ignore them, it's absolutely your free will to choose and implement what works best for you. Similarly, whatever, and however life that you want, you decide how important you want it to be. I have absolutely no say in that. The most crucial thing to consider out of all of this is not to regret what you didn't do for your own sake.

CHAPTER NINETY-TWO
PROVE TO YOURSELF

The question of self-worth is probably one that most of us get very perplexed about. If anything, we always fail to interpret it thoroughly because it is quite an abstract and ambiguous term. Narratively, despite its very obvious claim and definition, self-worth is essentially an integral sense of confidence and comfort that we feel with regards to the overall coherence of our own prioritized general specific and unique set of internal and external attributes, whether it is in regards of the collective congruence of our own abilities, circumstances, behaviors, beliefs, options, achievements, status, possessions, experiences, and even the people that we surround ourselves with. In other words, all the personally necessary elements that generate an immense sense of security within our daily lives. As human beings, we all have our own set of intrinsic and extrinsic motivations, thus allowing them to have a great impact on our behaviors, resource allocation, and decision making. However, generally these motives can always change or fluctuate depending on a person's imminent circumstances and priorities at a given moment, even their current emotional needs. That is why it is extremely hard for us to judge what are the things that makes us feel the best and most self-actualizing we can possibly be? One day you may prioritize your material possessions the most. The next day, week, month, or year, you may prioritize the people you surround yourselves with the most. For most people, it is constantly changing. That is why we always have a hard time in determining the right attributes and motives to attach our identities optimally and healthily to, plus certain attributes and motives are out of your control as they can come and go as they please, such as your friends and colleagues know. Most of you gentlemen in the self-improvement world would already know that it is always the wisest and most logical decision to attach yourself significantly more to those attributes and motives that you have for control over mainly your abilities, achievements, experiences, attitudes and behaviors or habits as they always have a positive direct correlation or impact with the amount of efforts and resources you invest into them, especially as a man where the majority of our pride comes through our body of work. However, despite our firm and thorough acknowledgement of this, some of us are still finding it's rather hard to commit to what's cultivating or improving them to elevate our sense of self-worth, all because of one single phenomenon. Doubt, doubt is simply the feelings of hesitancy due to the fear of uncertainty, and it is very normal for all of us to feel this way before any big commitment and or risk taking. We hate the idea of failure, humiliation, ridicule, and further pain and suffering because it will only demoralize us further and prompt us to discredit ourselves even more. However, doubt will also cause the birth of self-sabotage and self-deprecation as your fear of commitments will result in new attempting to distract yourself away from its for as long as possible that oi you, procrastinate and make excuses along the way for your own lack of significance because you don't even want to act or take chances to turn things around for the better. Eventually, you'll turn everything that you fear a lot worse practically. Now, assuming that at a particular moment before a big commitment, you have a very low to barely average sense of self-worth, in which case your self-worth will entirely depend on these two factors. Number one, your sense of conviction, and number two, your recollection of past successes. Remember, confidence always comes from your assurance and or reassurance that you can achieve success and or repeat success.

Now, some people just purely have that immense sense of belief in themselves even though they haven't yet cultivated or achieved anything of significance or value. Some may say that they are entirely delusional. Some may say it's their belief system that has been taught by their parents since their adolescent years, or the one that they've developed themselves as they grow up. Some may say, is their ability to visualize what is technically and physically possible, but regardless of that, it is simply them having an impeccable assurance or reassurance in their own current capabilities or lack of them to do whatever that is necessary in order to eventually succeed in their commitments. Basically, they just wholeheartedly believe that they can succeed despite their suboptimal circumstances. If any of you gentlemen genuinely have this natural enigmatic confidence, I really want to know where you get them from. Now, for the most of us, we fall onto the latter. We don't have that prodigious level of conviction from the get-go. Most of us have to have practical evidences and or recollection of them to heavily assist us in mustering convincing and assuring ourselves of our own capabilities towards any commitment such as past moments where you quote unquote rise to the occasion like performing really well in a football game, getting commended for your public speaking or getting yourselves out of a sticky situation, moments of high pressure and high stakes where you're just able to perform with merit and made you currently think. If I was able to do that, which I was initially scared and unsure of, why can't I do it again with this one? I found a way then I will find a way now, but what about if you don't have any sense of conviction and or any record of past successes to help you assure yourself? What if you have absolutely no sense of self-worth whatsoever in your mind is only filled with waves and waves of doubt and uncertainty? What should you do then? Well, there is only one way left, and that is to stop thinking, put yourself out there or get yourself in there and commit yourself entirely because your back is completely against the war, and you have absolutely nothing to fall back to. You have absolutely nothing left to rely on other than your last drop of faith in your functionality, which you rarely utilize to its full potential to viscerally prove yourself by diving deep and constantly adapting and adjusting yourself throughout the commitment while defying constant doubts simultaneously. In fact, for those of you who did have past moments where you rose to the occasion, I guarantee that you too did not have time to plan, think, or worry, and just did it anyway because overthinking will only amplify your doubts and let your unnecessarily dire imaginations run wild. The more uncertain you become, the more careless and sloppier you become. Thus, the more likely you will fail or choke, commit and give absolutely everything you have. Leave no stones unturned and spare, no efforts. Prove to yourself that you can do it and the level of confidence and eventually security in your own identity will skyrocket. Any insecurities you have will eventually be compensated and overshadowed by your immense level of certainty in your own possibilities. Shift your attitude and narrative towards commitment from will I make it, or will everything be worthwhile into quote unquote? Let's find out. Fill your demeanor with enthusiasm and curiosity instead of skepticism and uncertainty, succeed or fail. It's a matter for a much later time to worry about. Even if you eventually fail, which I highly doubt you would, if you give it absolutely everything you've got, you'll still gain something in the end, tremendously valuable experience. Self-worth for most of us, does not come by itself just like muscle intelligence or anything with valuable integrity. You have to build it over time to eventually justify your capacity, capabilities, flaws, and limitations as a human being. If you are not naturally gifted or born with confidence or taught from an early age how to build confidence and self-worth, stop begging to have it. Stop looking for instant hacks to cope and pretentious masks to wear in front of everyone. Acquire it, build it, and maintain it.

CHAPTER NINETY-THREE

THE DANGERS OF PERFECTIONISM

Now as men who are quote unquote pursuing excellence, it is considered important to hold ourselves to a high standard and also demand more from us in order to cultivate our abilities, character, and wisdom into a new dimension of understanding and mastery. Putting in long hours of work and immeasurable level of focus and consistency to attain desirable results while also upholding our level of satisfaction on a significant metric of merit can be both frustrating and taxing on both our physical and mental wellbeing. And at the same time, especially for those of us who are highly driven and ambitious individuals, inadvertently will cause us to slowly develop a very critical attitude towards our own set of personal goals and objectives, meaning we are unconsciously and slowly turning into someone who ruthlessly and selfishly puts objective performance on top of everything else i e, a perfectionist. Now of course, there is nothing wrong with being objectively focused or driven. In fact, it is what we must prioritize as young men, especially regarding our own burden of performance. Being a mild perfectionist is always tolerable as long as you don't escalate it to the point where it starts to cost you your own and others' wellbeing. Because when you elevate or transform that perfectionist attitude or rather ignorantly, let that perfectionist attitude catapults into a much more violent, rampant and unhinged state i.e. becoming a hyper perfectionist, you'll quickly reach a point of diminishing returns and instead will inevitably cause you to disrupt your own momentum, towards achieving your objectives, and even derail you completely and catastrophically from them, primarily through completely exhausting yourself or burning yourself out and pushing other people away due to your overly demanding perspectives or unrealistic expectations. Now, having said all of that, a hyper perfectionist's extreme need for total and ultimate control is not always formed during young adulthoods. Instead, it actually often stems from their troubled past within their family backgrounds. Children whose parents heavily and extensively criticize or punishes them from making the smallest of mistakes during their adolescent years will often end up becoming highly anxious and afraid of making mistakes as they will associate or register the occurrence of mistakes as unacceptable and undesirable, thus making them highly sensitive or critical of themselves and others towards making mistakes and will try their absolute best to avoid them or prevent them from happening. Also, children who've developed massive amounts of trust issues early on in their lives due to their parents' in capability and unreliability to give them what they need with regards to protection, provision, guidance, and affection will eventually develop dependency issues where they just can't bring themselves to trust anyone and will often have to oversee and micromanage everything and everyone in order to bring circumstances to their favor, which will often end up in them developing an overreliance on themselves, forcing

Such individuals Will find it extremely hard to control themselves or hide any emotional cripple. When uncontrollable circumstances hit them and goes completely against their ideals, you'll often spot a very obvious look of disappointment, annoyance, and irritation on their facial expressions. The most damaging effect of being a hyper perfectionist or extreme perfectionist is that you will make other people hired, resent you from being a literal tyrant, especially when it comes to running a business with a fair number of employees. People need to be given respect, time, and their own space to perform. And if you are constantly nagging them, pinpointing them, demanding unreasonable expectations from them, and abusing them even for the smallest and most unnecessary of mistakes borderline outside of objectivity, they will naturally become more hesitant and paranoid, which as we all know is absolutely detrimental when it comes to performance and will increase the likelihood for them to make even more mistakes. Everything will turn to chaos as you are never ever satisfied with anything, and people will slowly and eventually turn their backs on you and evil rebel against you to the point where they could plan your downfall. And yes, I've seen it with my own two eyes as my ex-boss was a hyper perfectionist and also a boss favorite, and every single employee of every department from finance to promotion to legal to tax or publicly admitted to one another, that they resent her for being an extreme control freak, emotional wreck, and an abusive dictator as literally everything. And I mean everything must flow through and be decided by her perspectives and judgments. Even stir as little as taking a bathroom break must be no longer than five minutes for every employee, otherwise a fine will be imposed on their paychecks.

I'm not kidding. There is literally a security guard who was originally placed on the entrance to the office was instead placed in front of the toilet that knocks on your door to remind you that your time is running out. How is a man supposed to enjoy and relish the satisfying sensation of dumping his big old number twos mate, you have no time to properly clean up your ass. It's ridiculous. And sure, criticizing one employee for a mistake he'd done from missing a variable in the marketing budget report and demanding or expecting more from him is fairly acceptable, but calling him a worthless pig whose mother didn't love him and an in that scoundrel with no future is actually crossing the line mate, it has nothing to do with the mistake he's done no more. It's all just personal superiority complex. She eventually resigned because office politics were unanimously not in favor of her being the director of the company. And I expected that as even the leaders of each department who were mutual friends with the owner of the company were resentful of her and the owner of the company eventually knows about her rampant shenanigans through relentless rally of word of mouth. Now, the purpose of this chapter is not to shit on perfectionists because I'm going to be honest, I'm a bit of one myself, but as for what I always preach to create a vivid awareness of your own discrepancies and evolution as a man gentleman, because as you pursue excellence and as you accumulate progress and results as much as you think you know and understand yourself to a high extent, there are always those small incremental complexities in your character that you may have not got a full grasp on yet, that you should make the effort to understand where they are coming from. There is always a high possibility that because of your arrogance in your own sense of autonomy, it can often lead to you becoming negligent through overlooking and ignoring your own selfish nature, completely taking over your thoughts and behaviors, which is actually very common as you grow in confidence. That is why having high awareness and being able to catch yourself slipping away will always be your best defense against self-sabotage and self-derailment. We human beings are extremely complex creatures. No matter how civilized or moralistically and ethically sound we think we are, there are always those dark, subdued, but significantly impactful qualities within us that will make us question our own integrity and the contemplation of penance or atonement or redemption due to us demonstrating those qualities. And you know what? It's completely okay as long as we are humble enough to admit their presence and be willing to improve our sense of authority over them.

CHAPTER NINETY-FOUR
EMOTIONAL SENSITIVITY

Everyone on average is a lot more emotionally expressive, and courageously vulnerable, or in other words, easily provoked or offended towards misdemeanor and wildly insecure of our own shortcomings in both our circumstances and identity. Most of us literally have the emotional tolerance level of a toddler getting his favorite teddy bear ripped off due to his own excitement. We just can't take jokes or sarcasm that lightly anymore. We apparently can't just ignore online trolls, and we always have to prove our point forcefully and often explicitly to someone for verbally ridiculing us online. We've become too soft, fragile, brittle, frail, flimsy, and thin skinned. The way civilization has evolved towards peaceful and taint domestication, where the introduction and implementation of technology in our lives is catered relentlessly towards ease of access, complacency, and convenience, or in other words, inadvertently invigorating and incentivizing laziness, or inaction for society. Having a spoiled unconditioned or unqualified background where all manners of adversity and necessary qualities that an individual has to develop during their upbringings, like taking full responsibility and accountability is all being overly handled by their overly involving parents, or worse being entirely untaught or unencouraged by their overly involving parents or due to the absence of them the age of emotionalism. Arguably one of the most well-known, discussed and debated topic of the modern age of centrism, where we're taught and encouraged to be in touch with our emotions and to freely express them at our will however, we want without the necessity of developing the ability to objectively decide the safest and most productive way to do such a thing. Seriously, this is how we as a fully functioning society have managed to produce online death threats, midnight stabbers and school shooters these days, and of course, genetical disposition as the first law of behavioral genetics said, all human behavioral traits are heritable or partially heritable. Now, this can be used by many of you as the most effective, apparent excuse for one's own hypersensitivity. I was born with it. There is nothing I can do about it. But that doesn't change the fact that you can bring yourself to become highly aware of it and do your best to develop ways to try and control it in order to mitigate its effects. Now, those are the general reasons that all of us are somewhat familiar with, but now let's discuss the more intimate and personal reasons that caused us to become so easily enticed towards emotional reaction and outbursts, and let's just get straight to the point, shall we? It's because we invest too much of our identities and egos respectively, into both our underlying insecurities and our personalized belief sets. Coupled with emotionalism in today's age of social media, we have been brought way more visceral clarity of our own weaknesses, discrepancies, or Faults than ever before.

As the more connected we've become, the more exposed and antagonistic we've also become, like I've said before, human beings have no choice but to make comparisons with one another in order to make further objective sense to the judgment of our status and circumstances. And when we sense that these from ourselves and from others surrounding us are not optimal to our state of autonomy, we either try to find ways to fix the issue or we go on the defensive to protect our self-esteem. The latter is what is meant by quote unquote, taking it personally often by trying to overly justify and denying our own weaknesses and or trying to attack and cripple other sense of autonomy and self-esteem to draw attention away from our own concealed issues. We hate the feelings of inferiority, disposability, and unfamiliarity or lack of control that our weaknesses will expose us to because it's innately makes us feel like outcasts or the least required or valuable for the tribe. And we all know that human beings absolutely hate the feeling of being isolated or being the only one out when it comes to our specific insecurities. We all have our own fair share of them.

We try to hide it as best as we can so that other people won't utilize them against us and make us food for their equally brittle sense of self-esteem. Understand first and foremost that you are not alone in this other people, and I mean every single person also have their own collection of underlying issues just like you, that you can sense if you are careful enough to spot the leakage often through the sudden change in their facial expressions when a specific attribute is being discussed. Now, the problem with hiding these insecurities or trying to ignore them completely is that you never really get to know the full honest extent of their effect on your mental state until you get exposed for them or someone called you out on them. What we resist will always persist, and the more you resist them, the more potent their effects will be on you because you don't have any psychological method to deal with that particular feeling of crisis, thus getting you unconsciously and imminently invested into them to desperately figure out a solution to your crippled autonomy. And when you can't, it's resulted into a feeling of personal attack because it's the easiest way out to attack or blame someone or something in order to forget our own issues. The only way you can eventually come to terms with your insecurities is to either be completely honest with yourself and peacefully realize that there is nothing you can do about them, mostly reserved for insecurities that you can't control like your height and troubled past, and or find a way or multiple ways to compensate for them, either by finding substitute qualities or attributes to cultivate on to eventually overshadow them or simply maximizing what you can get out of them by turning them as productive as possible, like going to the gym to get bigger.

When it comes to our belief sets, it's not just about religions, agendas, and political movements that we firmly adhere ourselves to, but also our habits, interests, values, lifestyles, and perspectives towards many circumstances. We attach ourselves heavily on these belief sets because they give us structure and hope for a better life in the future. In other words, tremendous ego investments towards Solipsism helping us tremendously in our sense of confidence, authority, and optimism. And when we find out, or most of the times others find out for us or criticizes us, that there are prices to pay and imperfections lingering with our belief sets. You guessed it. We go full on defensive to desperately prove that we are absolutes. In the end, you're only going to tie yourself out endlessly trying to convince everyone that you are the right one. The only way to let this go is to fully understand and accept that every single person we look at the world from different lenses or ever so slightly different lenses, and they will always have their own unique perspectives and judgments towards everything. However, without being said, we must never become mentally too rigid and adamant towards our belief sets because they will cause us to become diabolically, insistent, getting us to become even more sensitive and critical towards opposing views. We always want to understand things from different perspectives as they will provide us with more information to better solidify our judgments, which will eventually make us more confident in seeing how circumstances actually function. Only time will eventually unravel who is in the right and who is in the wrong. My only advice to you is to adhere yourself as much as possible towards objective truth and reality, the practical causes, and effects. So, in the end, taking things personally is all about optimizing your level of awareness or ignorance towards your own fierce and the level of flexibility or rigidity towards your ideals. Unfortunately, in this day of age of constantly chasing dopamine, such a task will be too much for the new generation to fathom and take seriously until a die, a consequence before them due to their own impulsivity. So, I personally think it will only get much worse from here on out.

CHAPTER NINETY-FIVE
INSIDE THE MIND OF A QUITTER

Like most major practical habits and character traits that human beings have developed throughout the duration of their life so far quitting, or in this case a quitter, has his or her own origin story. Some people might say that being a quitter or not a quitter is all inborn, that it's a quality that is just cherry picked by God and randomly instilled to those who are unlucky as a former predisposed reaction for us to respond to whenever we face or felt a significant amount of circumstantial distress. That might play some minor role in its genesis. But if we're honest, again, like most practical habits and trades, it's mostly having to do with our environments and our conditionings during our upbringings in case of the quitter or quitters during their childhood. First and foremost, they severely lack the much needed optimistic or enthusiastic support and encouragement from their parents. Whatever endeavors they've developed a profound level of interest in curiosity in their pessimistic and defeatist parents always stop them on their tracks and tell them to turn back mostly through excessive, even borderline unnecessary despondent and consequential thinking. Like for example, if one wants to try out martial arts, their parents would say something like, you are only going to hurt yourself doing such things, or it's too hard and brutal for someone like you, whenever there are major difficulties and adversities, their parents always tell them to conceit or let go of their persistence and discourage them from further trying through disheartening words such as You're not going to make it sun, or you're just not count out for this steer. This form of conditioning from their overly protective and controlling parents pretty much instill the foundational narrative that the quitter will subconsciously abide by. By default, the quitter will resort towards yielding and forfeiting as the quote unquote right or optimal choice for any adversity that he or she faces.

The lack of experience within struggles, failures, and eventual prevailing or triumphs during once upbringings will result in once hesitancy reluctance and lack of optimism to even try and push themselves to overcome his or her struggles and will become extremely shortsighted when pursuing goals and objectives, they secretly desire. Their lack of support and encouragement from their parents will also result in them secretly and desperately hoping that people would approve of them and validate them through their good deeds of extensive people pleasing. And speaking of shortsightedness, we've come to the second point, which is due to their shortsightedness or lack of training or experience in fast sighter perspectives, they will lack the ability to vividly form conceivable clarity in visualizing their goals and carefully compartmentalize the necessary steps or game plan for both sooner and later circumstances to eventually get there. Because obviously for everyone without a clear plan or at least some form of tangible or plausible pathways to follow and adhere to, we will all lack the confidence and assurance to even start most of the time. You'll only end up being able to and somewhat feeling excited through solely visualizing the end goal and pretentiously experiencing the pleasures or awards of it, but absolutely have no idea of what to do next. Thus, turning your imaginary and short-lived enthusiasm into a whirlwind of anxiety, uncertainty, dread, and eventually pessimistic despair, and again, due to a quitter, shortsightedness and the default result to yielding, they will inevitably and miserably let themselves flow with the momentum of their negative thoughts and emotions without even considering the future consequences of their actions, or in this case, inaction, which are the sense of emptiness and purposelessness. A quitter's detrimental lack of capacity in persistence, grit, and tenacity will inevitably culminate in one's own shortage or even complete absence of tangible and noticeable progress or results in the endeavor.

And without any vivid indication of them moving any closer towards their goals and desires, or rather extensively stagnating or regressing further away from their goals and desires, they will eventually lose grasp of their vision completely and any form of hopes and aspirations to even bring themselves to think otherwise, which will then ultimately transform their mental narrative completely into an existential nihilistic perspective where they will consider every form of struggle, adversity, challenges, or even daily tasks as a pointless and meaningless attempt to endure for every single person that exists in this world. Shifting the blame entirely from their own incapability to turn thoughts into actions and actions into results towards the seemingly miserable and unfortunate occurrence that is the human life or existence. Revoltingly discrediting other people's achievements and loathing, discouraging other people's efforts towards achieving their desires to desperately cope for their own self-imposed insignificance and irrelevancy, leaving them to become empty shells of once worse individuals that are full of potentials to be discovered. Now, I want to utilize the last part of this chapter to say something important. For those of you who can resonate significantly through all I've just said and currently are in the state and condition that I've just described, I e being a quitter, the true definition of a quote unquote, pointless and meaningless life is simply existing, and that is you right now, just existing and letting life takes you wherever it wants, like a speck of dust randomly drifting in the wind. Life is meant to be lived. And when I say lived, I mean to be explored, experienced, expanded, evolved, and enjoyed with the people you value and care about. A meaningful life or a fulfilled life is all about doing all that you want to do and can possibly do to make it worthwhile as much as possible.

And all of those takes effort to eventually be made palpable. Everything in life is deserved and earned, not given, and promised. It's ultimately a choice to make. Everyone has their own share of misfortunes, but what doesn't kill you can be transformed into something that further excels you. As long as you exist. It's never entirely pointless your life. It doesn't always have to be grand or extravagant. In actuality, it can be as simple and conventional as you want it to be, as in death. It only needs for you to be able to answer one question in the end. Have you done anything that is sincerely, purposefully, and objectively right?

As I come to the end of this book, I am filled with a sense of gratitude and fulfillment. It has been an honor to share my thoughts and experiences with you, the reader. I hope that the words written within these pages have provided some form of value and insight into your own life.

Throughout this book, I have explored various topics related to personal growth, including mindset, habits, relationships, and purpose. I have shared my own struggles and triumphs, as well as the lessons that I have learned along the way. My hope is that by sharing these experiences, I have helped you to navigate your own journey towards a more fulfilling and purposeful life.

As human beings, we all have the capacity to grow and change. We can choose to cultivate a growth mindset, adopt positive habits, and build meaningful relationships. We can discover our purpose and pursue it with passion and conviction.

BONUS LESSONS

Oh gentlemen, I hope you have come far in your journey, by the time that you read this. I wrote this book within 3 months, but I wrote these bonus lessons with only 17 years old. They were intended to be small, concise, blog posts – so please forgive their briefness. I wrote the book very quickly and with very little effort. It is very important to note that their briefness does not take away from their monumental importance and significance, and the impact they can have on your hopefully already profound life.
And please, do not forget to leave an honest review.

All lessons contained herein were previously reviewed by my 53-year-old friend, and he commended them for their profoundness and truthfulness.

Why A Woman Saying, "I Love You" Doesn't Mean Sh*t

It is actually really simple; because words can so easily and simply be manipulated, censored, twisted, and also held back, whereas our actions are more instinctually & neurologically connected with our natural, primal, innate impulses as well as desires.
This is also why we, unconsciously, often shake our legs when we are either nervous or uneasy or feel distressed. It is a major stressor.
This is why we unconsciously look around ourselves when are bored or worried.
Naturally, this, in a relationship, is the very same case. Again, this is a major stressor and therefore a red flag.

Of course, she can say "I love you so much" to you gentlemen and yet say them with a completely imitated, fake, or even dead tone while refusing to look you in the eyes, only giving you half-assed hugs, kisses & overall general affection.
You know what I mean - hugs that felt and feel as light as your own towel hugging you after a long and intense workout session and

kisses that felt just as weak as a needle's sting at the Doctor's Office. Yeah, I know how it feels, and so do you.

Her attitude and especially her behavior are what actually matters and what matters most. In other words, how they actually act, especially in your presence.

So, ask yourself this:

Do they show real, genuine, loving desire & excitement?

Do they always smile while looking you deep into your eyes?

Are they willing to extend infinitely to spend more time with you that you may not even crave?

Do they kiss & hug you like glue on a piece of paper?

Well, you gentlemen, this is what truly and actually matters and what you gentlemen should always be paying attention to in your Partner. Do not listen to a bunch of empty, meaningless words that are not really and actually meant. Know what truly counts, and this is how you know to tell a real relationship apart from a false one.

Why You Two as A Couple Should NOT Stay Together in Your 20s Ever

This is one that is, in essence, also quite simple. It is because your never-ending mutual availability will rapidly eat away at your mutual desires for real physical intimacy, not limited to Sex.
Your mutual & natural Commonality will eventually spawn contempt, boredom, irritability, laziness, and dysfunctionality between you two as a Female-Male Couple.

Therefore, through your and her daily Commonality both of you will quite quickly be interested or even tempted to introduce something new, some kind of stimulation into your Relationship to mix things up a little. Especially today, in Modern Day's highly stimulated, active, and degraded & weak Cycle you are living in. Indeed, this is where all of your unnecessary dramas, arguments, and even fights stem from, which will eventually run your relationship - into the ground. You both will start to criticize each other needlessly, rub up against each other creating hostile tension, and you will eventually start to take each other for absolutely granted while your mutual easiness and accessibility deters your sex-life which births a sense of appreciation.

As young, active, and energetically passionate men and women, you both need time to develop your own spaces, to gain experience, and to grow individually, so as to when you eventually do meet and become a male-female couple and connect, you can share your knowledge and experience to grow together and create a stronger bond, which is much, much deeper and far more significant. Do not let your doubts conquer you, take this advice.

That is why you both need to have your own space, as absence breeds great longing, and increases your yearning to be physically together with each other, mutually as a couple.

How to Kill Your Depression!

Depression is caused by 3 Things:

1. Your past

You either cannot move on from your Past into the Present,

2. Present

You are frustrated or unsatisfied in any way by your Situation in the Present

3. Future

And you are unconfident of your ability to fix your bleak future.

Most people deeply dwell on these things far too much and therefore further amplify their own mental as well as physical State of Decay by self-inflicted deprecation & heavy discouragement through listening to sad music and simply drowning themselves physically & mentally in different things such as alcohol to seemingly numb the pain, which as we know and all experienced in the past, will only make things far worse.

That is because you are just extending your state of decay by stagnating and regressing. So, in order to get rid of them, you have to continuously progress and enter a full state of non-stop progression. This is why this Book is here. This is why you are reading this book. Naturally, Humans search for growth - In order to achieve that, you must engage in activities that promote your self-esteem and self-growth, aka self-actualization.

In other words, if you want to really get rid of Depression within yourself, just commit yourself truly to activities that will rip you out of your state of decay, and into a state of progression to bring you closer to manifesting the goals and the future you desire. Picture learning woodworking, hiking, going to the gym, or even all three.